A Life Less Stressed

The five pillars of health and wellness

Ron Ehrlich

SCRIBE

Melbourne • London

Scribe Publications
2 John Street, Clerkenwell, London, WC1N 2ES, United Kingdom
18–20 Edward St, Brunswick, Victoria 3056, Australia

First published by Scribe 2018

Neither the publisher nor the author is engaged in rendering professional
advice or services to the individual reader. The ideas, procedures, and suggestions
contained in this book are not intended as a substitute for consulting with your
physician. All matters regarding your health require medical supervision.
Neither the author nor the publisher shall be liable or responsible for any
loss or damage allegedly arising from any information or suggestion in this book.

Patients' names, identifying characteristics, and certain other details regarding
their stories have been changed to protect their confidentiality.

Typeset in 11.5/16.75 pt Adobe Garamond Pro by the publishers

Printed and bound in the UK by CPI Group (UK) Ltd, Croydon CR0 4YY

Scribe Publications is committed to the sustainable use of natural resources and the use of
paper products made responsibly from those resources.

9781911344834 (UK edition)
9781925322491 (ANZ edition)
9781925548792 (e-book)

A CiP record for this title is available from the British Library and the National Library
of Australia.

scribepublications.co.uk
scribepublications.com.au

Contents

Key Concepts Defined

Introduction

Whenever I mention I have written a book about stress, almost everyone gives a familiar sigh and says: 'I need a book like that!' The fact that you are reading this now means you, too, can relate. Chances are you have picked up this book because you also feel stress is affecting your life and, ultimately, your health. There seems to be almost universal agreement that stress has become ubiquitous in our modern world.

Over the last 10,000 years, we have moved through the agricultural revolution, the scientific revolution, and the industrial revolution. Each one has posed huge challenges and changes for us, both as individuals and as societies. Today, we live in the technological age, an era of globalisation, economically, politically, and culturally. We find ourselves in a time when corporations exert influence on politics, governments, our environment, and even our health — and whether we realise it or not, that influence is unprecedented.

We are living in challenging times, and many people are justifiably feeling let down by big business. The last 40 years have delivered huge financial gains for global corporations — to less than the top 1 per cent of the global population. And while many in the developing world have been lifted out of poverty, many in the developed world have seen no benefit from this economic growth; there has been no 'trickle-down' effect. Instead, lifestyle improvements have been achieved and maintained through unprecedented access to credit, through higher personal debt, and by working harder than ever.

There was a time prior to globalisation, particularly in Australia, the United Kingdom, and Europe, when education and healthcare were free for everyone, irrespective of social class. In Australia, for example, the government owned the major banks, telecommunication and postal services, and water, electricity, and gas utilities — and we as taxpayers benefited from this.

Today, these same institutions have been sold off, privatised, and listed on the stock exchange. In a strange twist of economic logic, we can now invest in these very companies and some of us even go to the extent of borrowing money to buy shares in services we all once 'owned'. As we are encouraged to be good consumers rather than good citizens, the gap between rich and poor has never been greater.

It's no coincidence that 50 years ago, chronic degenerative diseases, autoimmune diseases, and mental-health conditions were not the problems they are today. Over the last four decades, health messages have been confusing and often contradictory, while even basics such as our food, our health, and the health of our planet have become commodities.

I can still remember a time when the technological revolution we now find ourselves in promised more leisure time and a golden age for all. And yet, we all seem to be eternally 'busy', with no chance to escape emails, news cycles, and constant engagement through an ever-increasing range of social-media platforms. As the social, economic, and political pendulum swings, we have certainly overshot the mark. What happened to that promise? I am still an optimist and believe the 'golden age' is achievable, but time is running out and things have to change. Rather than measuring the success of a country or community in purely economic terms, we need to place the health of individuals, communities, and the environment as the central measure of a successful and sustainable society.

People today are stressed

In fact, life, it seems, has never been more stressful. I doubt whether those who have endured the horrors of war, economic depression, or famine would agree, yet our perception of what we as individuals consider stressful is relative — and that perception is real and (as you will see) has an impact on our health.

One thing is certain: today, people of all ages are exposed to more outside influence and potential stress than ever before — uncounted chemicals in our food, homes, and environment; foods that our ancestors wouldn't recognise as food; electromagnetic radiation in our pockets, offices, and homes; access to more information than existed even a few years ago; and a 24/7 news-and-entertainment feed together with an unrelenting torrent of social-media updates.

We hear about every disaster or murder in each far-flung corner of the world at the very moment it happens. It's hard to believe that we live in the most peaceful time in human history. The wars of the first half of the 20th century could see tens of thousands of people killed in a single day — casualties from those conflicts ran into the tens of millions. The terror attacks we are so afraid of, that we hear about in almost every news cycle, are actually fewer than occurred in the 1970s. Just as we have access to each attack or disaster in the palm of our hands, it also gives each attack an immediacy and intimacy that is unique in our human experience, making life seem even more stressful.

According to the World Health Organisation (WHO), in 2012 globally 120,000 people died in war or military conflict, 800,000 committed suicide, while 1.5 million people died of diabetes.[1] Going by the evidence, it would seem we are at greater risk from harming ourselves than being harmed by terrorists — with sugar being the greatest danger of all.

While we congratulate ourselves on how long we are living, preventable chronic degenerative diseases are reaching epidemic proportions, affecting more people than ever before and at ever-younger ages. If our children are the 'canaries in the coal mine', things are looking bleak. Theirs may be the first generation where life expectancy is reduced compared to that of their parents.

Our environment is also clearly in crisis, and our health is inseparable from the health of the planet. With our growing population, climate change, and soil degradation, we are surrounded by environmental factors that are adding to the stress we face on a daily basis. Yet most of us are unaware of the potential for these stresses to affect our health and wellbeing, both physically and mentally.

Add to this the personal complexity of the world in which we live, a world where we can have hundreds of 'friends' and be 'liked' by thousands, and yet still feel lonely, isolated, and stressed.

Arguably, there has never been a more important time in human history for us to build resilience and take control of our own health; and while we are at it, the health of our entire planet.

DISEASES DEFINED

Throughout this book, I make reference to disease. Whether I'm referring to chronic degenerative diseases, autoimmune diseases, infectious diseases, or even mental illness, my aim is to identify causes and build resilience, so this is a good time to offer some definitions.

Infectious diseases are defined as disorders caused by other organisms — such as bacteria, viruses, fungi, or parasites. Many organisms live in and on our bodies; they're normally harmless or even helpful, but, under certain conditions, some organisms cause disease. Some infectious diseases can be passed from person to person, some are transmitted by bites from insects or animals, while others are acquired by ingesting contaminated food or water or being exposed to organisms in the environment. Infectious diseases tend to be *acute*, meaning that they are brief and severe.

Historically, humans have been affected mainly by infectious diseases. With clean water, sanitation, and antibiotic use, the risk of infectious disease in developed countries has significantly diminished, at least for the time being. Antibiotic resistance in the future from overuse in both human and animal medication poses a significant threat to our health.

Degenerative diseases are non-infectious disorders characterised by progressive disability. Many degenerative diseases are *chronic*, meaning that they persist for a long time, perhaps even for the rest of the sufferer's life. Although people may not die as a direct result of degenerative diseases, their symptoms usually grow more disabling and they often die due to complications of their disorders.

Chronic degenerative disease is now the greatest challenge to health in developed countries, and is the result of a continuous process of cell changes affecting tissues (e.g. muscles, nerves, bone, joints, blood) or organs (e.g. heart, lung, kidney, brain, skin, eyes, ears) causing them to increasingly deteriorate over time. These changes may be due to normal bodily wear or lifestyle choices involving postural, nutritional, or environmental factors.

The common denominator in every chronic degenerative disease is chronic inflammation.

Some examples of chronic degenerative disease include cardiovascular disease, cancer, type 2 diabetes, osteoarthritis, and osteoporosis.

Autoimmune disease is where the body produces antibodies that attack its own tissues, leading to the deterioration and in some cases the destruction of such tissue. Autoimmune diseases can affect almost any part of the body, and the classic sign of an autoimmune disease is inflammation, which can cause redness, heat, pain, and swelling. Today, there are over 80 recognised autoimmune conditions, including coeliac disease, inflammatory bowel disease, Graves' disease (overactive thyroid), Hashimoto's disease (underactive thyroid), rheumatoid arthritis, type 1 diabetes, multiple sclerosis, and Parkinson's disease.

A Life Less Stressed: the five pillars of health and wellness is a call to action

This book is a starting point from which to develop a broader understanding of the many stresses in our modern world and how they can compromise our physical and mental health and wellbeing. It is also a guide on how to build resilience and create a healthier, happier you.

In the first part of this book, I want to offer a perspective on how we approach healthcare in our modern world, and to explore some of those corporate influences I mentioned. The modern approach is often not what you would expect or hope, but it's important to understand.

While the world we live in has become more complex and stressful, as you read on you will discover that, ironically, the solutions to these issues are remarkably simple to achieve.

If you are expecting positive changes in your health to come from above — from government health initiatives, professional health organisations, the food and pharmaceutical industries, or even universities — you may be waiting a long time. The changes must come from you. Most importantly, you must start by recognising the factors that can cause us stress. Recognising those means you can make informed decisions, build resilience, and take control of your own health.

Our chronically stressed health system

Of course, if you are faced with a medical emergency or health crisis, there is no better place to be treated than within the western medical model. The skill, knowledge, and ingenuity of our healthcare professionals are often nothing short of miraculous, restoring function and saving lives. Like many of you, my own family has faced health crises where modern medicine has literally been a lifesaver.

However, beyond this crisis management, our healthcare system has largely become a chronic-disease management system. Inside it, individuals often lurch between health crisis and chronic degenerative disease, or may suddenly find they are suffering from both at great cost.

6

We are often reminded that if current trends continue, the financial cost of our healthcare system in the future will be unsustainable — but surely the human cost in both lost potential and life itself dwarfs any financial considerations?

From an evolutionary perspective, our stress response — our body's response to immediate danger — has always acted as our first line of defence. The same is true of inflammation, our body's first line of defence against infection or physical trauma. Yet in our modern lives, inflammation and stress all too often serve us poorly or, worse, actively harm us.

I think we all acknowledge that stress affects our lives and has an impact on our health each and every day, but how do we actually define 'stress' and how exactly does stress affect us? To know, identify, and understand those things that have the potential to add stress to your body and mind is an important step in personally taking control of your own wellbeing. In order to fix something, we first need to know what the problem is. And we do seem to have problems globally, nationally, locally, individually, and even, as you will see, microscopically — and these problems affect us all. Put simply, we need to think holistically.

INFLAMMATION DEFINED

Inflammation is the body's first line of defence, an important part of the complex biological response to harmful stimuli, such as pathogens (infections), damaged cells (caused by trauma or accident), or toxins and irritants. It is a protective response of the immune system, including not only the white blood cells and antibodies you may have heard of, but also a wide variety of other cells and molecules.

As with disease, inflammation is classified into acute inflammation, which occurs over seconds, minutes, hours, and days, and chronic inflammation, which occurs over longer times and may go on for years.

Acute inflammation is usually associated with an infection or injury, and often involves redness and swelling. You know when you have an acute inflammation. There are two main processes: increased blood flow due to dilation (expansion) of blood vessels supplying the region; and increased permeability of the capillaries, allowing fluid and immune-system components to move into the surrounding tissue.

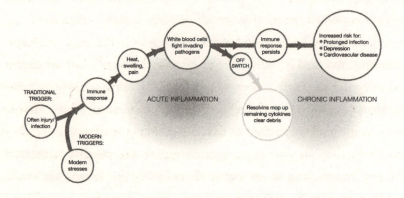

From an evolutionary perspective, inflammation has always been a crucial response for fighting off injury or infection, but if it persists it moves from acute to chronic inflammation and chronic disease follows. Modern stresses now contribute to chronic inflammation.

Chronic inflammation refers to a prolonged inflammatory response where the original assault has not been resolved. In fact, the triggers of that inflammatory response may still be present and the number of triggers may even have increased. You may have no idea that you have a chronic inflammation. Chronic inflammation is characterised by a progressive change in the type of cells present at the site of inflammation, affecting normal function. It is also characterised by simultaneous destruction and repair of the tissue involved in the inflammatory process.

Many of the features of acute inflammation continue as the inflammation becomes chronic, including increased blood flow and increased capillary permeability. Accumulation of white blood cells also continues, but the composition of the cells changes.

A large part of this book is about what triggers chronic inflammation.

What does thinking 'holistically' mean?

A Life Less Stressed: the five pillars of health and wellness is the result of over 35 years of clinical practice, encompassing a professional and personal journey towards a holistic perspective. The most common question I am asked is, 'What is the difference between a holistic dentist and a regular dentist?' The answer is simple. Dentists primarily focus on the oral cavity, the teeth and gums. As a 'holistic dentist', I primarily focus on the person attached to those teeth and gums, recognising they also have a nervous system, a digestive system, a respiratory system, an immune system, and much more. Recognising this means I'm aware that I am treating a whole person and that I'm aware that everything I do as a dentist has the potential to have an impact on that whole person.

For me, looking at life 'holistically' means: recognising the interconnected way the world works; keeping an open mind to the ambiguities and complexities of life; acknowledging there are aspects of our lives that lack certainty; and realising there is a great deal we are yet to learn. Finally, it means understanding that nothing exists in isolation. It is an all-encompassing way of viewing the whole world and our place in it.

So are you a 'holistic' citizen? Do you focus only on yourself and what gives you pleasure, or do you recognise that you are part of something much bigger? Do you realise that your own health, the health of your family and friends, and the health of our planet are intimately linked? The decisions you make every day play an important role in maintaining the quality of the environment, which we rely on to nourish and sustain us now and for our future generations. You, and each of the decisions you make, directly affect our environment; you are the most critical part of the food cycle.

We are all connected — every organism and every atom that make up our planet — and so we are all affected. Decisions that we make and that are made for us affect us all in some way.

Our relationship with the world that we can clearly see is challenging enough, but there is another, microscopic world we need to deal with: one we cannot see and have little understanding of, one that is proving to be even more important to our overall wellbeing. There is a synergy between microbes in the soil and the quality of the plants and animals that we grow in and on those soils in order to nourish us. Similarly, there is a synergy with the microbes that we share our bodies with that needs to be further explored, understood, and, above all, respected.

Just as microbes in the soil confer disease-resistance, resilience, and nutrients to the foods that grow in and on them, the microbes in our body also confer disease-resistance, immunity, and essential nutrients. We need to nurture and respect those 'friendly' microbes in both the soil and our bodies; they vastly outnumber the 'harmful' bacteria we have become so preoccupied with.

Over the past century, we have taken an adversarial approach to microbes, leading to an 'us-and-them' approach. But as we learn more about the importance of microbes, we are beginning to understand that the situation is far more complicated.

Respecting the role of microbes and nurturing our relationship with them is vital for our own individual health and that of our entire planet. It's a timely global metaphor for us all: learning to live in harmony with each other; the good far outnumbering the bad; and the benefits to all when we nurture a vital synergistic relationship.

Far from viewing the earth in a holistic way, we have built our understanding of the world in a linear, reductionist way. With increasing specialisation, we seem to be learning more and more about less and less, forgetting that each one of us is in fact a whole person reliant on our whole world. When it comes to our health, our food, the air we breathe, and our planet, too often our focus is narrow and short-term, driven by financial gain rather than health and sustainability.

For both diagnosis and treatment, the current western medical model typically follows a reductionist, symptom-based view of health. So, if you have a bacterial infection, it is treated with antibiotics; if you present to a doctor with depression, you will most likely be prescribed an antidepressant; if you have trouble sleeping, you will be given a sleeping pill; and so on. The problem is that patients often present with all of these symptoms, each with its own medication — these patients need to be looked at as a whole, not in isolated pieces. Focusing on underlying causes rather than managing single diseases may actually produce cures for many of those seemingly unrelated mental and physical ailments that are so easily compartmentalised into various medical specialities and pharmaceutical medications.

Our chemical, food, health, and pharmaceutical systems are highly profitable economic models, which literally feed one another. A poorly regulated chemical industry produces fertilisers, pesticides, insecticides, herbicides, and fungicides, all introduced into the food chain; the food industry provides highly processed, high-calorie, nutrient-poor, and seemingly cheap food; and the health and pharmaceutical industries manage the inevitable disease this way of life delivers. A perfect economic supermodel, generating billions of dollars in profits. But it is clearly not a very good health model. Something has to change, and that change starts with you.

If we are taking a long-term, sustainable, holistic approach, then a paradigm shift is worth exploring and embracing. When it comes to healthcare, looking for cures and not customers should be the focus; when it comes to the environment, empowering citizens who think holistically as opposed to encouraging consumers who think only about what's put in front of them is surely better for us all. We need to think in an integrative, holistic way about our world, our bodies, and how the two are interconnected. This book is an exploration of stresses, a way of looking and thinking about the things that can challenge our physical and mental wellbeing — and it provides a simple approach to dealing with those challenges.

I don't want to pretend it's a book that has all the answers, but, in my 35 years of using this model professionally and personally, I've found it an excellent framework for asking all the right questions.

For me, this story starts at the beginning of my career

I had only been a dentist for a few years when a patient came in with a crown that had been done five years earlier and had never quite settled. It was occasionally painful when chewing and often sensitive to cold. I determined that the patient's bite was probably the cause and simply adjusted the heavier contact on the crown. Within a day, the pain and sensitivity had settled, but the patient reported months later that the stress-related headaches, which he had 'coincidentally' been suffering from several times a week for the last five years, had also disappeared. This intrigued me and so I started asking questions — was this coincidence or could dental problems cause these common 'stress-related headaches'?

That was in 1980. At the time, the dental profession was realising that the jaw joints (the temporomandibular joints, or TMJs) together with the way the upper and lower teeth connected (the occlusion) was a significant and often-undiagnosed cause of these common stress-related (or tension-type) headaches. As we were dentists, it was referred to as TMJ dysfunction, with a focus on achieving a well-balanced occlusion. I was excited and had to learn more.

At some point in their lives, at least half the population will suffer from tension-type headaches. Given that over 90 per cent of the population also has a less-than-ideal occlusion, and many also have clicking in their jaw joints, this was potentially a big thing, certainly for the growth of my practice. At the time, armed with my new knowledge, I rather excitedly thought there must be many more people who would benefit from my help.

Over the last 35 years, I have successfully treated many patients for chronic headaches and neck aches, which I look at in greater detail in Chapter 8: Dental Stress and Chapter 9: Postural Stress.

However, there was one question that challenged my excitement: why was it that there were many other people with imbalances in their occlusion and TMJs who didn't ever get headaches? Clearly there was more to this stress-related pain problem than just a dental biomechanical imbalance. In 1983, I attended a program run by a holistic dental practitioner from the United States who introduced me to a unique model of stress, identifying emotional, nutritional, environmental, postural, and, yes, also dental stresses that contribute to these chronic, stress-related, tension-type headaches.

The program was a life-changer for me and provided me with a more holistic structure or philosophy to explore health from then on. It empowered me to explore my suspicions: that these other stresses actually existed, interacted with one another, and could not only have an impact on chronic headaches, but on an individual's general health as well.

It was while looking at the nutritional aspects of health and stress that I discovered the work of Weston A. Price, who, over 80 years ago, conducted what must still be considered the most unique and important investigations into health, nutrition, and physical degeneration and disease. In fact, his findings are even more relevant today than when they were done all those years ago. What made this especially relevant and even more exciting for me was that Price was a dentist himself. His search began as a quest to find out what actually caused tooth decay, which at the time was rampant in the western world. Price found the answers he was looking for and much more.

Throughout this book, you will see how Price's studies illustrate the connection between diet, dental health, and degenerative disease. I use his research and my own clinical observations to show you how problems in nutrition manifest themselves in both our mental and physical wellbeing, and, through this understanding, hopefully help propel you towards better health and wellness.

For me, understanding health is personal

If you want to do something stressful, write a book. If you want do something even more stressful, write a book about stress. While researching this book, I uncovered some uncomfortable facts. One of those was that one in two men and one in three women will contract cancer by the age of 60. I knew several 60-year-old men and women, and some did indeed have cancer. Fortunately, most didn't, but the statistic worried me.

In 2015, as I was celebrating my own 60th birthday, I was diagnosed with prostate cancer. Given all that I had read over the years on the various subjects I cover in the book, it didn't come as a huge surprise, but I'll have to admit I was a little disappointed. Was it nature or nurture, genetics or epigenetics?

It certainly gave me a new-found respect for family history. All of my professional life, I have been taking health and medical histories of my patients, but I have never taken 'family history' as seriously as I do now. My uncle had prostate cancer at 60 and so did my brother at the same age.

The book I was writing — this book — started to become more personal. I wish I could say *A Life Less Stressed* is autobiographical. It's definitely not. It's aspirational, for me now more than ever.

When a 'crisis' occurred, I was extremely grateful for the skill and expertise that dealt with the immediate issue at hand. But there were so many issues beyond that. Prostate cancer is a complex set of issues, as are most chronic diseases, mental and physical. What are the causes? How should it be treated? Is a particular treatment worse than the disease? How to do I improve outcomes and reduce further risk? No medical professional can take charge of your health, even if you wish they could. When it came to my health and wellness, I chose to take charge and to ask to be treated as a whole person — and to this point in time, that has worked very well for me.

It's a work in progress.

An overview

At the risk of compartmentalising stress and health and approaching it in a linear and reductionist way, I have divided this book into three parts for ease of use and easy reference:

- Part 1: Understanding Public Health Messages
- Part 2: Redefining Stress
- Part 3: Taking Control of Your Health.

In Part 1, I offer a snapshot of our approach to health, and address why so many health messages are confusing. The question is what has gone wrong and why? The ultimate purpose of the book is to empower you to take control of your own health. But to accomplish this purpose, I believe it's important to give you a broader perspective of some of the issues surrounding healthcare today.

In Part 2, I explore key stresses that have an impact on our daily lives and our overall wellbeing. While everyone acknowledges that stress plays an important role in life, affecting us all in a variety of ways, what do we actually mean by 'stress'? Here, I will refine and broaden the definition of stress and its effects. You may well find this section confronting, but with knowledge comes power: the power to identify, understand, and, ultimately, make informed and wise choices. I look at stress as a combination of five factors, all of which have the potential to compromise your health:

- Emotional Stress
- Nutritional Stress
- Environmental Stress
- Dental Stress
- Postural Stress.

In Part 3, I outline some remarkably simple steps that can help to negate those stresses. I explore the five pillars of health that build physical, mental, and emotional resilience, helping us deal with the many challenges of our modern world:

- Sleep
- Breathing
- Nutrition
- Movement
- Thought.

There is an important point I need to make. Even though I have divided the book into parts and chapters and sections, the stresses and pillars are inseparable and interrelated. Information about some conditions and solutions will appear across multiple chapters, underlining the holistic message.

Since you only get one chance at life, fulfilling your potential should surely be your highest goal. Central to achieving that potential is good health — good health for you as an individual and for your family, your workplace, and your community. When you're in good health, you have a strong foundation from which to achieve and fulfil your potential.

In order for change to occur, here is a fundamental question. Putting aside genetics for a moment, do you believe that primarily you control your life or do you believe that something else controls it? This is sometimes referred to as a 'locus of control'. A person with an *internal locus of control* believes that he or she can influence events and their outcomes, while someone with an *external locus of control* blames outside forces for everything. Obviously, this is not black-and-white, but a spectrum.

But when it comes to your health, I believe it is far too important to entrust to someone else. This book is intended as a call to action, to encourage you to take control of your health, build resilience, and be the best you can be.

Be well.

PART 1

Understanding Public Health Messages

CHAPTER 1

An Integrative, Holistic Approach to Health

Modern medicine is amazing. It saves millions of lives and deals with a wide range of crises, including trauma, loss of function, and loss of body parts. It overcomes disease, repairs the body, and certainly prolongs life. I admire and applaud the intelligence, skill, and ingenuity of those who dedicate their professional lives to its practice. During a medical crisis, there's no better place to be than in the hands of a skilled medical practitioner — something I've been privileged to witness myself, and many times with friends and family. Here are two examples of the wonders of modern medicine, one young, one old:

- **A one-week-old baby.** Several years ago, a dear family friend gave birth to a gorgeous baby boy. Within the first week of his life, it became clear something wasn't right, and he was diagnosed with a congenital heart condition requiring open-heart surgery. This kind of surgery is amazing enough when performed on an adult but even more impressive when done on a one-week-old baby. The surgery was a success, and Harry is now a thriving, healthy, and boisterous four-year-old.

- **An 88-year-old woman.** For some years, my mother suffered from shortness of breath, making her life difficult and often leaving her very anxious. Her cardiologist knew her aortic heart valve was faulty, but, given her advanced age of 88, open-heart surgery was not an option. He suggested a revolutionary procedure in which a synthetic aortic valve would be passed through a major artery in her leg. After the procedure, my mother suffered some complications and spent time in intensive care with a nurse at her side 24 hours a day for ten days. The level of care was nothing short of astounding. Despite the setback, the great news was she recovered and enjoyed life for a further five years before passing away just short of her 93rd birthday.

As these stories illustrate, *modern* medicine saves and prolongs lives, both young and old — there are millions of examples of this around the world every day.

However, there is a problem with what we call *western* medicine — a system in which medical practitioners are encouraged to use an 'evidence-based' approach to treat the symptoms and chronic diseases patients present with, primarily using prescription medications, surgery, or even radiation. Today, we are confronted by an epidemic of largely preventable chronic degenerative diseases and a problem with the way western medicine treats and manages these diseases.

Compartmentalising the body

Western medicine is about specialisation. It compartmentalises the body into increasingly smaller parts. Dentistry is a great example of 'compartmentalising' to an extreme. For a general dentist, treatments focus on the mouth, teeth, and gums, with other dental specialists narrowing that even more. Periodontists focus only on the gums, and endodontists focus on the nerves inside an individual tooth. It doesn't get more specialised or compartmentalised than that. For medical doctors, it's the same; orthopaedic surgeons, for instance, often specialise in either knees, hips, hands, shoulders, or backs.

So while medical or dental practitioners are all highly skilled, it can be easy for them to forget they are looking after a complete human being.

As western medicine becomes more specialised, we seem to be learning more and more about less and less. The same could be said for any area of specialisation, and it's easy to forget not only that we are always dealing with a 'whole' person, but also that we live on a 'whole' planet.

How did science in general (and the medical system in particular) reach this point of an ever-narrowing focus? The western approach to science and medicine was massively influenced by the 17th-century philosopher and mathematician Rene Descartes. At the time, healthcare and medicine lacked a great deal of knowledge and structure, so he introduced several concepts that shaped the way medicine is approached and his principles affect the way medicine is practised to this very day. Descartes proposed the following:

- **To understand the human body, break it into its smallest parts, like a machine.** This was important at a time when little was known about the workings of the human body and the process of disease. In order to understand how the whole person works, he proposed we need to understand its parts.
- **For a treatment to be significant, it needs to be reproducible and predictable.** Results have to be statistically significant. Today, the gold standard is evidence-based medicine in which randomised control studies and meta-analysis of many studies are used. While there's no question that this is an important guiding principle (particularly if you want to show how one drug might work when compared with a placebo or sugar pill), it has its limitations in the complex clinical situation of treating degenerative diseases, as it is difficult in the real world to isolate just one factor at a time affecting the health of a human being.
- **The mind and body are separate.** Descartes may actually have been trying to appease the powerful influence of the 17th-century church, but this principle encouraged the concept of dualism, separating the mind and body. This had a dramatic effect on our approach to diseases, both physical and mental. We now know that

mind and body are intimately connected and affect each other. They are inseparable, but this seemingly obvious fact is only just starting to be acknowledged by western medicine.

The reductionist model

The western medical model takes a reductionist view of health in both diagnosis and treatment. It usually follows this pattern: a patient presents with a symptom (A), which, once identified, is then managed with medication (B), which may have a side effect or there may be another seemingly unrelated symptom (C), which requires another medication (D), which in turn may have another side effect or there may be yet another symptom (E), and so on.

For example, if you have inflammation, you are given an anti-inflammatory; infections are treated separately, as are acute mental-health or sleeping problems; if you have reflux or heartburn, an antacid or proton-pump inhibitor will manage the problem; et cetera. Each of the prescribed medications has side effects: an anti-inflammatory may compromise heart health; an antibiotic affects the gut flora and overall immunity; an antidepressant may cause anxiety, suicidal thoughts, or poor sleep; a sleeping tablet may get you to sleep but not provide you with the refreshing sleep you require; and a proton-pump inhibitor may predispose you to weaker bone structure and osteoporosis. It's not unusual for a patient to present with a complex array of all of these symptoms, each with its own medication, each with its own side effect.

Chronic inflammation, depression, anxiety, insomnia, and over 80 autoimmune diseases are seldom cured by a simple medication. The majority of chronic degenerative diseases today are managed, not cured. The cause of the problem is rarely addressed unless a more integrative, holistic approach is taken.

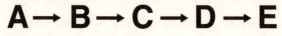

Figure 1-1. The reductionist linear view of health: a series of symptoms to be managed.

The pharmaceutical industry

The global pharmaceutical industry is conservatively estimated to be worth US$300 billion a year,[1] and, according to a recent report, this figure could reach US$1.6 trillion by 2020.[2] Prescription drugs are the backbone of western medical practice.

According to the World Health Organisation (WHO) and Health Action International (HAI), pharmaceutical companies spend twice as much on marketing as they do on research and development.[3] HAI argues that 'there is an inherent conflict of interest between the legitimate business goals of manufacturers and their responsibility to their shareholders compared with the social, medical and economic needs of providers (medical practitioners) and the public to select and use the drugs in the most effective ways'.[4] Put simply: company profits outweigh health; managing a disease is economically more profitable than curing a disease. This is particularly true when a drug company is the main source of research, assessing the efficacy and side effects of their own products, as is often the case.

Drugs play an important part in managing disease, but should this be the ultimate goal of a healthcare system? Or should we inform and empower people to understand that chronic disease isn't inevitable and that there are common themes running through many degenerative diseases, with genetic predisposition often determining how such a disease may present?

Integrative, holistic medicine — not a new-age concept, simply common sense

An integrative and holistic approach to health looks at the range of factors that might influence a condition. It considers a wide range of stresses that may have thrown the body out of balance and acknowledges the intimate connection between these different factors and the effect on both mind and body. It recognises that there is interplay between those stresses that have the potential to break us down; no single stress works in isolation.

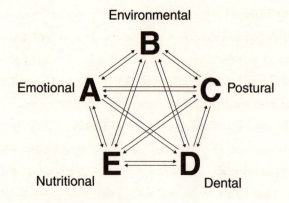

Figure 1-2. Five stresses that break us down.

An integrative, holistic approach also recognises the body's extraordinary ability to heal itself: it strives to restore a healthy balance. My approach is to build physical and mental resilience by focusing on the five pillars of health: sleep, breathing, nutrition, movement, and thought. Again, none work in isolation.

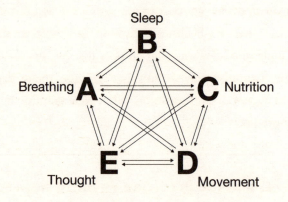

Figure 1-3. The five pillars of health and wellbeing.

In my weekly podcast, *The Good Doctors*, which I hosted for three years with holistic medical practitioner Dr Michelle Woolhouse, we explored health, wellness, and disease from a nutritional and environmental perspective. We looked at food from soil to plate, and the connections between mind and body. Our message is a simple one: it's all connected and we are all affected — taking control of your own health is the best 'alternative', enabling you to be the best that you can be.

As Michelle often said, 'An integrative, holistic approach to medicine is not alternative medicine, it is just good medicine; and that medicine is an art informed by science.' I couldn't agree more.

An incredible 60–70 per cent of all degenerative diseases have a nutritional or environmental cause,[5] and I would consider that a very conservative estimate. The medical profession has unwittingly presided over the greatest epidemic of chronic degenerative diseases of all time. I say 'unwittingly' because every medical practitioner I know wants the best for their patients, and many are just too busy to explore why so many health messages, standards of care, and treatments are influenced by industry rather than patients' health needs.

The fact that nutritional and environmental medicine is not an integral part of medical education in almost every university is a travesty. Medical practitioners are perfectly placed to be the champions for a healthcare system that:

- seeks to understand the cause of diseases
  (which are often multifactorial)
- focuses on empowering patients to be active participants
  in their own disease management
- aims for health and wellness of body and mind.

Imagine the far-reaching effects on the health of individuals and society if we had an integrative, holistic approach to those preventable chronic degenerative diseases — many of which have common causes. It would free up funding for urgent and proven global public health initiatives: making clean water and sanitation a right for all, providing funding of medical treatment for those with real health crises, caring for those with mental and physical disabilities, supporting their carers, and creating an inclusive, universal, and affordable healthcare system the entire world could be truly proud of. A healthcare system focused on health and wellness rather than chronic-disease management not only makes financial sense, but also, even more importantly, achieves huge benefits and gains in both human and environmental capital. The two are intimately linked — a theme running through this book.

Infectious diseases have been one of the greatest challenges to humans since we shifted from an isolated nomadic hunter-gatherer way of life where we numbered in the hundreds to a crowded agricultural/urban existence where thousands and then millions live in a confined space of a town or city. The introduction of clean water, sewerage, and sanitation has, without a doubt, been the greatest public health measure in history, although this simple public health intervention is still lacking in many parts of the world. Sadly, over one billion people don't have access to clean drinking water, and almost two-and-a-half billion live without adequate sanitation.[6] The impact of these simple, proven, cost-effective interventions on disease, particularly in the developing world, would be profound if we had a holistic approach to health worldwide.

According to the United Nations Food and Agriculture Organisation, about 795 million of the 7.3 billion people in the world (or one in nine) were suffering from chronic undernourishment in 2014–16. On the other hand, the WHO estimated in 2014 that more than 1.9 billion adults were overweight and that of these over 600 million were obese. The incidence of childhood obesity has more than doubled in the last 30 years, with over 41 million children under the age of five now considered obese. Our western lifestyle wastes financial, human, and environmental resources, creating mostly preventable diseases and requiring even more resources to manage those challenges. Food waste in western countries is a huge problem, too, as I will discuss in coming chapters.

I believe a big part of the problem is that our food, medicine, and healthcare over the last 40 years have become commodities in a market-driven, global economy. When we allow the economy to dictate our lives, when the major stakeholder is a shareholder rather than the community, when our governments, financial institutions, and media encourage us to be good consumers rather than responsible citizens, we lose sight of what is really important. When quarterly profit reports and the economic measure of gross domestic product (GDP) are drivers of 'good' policy and the measure of 'success', our individual and collective health suffers. If you are happy to be part of that system, there are chemical conglomerates, processed-food manufacturers, healthcare providers, and pharmaceutical companies waiting to greet you with open arms.

For those who don't see that as their own future, read on.

Chronic-disease management or health and wellness? Which model do you choose?

The foundations for chronic degenerative disease are in the many stresses we place ourselves under in our modern world. They are built on increased consumption of processed foods, sugar, and seed oils, along with exposure to thousands of poorly regulated chemicals and unprecedented levels of electromagnetic radiation. This epidemic of disease is further consolidated by an ever-broadening definition of what actually constitutes a 'disease' or the new term of 'pre-disease', often in order to capture a bigger market share.

I believe there are three key components in this chronic-disease-management economic model we find ourselves in today:

1. **Industrialised food production.** Industry produces highly processed, calorie-rich, nutrient-poor, and seemingly cheap food made for convenience and profit rather than health, together with exposure to thousands of poorly regulated chemicals in everyday life that we naively assume have been thoroughly tested for potential health problems. We are told it's the only way to feed the planet, but when viewed from a global, integrative, holistic perspective, adding in the real environmental

and health costs, together with food waste and the poor use of our precious resources, we are paying a very high price for this supposedly cheap food. These are issues I cover in Chapter 6: Nutritional Stress and Chapter 7: Environmental Stress, while I offer some guidelines in Chapter 12: Nutrition.

2. **Medicalising and pathologising conditions.** Throwing the 'net' out wider creates more 'patients' or customers by changing and broadening the definition of disease and introducing the idea of a 'pre-disease'. People who once believed they were healthy are now defined as ill or likely to be ill and in need of management — which usually means medication for a lifetime. Normal blood pressure, bone density, cholesterol, and mental health are just some examples. You may have once been 'shy', but now you could be diagnosed with 'social anxiety disorder' and be prescribed medication to manage this 'condition'. By creating 'pre-diseases', the potential market is made bigger, creating consumers for healthcare and pharmaceutical services, which may require a lifetime of management. There are many conditions I could draw on, but I will focus on mental health and cholesterol in Chapter 3: Big Pharma, Big Profits.

3. **The marketing of evidence-based medicine to manage chronic disease.** Lobby groups and so-called 'thought leaders' are sponsored or supported by those global food and pharmaceutical companies. It means they often are instrumental in establishing a 'standard of care' and 'practice guidelines' that influence the delivery of 'healthcare' in medical practices. The ideal business model for a pharmaceutical company is one in which more drugs are sold to more people for as long as possible, without either killing or curing them. The economic returns to shareholders are achieved by creating customers, not cures. Good health may make sense, but it does not make dollars. As you will also see in the coming chapters, while the term 'evidence-based medicine' reassuringly prefaces many health messages, sadly science today is not as foolproof as you might expect.

Why are health messages so confusing?

I believe the key to taking control of your own health is first to understand how commercial interests distort public health messages and how the 'science' of evidence-based medicine too often resembles evidence-based marketing. Once you have an awareness of the global influences on healthcare and the many conflicts of interest, you'll be empowered to take control of your health and wellness. Your health is just too important to leave to someone else.

If this information about 'conflicts of interest' is new to you, it may be shocking. It's a story that's easy to miss but difficult to ignore. I present it as a starting point on a journey to empower you to take control — by making everyday choices that are good for your health and that of our planet.

But first, let's take a closer look at public health messages and get a better understanding of why they are being broadcast and by whom. It's a subject that has fascinated me over the last two decades and hopefully will help you wade through the avalanche of health messages we face on a daily basis.

Should I be drinking milk for calcium and strong bones?

Low-carb or high-carb?

Grains are good for you?

I thought the Food Pyramid was healthy?

Should I be taking supplements?

Should I avoid all grains?

How do they define who is sick?

Low-fat or high-fat?

Confused?

Do dairy products cause health problems?

What is normal blood pressure?

Should we all be on statins?

Why is there so much cancer?

Is having high cholesterol a disease?

Why are so many of us on multiple medications? Are they safe?

Who sets guidelines for healthcare?

Should we all be lowering our cholesterol levels?

CHAPTER 2

A Personal Journey

You can either accept what authorities tell you or you can question them. When it comes to health and the environment, something that affects us all on a very personal level, listening to 'experts' can be confusing, not only for the public but also for health practitioners. Could there be something else going on besides simply presenting the facts? It's time to question.

When considering an 'expert opinion', we also need to factor in that person's possible link to commercial interests, marketing, professional reputations, and, of course, let's not underestimate the ego of health professionals themselves and their organisations. If you are going to accept responsibility for your own health and truly take control, then the stories of how public health messages are developed and influenced along with how diseases are defined and managed are important ones to hear.

My own journey in questioning authorities started in my practice many years ago, with one of the most toxic elements known to man — mercury. This element can destroy nerve function and compromise immune systems, muscle strength, moods, and the ability to think clearly; it has the potential to adversely affect every system in the human body.

When I studied dentistry at one of the most respected dental schools in Australia, we were taught that dental amalgam was the best available filling material. As dentists focused on providing the best, most affordable solution to restoring a tooth, our teachers were right, particularly at that time in the history of dental filling materials. Dental amalgam is relatively straightforward to place, and long lasting. The fact that the material should be more accurately described as 'dental mercury amalgam' didn't occur to me even though the material was actually 50 per cent mercury, with the other 50 per cent a combination of silver, tin, zinc, and copper. When I graduated in 1979, I never queried this. After all, this was university, and I was being taught by professors. I never even considered questioning their authority.

As amazing as it seems to me now, it didn't occur to me, nor to any of my fellow students, that placing this known highly toxic material into a human body could be a problem. After all, I wanted to be a dentist, focused on restoring teeth, and that's what I was learning how to do. We were reassuringly taught that this particular form of mercury didn't pose any health risks as it was 'locked in' to the filling and didn't escape into the rest of the body. At university, we had a lot to learn, and questioning established practices was not part of our training, or even our thought processes. For me, the questioning would come later.

Perhaps the same is true in the study of medicine? A dean of Harvard Medical School, Charles Sidney Burwell, once told a class: 'Half of what we are going to teach you is wrong, and half of it is right. Our problem is that we don't know which half is which.'[1] A humbling and sobering reminder that school is actually just the beginning of our lifetime learning experience as health professionals.

It wasn't only my university that was promoting dental mercury amalgam fillings, but also organisations such as the Australian National Health and Medical Research Council (NHMRC), the USA's Food and Drug Administration (FDA), and every dental association around the world. All endorsed this same position: dental mercury amalgam fillings posed no threat to human health, as mercury was locked in to the filling.

In 1979, I thought the word 'holistic' may have been derived from the word 'hole' — and that was what I was fixing: holes in teeth. It seemed a good fit. By 1983, having started to treat people for chronic headaches and jaw problems, I had started to think more holistically.

By early 1985, I had begun to work with several chiropractors to treat patients suffering from chronic headaches. These chiropractors encouraged me to read beyond the dental associations' journals, to consider the issue more carefully, more holistically, and to think logically about what I was taught and how I was practising.

What I soon learned surprised me on many levels. Mercury, in fact, continually escapes from the fillings I had been placing in people's mouths. It is then stored primarily in the kidneys, liver, and brain. It can be altered from a supposedly inert or 'safe' form to a more toxic form in the body and the environment through a process called methylation, making it active, after which it has the potential to adversely affect individuals as well as the environment. By mid-1985, I had stopped using it.

The leaders of a study group I was associated with at the time made a lengthy and well-referenced submission[2] to the NHMRC regarding its questionable position of completely endorsing dental mercury amalgam fillings and advising the public that they posed absolutely no concerns for human health.[3] We didn't succeed in getting them to change their public message. In 2002, however, almost 20 years after I first considered the issue, they changed their position somewhat, acknowledging that mercury did in fact leach out of the filling.[4] They now recommend that it should not be used in pregnant or breastfeeding women, people with kidney disease, or children. They also recommend that when removing dental mercury amalgam fillings, the dentist should do so cautiously, with the use of dental dam and a separate air source so patients won't inhale the mercury vapour when it's drilled out. They even point out that the so-called 'safe' form of mercury could be transformed into the more active form by methylation. Paradoxically, they finish by reassuring us that apart from all their recommendations, dental mercury amalgam is still perfectly safe and the material of choice. Should I have expected more?

Fast-forward to 2016: the World Dental Federation (FDI, a federation of approximately 200 national dental associations and specialist groups) became a signatory to the United Nations Environment Program's Minamata Convention, whose aim is to phase this toxic metal out of the environment.[5]

Encouragingly, the FDI acknowledges that mercury is an environmental hazard, and that if it enters the food chain, it poses health risks to humans. Yet its recommendation is that dental mercury amalgam remains the material of choice for restoring teeth. It is worth noting that it is against the law for a dentist who uses this material to dispose of any leftover dental mercury amalgam in the garbage, toilet, or sink. Leftover material must be disposed of as toxic waste — according to the representatives of 200 dental associations, the only place it is safe to store mercury is in a human being! To say I was disappointed is an understatement.

I tell this story because given what we know about toxic load on the body and the synergistic cumulative effects of exposure to several toxic substances (discussed in more detail in Chapter 7: Environmental Stress), one would hope the question of whether or not to implant mercury into a human body would be a 'no-brainer'. Sadly, and worryingly, it's not. As a public health message, dental mercury amalgam fillings are still endorsed by professional organisations and government regulatory bodies around the world. For me, this was the beginning of an exploration of many other confusing and contradictory health messages.

Whether we are talking about climate change, cholesterol, low-fat vs high-fat, saturated fat, gluten, sugar, dairy products, low-carb vs high-carb, chemicals in our foods and environment, the safety of our phones, water fluoridation, the use and effectiveness of various medications or surgical procedures, how we actually define diseases, or the latest breakthrough, superfood, or supplement — we are constantly bombarded by public health messages, and we need to put them in context.

Once you start to ask the questions, sadly, you will realise the answers do not always place the health of the individual or the planet as the number one priority.

Allan Savory, holistic land-management specialist and a personal hero of mine, said, when interviewed on *The Good Doctors* podcast: 'Large organisations are slow to take on new information, lack common sense, and often lack humanity. If you are expecting change to come from them, you will be disappointed. The change has to come from the ground up, from you and me.'[6]

These words reverberated for me as I thought about the 30 years that have passed since I explored the literature on mercury in fillings and used my common sense.

If change is indeed to come from the ground up, from you and me, we need some guiding principles. Ultimately, the choices we make and how we spend our money, individually and collectively, is our greatest tool.

CHAPTER 3

Big Pharma, Big Profits

If knowledge is power, then doubt and confusion can equally become disempowering. As I've mentioned, public health and indeed environmental messages are notoriously confusing and often contradictory, creating doubt and uncertainty. The purpose of this book is to empower you, so I need to discuss what influences many of those health messages — and sadly, good health, for our planet and for us, is not always the primary objective.

Since 1980 and the emergence of so-called economic rationalism — with its focus on financial deregulation and a market-driven global economy — profit and shareholder dividends have become the way in which the 'health' of an economy, and often a country, is measured. The food and pharmaceutical industries are now multi-trillion-dollar businesses. Their primary goal is increased sales resulting in profit for their main stakeholders: company directors and shareholders.

In recent years, these industries have sponsored thought leaders and research, successfully utilising what is now referred to as the Tobacco Playbook.[1] This is a reference to the actions of the tobacco industry starting in the 1950s, when, even though the health risks of smoking were already scientifically proven, the might of the industry and its lobby groups helped persuade governments and their health agencies to hold off on admitting to this for decades. Parallels can be drawn with today's 'health' industry. The controversies surrounding tobacco use, regulations, and public health warnings provided a template for subsequent health, environmental, and climate change issues, which are clearly outlined by Harvard science-historian Naomi Oreskes in her book *Merchants of Doubt*.[2]

There is an obvious conflict of interest between public health and wellness on the one hand, and delivering maximum financial return in processed food and pharmaceuticals on the other. Yet the influence of these industries on health and wellness is profound. In fact, one could argue that good health and corporate profit, in these industries at least, are mutually exclusive. A healthy population by definition would not eat processed food, nor need medications to manage the inevitable illness. This hasn't stopped these companies from exerting influence on health organisations, universities, journals, regulatory bodies, and government policy. The evidence of influence speaks for itself.

The marketing and management of chronic diseases has also reached a level of sophistication that is easy to miss, for patient and practitioner alike. When you buy a car, TV, or mobile phone, you know you are being marketed to because you expect each manufacturer to claim they have the best product. Yet what is the most effective way for any company to market a commodity? When the consumer doesn't realise they are being marketed to. An excellent example is the presence of a 'low-fat' label on a food product or a Heart Foundation tick, both of which have become synonymous with a healthy product, even if that food is laden with sugar, preservatives, and additives.

Even more powerful is when the provider of a commodity (in the case of pharmaceuticals, the medical profession) doesn't realise that they themselves are doing the marketing, often unwittingly drawing on 'evidence' conveniently provided to them by manufacturers of those very same products.

As marketing and branding guru Vince Parry, a 30-year veteran of the communications industry who has worked closely with many global pharmaceutical companies, outlines in his article 'The Art of Branding a Condition': 'Healthcare marketers are taking the concept of "branding a condition *(disease)*" to new levels of sophistication. Done appropriately, this type of branding helps keep both the brand managers *(from the pharmaceutical industry)* and the clinical community *(healthcare workers)* focused on a single story with a problem/solution structure.'[3] In other words, brand a new disease (high cholesterol) or rebrand an old one (heartburn) and then market a pharmaceutical to manage the disease, preferably for a lifetime; increase the number of people defined as having a disease, and profit is assured.

Globally, US$6.5 trillion is spent on healthcare.[4] According to Bloomberg, Australia ranks third in a list of the world's 40 healthiest countries.[5] According to an Australian government report, Australians spent AU$154.6 billion (AU$6,639 per person) in 2013–14 on healthcare, which constitutes 9.8 per cent of the nation's gross domestic product (GDP).[6] Despite our high ranking, we still have a healthcare crisis in this country. We are constantly reminded that these costs will escalate and are financially unsustainable, and this is without even considering the human cost in lost potential.

Does spending more money on healthcare in general (and pharmaceuticals in particular) lead to better real 'health' outcomes for individuals and communities? The United States has the biggest health spend globally at US$2.7 trillion (US$8,362 per person) annually. This accounts for almost 18 per cent of their GDP. The US is ranked 33rd on that Bloomberg list. As US Democratic senator Tom Harkin observed: 'With all that we have spent, why are we so sick? America's health care system is in crisis precisely because we systematically neglect wellness and prevention.'

The global spend on medicines is estimated to grow to US$1.6 trillion by 2020. Even though the US makes up only 5 per cent of the world's population, it consumes almost 50 per cent of the world's pharmaceuticals. In his book *Overdosed America*, John Abramson, who lectures in public health policy at Harvard Medical School, reveals the ways in which drug companies have misrepresented statistical evidence on pharmaceutical effectiveness in dealing with chronic diseases, misled doctors, and compromised health.[7] He says that the current crisis in American medicine lies in the commercialisation of medical knowledge.

But there is some good news — the best independent scientific evidence clearly shows that reclaiming responsibility for your own health is more effective than taking the latest 'blockbuster drug'. According to the WHO, the solution is remarkably straightforward: 'Chronic diseases are largely preventable, lifestyle-related conditions, resulting in billions of dollars of potentially avoidable healthcare spending and untold personal cost.'[8] Good health shouldn't be complicated, and that is largely the message of this book.

Creating doubt and confusion undermines our confidence when making decisions about our own health, the health of our dependents, and that of our environment. But in the name of profit, maybe that's the point, and our health pays the price.

The influence of the food and pharmaceutical industries on research, professional health organisations, regulatory bodies, and government policy has significantly contributed to poor health outcomes for global populations. I will deal with the issues surrounding the food industry's influence on health messages in the next chapter, but first I want ask a fundamental question.

How healthy are we?

Heart disease is so prevalent these days, it's hard to imagine a time when it was both less understood and less common. But a century ago, it was a relatively rare event. In the space of 100 years, it has become the world's number one killer. The incidence of heart disease increased so sharply between 1930 and 1967 that the WHO called it the world's most serious epidemic. One reason for the increase in heart disease might be that we're living for longer, but that's not the entire story.

After heart disease, the second biggest killer is cancer. Again, the fact we are living longer is often offered as the reason for its prevalence. However, since 1975, when President Nixon declared the 'war on cancer', there has been a 25–30 per cent increase in cancer rates, even allowing for gains in lifespan.[9]

And consider autoimmune conditions. You don't have to be old to contract an autoimmune disease, and they are now among the leading causes of death for young and middle-aged women in the United States. Researchers believe the increase in autoimmune diseases is related to genetic and environmental factors.[10] While genes may explain a disposition, the environment, diet, and lifestyle have clearly triggered the response. Though not enough is known about those triggers, with 50 million Americans currently living with an autoimmune disease, discovering the causes should be a priority! I'll deal with some of those issues in Chapter 7: Environmental Stress and Chapter 6: Nutritional Stress, while I offer some guidelines in Chapter 12: Nutrition.

With all the advances in medicine, what explains the increase in non-infectious, chronic degenerative diseases, which account for an estimated 72 per cent of the global burden of illness in adults aged 30 years and over?[11] Thirty is hardly old age, and, while we congratulate ourselves on living longer, how are our children faring? Take a look at these alarming statistics:

- one in three children in Australia has allergies[12]
- one in four suffers from asthma
- the rate of child cancer increased by 15 per cent from 1983 to 2006 (while in the USA, it's increased by 36 per cent since 1975)[13]
- diabetes, obesity, and depression have increased dramatically in the last 20 years
- one in ten Australian children has been diagnosed with attention-deficit hyperactivity disorder (ADHD)[14]
- one in 100 Australian children has been diagnosed with autism (in parts of the US, the figure is one in 50, which is alarming in itself, but particularly when compared to 1975 figures of one in 5,000 diagnosed with the condition).[15]

Are we *all* sick? Do we *all* need medication?

It would seem the answer is yes *and* no. Yes: heart attacks, cancer, diabetes, and autoimmune diseases are certainly on the rise. But also, no: many 'diseases' are either just normal function, or newly defined 'pre-diseases', opportunistically targeted and marketed by Big Pharma. And so the real crisis, dealing with preventable diseases, isn't being addressed, while the 'health' crisis makes money.

The more people who can be defined as sick (or at risk of being sick), the greater the market for selling products to manage those 'diseases' and 'pre-diseases'. How pharmaceutical companies have influenced the definition of 'disease' and the subsequent, often-lifelong management of that disease has become big business. Let's look at two examples.

Mental health

Mental health is a huge and growing issue in our society, and its impact on our general health and wellbeing is significant. Mental health is defined as a state of wellbeing in which individuals can cope with the normal stresses of life, work productively and fruitfully, and contribute to their community. Mental illness, on the other hand, describes a number of diagnosable disorders that can significantly interfere with a person's cognitive, emotional, or social abilities.[16]

According to a 2007 report, almost half (45 per cent, or 7.3 million) of Australians aged 16–85 reported that they have met the criteria for mental illness at some point in their lives, with one in five (3.2 million) reporting they had experienced some symptoms in the last 12 months.[17]

The financial cost of mental illness has been estimated to be anywhere between AU$20 billion per year (taking into account loss of productivity and labour force participation)[18] and a massive AU$155.5 billion per year (taking into account a more-complex model of collective wellbeing from a social, political, and economic perspective).[19] Whichever way the financial cost is calculated, it's a huge social and personal problem, with the human cost dwarfing all of those financial considerations.

There are many factors influencing mental health, and I will cover some of these in Part 2 and Part 3 of this book, but, needless to say, these are affecting more and more people in countries around the world. Yet how mental health is defined and subsequently managed is also an important component.

However, the current criteria for diagnosing mental-health disorders has thrown the net far and wide, creating patients — customers for drugs — with questionable efficacy but significant side effects. The *Diagnostic and Statistical Manual of Mental Disorders* (*DSM*) was first published by the American Psychiatric Association in 1952 and was just 100 pages long and listed 106 mental disorders. The latest version, *DSM-5*, published in 2013, is a staggering 1,000 pages in length, lists almost 300 mental disorders, and is considered by some to be the gold standard for diagnosing mental disorders.[20] While this latest publication has been embraced by many psychiatric authorities, it has at the same time been widely criticised for broadening the definition of mental illness to the point at which one could justifiably ask, 'Is anyone normal?'[21]

People often feel happier and healthier in the summer, enjoying the warmth of the sun (particularly given the importance of vitamin D), but, today, if winter gets you down, you could be diagnosed with 'seasonal affective disorder'. It is human nature to sometimes feel happy and sometimes sad, but now you may be diagnosed with bipolar disorder. The diagnosis of this condition prior to 1990 was uncommon but has since increased by 4,000 per cent. Children, too, are now diagnosed with bipolar disorder, everyone knows a child diagnosed with ADHD, and childhood depression has apparently doubled in the last 20 years, in line with the broader definitions contained in the ever-expanding DSM manuals. I can't help noting that more than half of the 28 members of the *DSM-5* task force had ties to the pharmaceutical industry.[22]

While I do not want to minimise or trivialise the real traumas people experience in life or question the reality of mental-health issues, today many people are diagnosed with a mental disorder 'by definition' and all too often prescribed psychotropic drugs, particularly antidepressants and anti-anxietics. This has spawned a US$80-billion-dollar-a-year industry in psychiatric medications, which don't cure anyone, and at best manage 'conditions' often for life and (far too often) come with unpleasant or potentially life-threatening side effects. Peter Gotzsche perhaps summarises it best in the title of his book *Deadly Medicines and Organised Crime: how big pharma has corrupted health care.*[23]

Deadly medicines and organised crime? What does this have to do with health?

According to Gotzsche, the very drugs that are supposedly keeping us alive, prescription medications, are also the third-most-common cause of death. He's well placed to make this claim: in 1993, he co-founded the Cochrane Collaboration, a network of 34,000 medical researchers in more than 100 countries, whose main task it is to assess scientific research critically.

Gotzsche himself is a specialist in internal medicine and professor of clinical-research design and analysis at the University of Copenhagen. He teaches how scientific research should be carried out properly and is one of the leaders in the field worldwide. He has published more than 70 scientific articles in the five major medical journals and has been cited more than 15,000 times by other researchers. So I feel happy to cite him here.

Gotzsche's book won first prize in the 'Basis of Medicine' category at the British Medical Association's 2014 book awards. One judge stated that the book 'should be compulsory reading for medical students and junior doctors to make them aware of these issues'. It doesn't look at what causes problems, how to overcome and cure illness, or how to maintain health and wellbeing. Instead, it reveals in detail something that is of grave concern to us all: how the pharmaceutical industry has developed a great model for profit, but not for health.

The book outlines numerous examples of pharmaceutical companies being fined for making false claims about a wide range of prescription medications. This is disturbing, to say the least. Here are just two examples:

- AstraZeneca paid US$520 million in 2010 to settle a fraud case involving the claims made about the antipsychotic drug Seroquel, which incidentally had made the company US$4.9 billion in 2009. The drug is prescribed for schizophrenia and bipolar disorder. The company had marketed the drug to children, war veterans, and the elderly for uses that were not approved, including the treatment of aggression, Alzheimer's, anger, anxiety, depression, dementia, post-traumatic stress disorder, and ADHD. While serious side effects, including suicidal behaviour, were known when the drug was introduced in 1997, it took until 2010 for fines to be issued.

- GlaxoSmithKline paid US$3 billion in 2011, making it the largest healthcare fraud in US history for its illegal marketing of the drugs Wellbutrin (antidepressant), Paxil (antidepressant), Advair (asthma drug), Avandia (diabetes drug), and Lamictal (epilepsy drug). In the case of Avandia, it claimed there were cardiovascular benefits, when in fact the drug caused a 20 per cent increase in cardiovascular deaths and a 50 per cent increase in cardiovascular disease. In the case of Paxil, a study done by the company and cited 184 times in the literature ignored the fact that when the drug was prescribed for children, they became suicidal in a disturbing number of cases.[24]

To put this in perspective, it's easy for drug companies to see these fines as just part of their marketing budget. For example, GlaxoSmithKline's 2011 fine, despite its size, represented only a portion of the profit GSK made on the drugs for which they were fined — Avandia alone brought in US$10.4 billion in sales during the years covered by the settlement. The companies are clearly unperturbed, often reoffending.

Every two years, the Access to Medicine Foundation publishes a detailed report on the activities of drug companies, both positive and negative. The 2014 report states: '18 out of 20 companies were the subject of settlements or fines for corrupt behaviour, unethical marketing or breaches of competition law. Collectively, companies were found to have been accountable for almost 100 separate breaches. The majority of these (89%) concerned improper marketing, bribery and corruption.'[25]

Company	Year	Fines (US$ million)	Type of crime
GlaxoSmithKline	2006	3,400	Tax evasion over 20 years
Pfizer	2009	2,300	Illegal marketing, bribery
Eli Lilly	2009	1,400	Illegal marketing
TAP Pharmaceuticals	2001	875	Overcharging government health programs
GlaxoSmithKline	2010	750	Poor manufacturing practices
Serono Lab	2005	704	Illegal marketing, bribery, monopoly practices
Merck	2008	650	Overcharging government health programs, bribery
Purdue Pharmacy	2007	601	Illegal marketing
Allergan	2010	600	Illegal marketing
AstraZeneca	2010	520	Illegal marketing
Bristol-Myers Squibb	2007	515	Illegal marketing, bribery, overcharging government health programs
Schering-Plough	2002	500	Poor manufacturing practices
Schering-Plough	2006	435	Illegal marketing, bribery, overcharging government health programs
Pfizer	2004	430	Illegal marketing
Cephalon	2008	425	Illegal marketing
Novartis	2010	423	Illegal marketing, bribery

AstraZeneca	2003	355		Overcharging government health programs
Schering-Plough	2004	345		Overcharging government health programs, bribery
Forest Laboratories	2010	313		Illegal marketing, concealing study findings, bribery, illegal distribution
Johnson & Johnson	2010	258		Illegal marketing

Figure 3-1. Top 20 largest pharmaceutical company settlements 1991–2010.[26]

When it comes to your health, are you happy to entrust it to these companies? I must agree with Gotzsche when he says, 'it's seductively easy to convince healthy people to take drugs they don't need for a disease they don't have'.

Creating a new disease — high cholesterol

Over the last 40 years, we have seen the demonisation of saturated animal fats, which have been an important part of the human diet for tens of thousands of years. We have also seen the demonisation of cholesterol. Yet it is an integral component of every cell in our body.[27] In fact, cholesterol is vital for the following:

- healthy cell membranes
- intracellular communication
- the production of many important steroid hormones
- bile-salt metabolism, which helps break down fats that we need to absorb for good health
- vitamin D production, which in itself is important in combating almost every degenerative disease
- dealing with toxins and stress.

How can something so important be such a problem?

In 2001, a panel of experts lowered the parameters for the healthy cholesterol range, which meant more people were diagnosed with a new 'disease'. But, as Ray Moynihan and Alan Cassels reveal in their book *Selling Sickness*, five of the 14 experts (including the panel's chair) had financial ties to pharmaceutical companies that manufactured cholesterol-lowering drugs, called statins.[28]

Another panel was convened in 2004. This time, eight of the nine experts were paid speakers, consultants, or researchers tied to major drug companies that manufactured statins. The committee chairman alone had professional associations with *several* drug companies. It branded a new condition, 'high cholesterol', and in the process medicalised a further 37 million people who were then prescribed cholesterol-lowering medications such as Crestor and Lipitor. A new disease was created, and a new term, 'blockbuster drug', was born, meaning a drug that generates annual sales of over $1 billion.

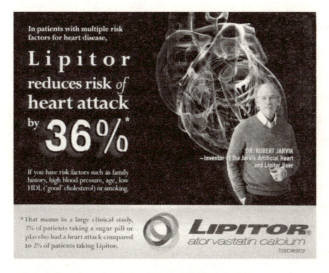

Figure 3-2. Lipitor advertisement in medical journals.

From 1996 to 2012, Lipitor became the world's bestselling drug, with more than US$120 billion in sales, and annual sales of US$7.7 billion.[29] If you were a busy medical practitioner faced with an epidemic of heart disease, and a medication was offered to you that promised to reduce the risk of heart attack by 36 per cent,[30] then it would be a difficult offer to ignore. Particularly if your waiting room was full and your consultations lasted between seven and 15 minutes. Reassuringly, for these doctors at least, there were also many articles published in respected peer-reviewed journals 'supporting and reinforcing' those claims. But how true, how upfront were these claims?

The fine print from the advertisement explains: 'That means in a large clinical study, 3% of patients taking a sugar pill or placebo had a heart attack compared to 2% of patients taking Lipitor.' I'll come to the 'trouble with science' in a moment, but let's look closer at that 36 per cent reduction in risk of heart attack.

To put it another way, what if I said to you the chance of you suffering a heart attack was actually 3 in 100, and by taking a statin medication, Lipitor, the risk lowered to 2 in 100? That is clearly a lot less impressive or compelling. Especially if I go on to tell you the statin drug's side effects might include muscle or nerve aches, pain in the arms and legs, impaired memory, and damage to liver function — would you still be as keen to take that statin medication? The improvement in the real or absolute risk from 3/100 to 2/100 (give or take a few decimal points) is also a 36 per cent improvement in the relative risk; using such terms is a clever and engaging marketing tool often used and designed to impress busy practitioners and an unsuspecting public.

Yet despite the focus on cholesterol and the huge increase in the number of people taking statins, heart disease remains the world's number one killer, which begs the obvious question: is high cholesterol a disease? If not, why bother taking statins other than to allow a practitioner to feel they are doing something proactive and measurable by monitoring your cholesterol level and — after prescribing you medication — showing you they have lowered it? It may be more complicated to explain that heart disease is a caused by a combination of diet, lifestyle, environmental factors, and genetics or family history, but clearly this is a message worth conveying. It's a message that's relevant to so many diseases, not just heart disease.

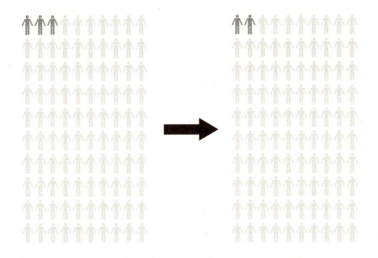

Figure 3-3. Relative reduction in risk of 36 per cent, represented as 'before and after' absolute risks.

Despite this and the range of side effects, I'm not calling for statins to be banned. In low doses, they do have an anti-inflammatory effect, and, in people who have a family history of heart problems, they may be of benefit. Obviously, consult a medical practitioner who is aware of and open to these facts (and aware of the power of nutrition, which I will discuss in Chapter 12: Nutrition).

Perhaps the last word should be left to the actual manufacturer of Lipitor, the world's highest-selling statin drug. This is Pfizer, one of the largest pharmaceutical companies in the world. They have sponsored literally millions of dollars' worth of research and spent even more money on marketing and education, particularly directed at the medical profession. In the information sheet that comes with each prescription of Lipitor, they provide the following caveat:

LIPITOR® (atorvastin calcium) is a prescription drug used with diet to lower cholesterol. LIPITOR is not for everyone, including those with liver disease or possible liver problems, women who are nursing, pregnant, or may become pregnant. LIPITOR has not been shown to prevent heart disease or heart attacks.

Just in case you missed the last line: Lipitor has *not* been shown to prevent heart disease or heart attacks.

Cholesterol and statins are big business, a lucrative market, and many researchers' and organisations' reputations have been built on this very topic. There is no shortage of 'evidence' published in peer-reviewed journals to continue this argument that we should all lower our cholesterol and therefore many of us should be on statins, and this will go on for many years. So this is a good time to explore the world of evidence-based medicine.

The trouble with science

Almost 75 per cent of US clinical trials in medicine are paid for by the pharmaceutical industry.[31] This in itself is of concern in an industry focused on customers not cures. It is worth noting that there is a significant difference between studies done by the companies themselves and those done by independent researchers.[32] This is reflected in the way in which 'key opinion leaders', sponsored by the pharmaceutical industries, are used to influence practitioners' approaches to healthcare. If you happen to attend a medical and dental conference, you might be surprised at how it resembles a trade fair. The practice of influencing health guidelines is another way drug companies help market their products, in addition to funding medical education and refresher courses.

Even more disturbing is that companies are not compelled to publish all clinical trials. Negative results are often not published, which has led to the global initiative AllTrials campaign, supported by over 600 organisations and companies. According to this initiative:

> *Thousands of clinical trials have not reported their results; some have
> not even been registered. Information on what was done and what was
> found in these trials could be lost forever to doctors and researchers,
> leading to bad treatment decisions, missed opportunities for good*

medicine, and trials being repeated. All trials past and present should be registered, and the full methods and the results reported. We call on governments, regulators and research bodies to implement measures to achieve this.[33]

Of course, these trials already occur with one outcome in mind: the 'treatment' or management of an ailment or disease through medication. The medical system is less likely to go looking for the reasons why an ailment or disease occurred in the first place, due to time constraints and both patients' and doctors' focus on a problem/solution structure.

Is good health conducive to company profits?

In his groundbreaking book *Bad Pharma*, British epidemiologist Ben Goldacre (who helped found the AllTrials campaign) gives many examples of the ways pharmaceutical companies use 'evidence-based' medicine to market their products:[34]

- Researchers at Harvard and Toronto Universities looked at over 500 trials across five major classes of drugs, including statins, antidepressants, and heartburn drugs. Eighty-five per cent of industry-funded studies were positive compared with only 50 per cent from independent studies.
- In 2007, researchers looked at every published trial that set out to explore the effects of a statin, other than just its ability to lower cholesterol. They wanted to explore the more important question: is there a health benefit? Of the 192 statin trials, industry-funded studies were 20 times more positive than independent trials.[35]
- In 2006, researchers looked into every trial of psychiatric drugs in four leading academic journals, finding 542 trials of such pharmaceuticals over a ten-year period; 78 per cent of industry-sponsored trials were positive compared with only 48 per cent of independent studies.[36]

- For antidepressants, industry-funded studies were four times more positive than those conducted independently.

In fact, it's often difficult to find research on the medical management of a disease that hasn't been sponsored by a drug company. Medical education and research has also changed significantly over the last 35 years, as is outlined by the former editor of the prestigious *New England Journal of Medicine*, Marcia Angell. She discusses several key factors:[37]

- **University medical-research units.** Most university departments nowadays need to be economically self-sufficient. One of the consequences of this shift is a pro-industry bias in medical research. The discovery of a drug to manage chronic disease is more profitable than finding a cure for that disease. In addition to academic institutions, this economic imperative affects professional bodies, medical journals (who rely on advertising revenue for their very existence), and even not-for-profit 'patient-advocacy' groups (too often sponsored by drug companies).

- **Changes in patent laws.** Historically, medical research was published in peer-reviewed journals. The research was reproduced and found to be either valid or not. Research was collaborative and cumulative. In the US, this changed with the Bayh-Dole Act of 1980, which allowed government-funded universities to patent discoveries.[38] This encouraged partnerships between universities and industry to create profitable medications. It led to the 'blockbuster drugs', including Lipitor (cholesterol), Plavix (blood clots), Nexium (reflux), Prozac, Abilfy (depression), Advair (asthma), Seroquel (bipolar, schizophrenia), Crestor (cholesterol), Cymbalta (depression), and Humira (autoimmune inflammation).[39] Again, a great economic model was born, but not necessarily a good health model.

- **Influence on regulatory bodies and governments.** As many regulatory bodies have had their funding cut, it has forced them to make closer ties with the very industries they are actually meant to regulate. The power of industry lobby groups on government policy has been all too evident in the world of finance and the environment, and health is no different.

Here's a basic but important question: considering that industry funds the vast majority of research on their own drugs, are industry-funded studies as reliable as independent research? Let me give you an example of how science can be used to protect a market position.

I just quoted you a 2007 study that concluded 'Of the 192 statin trials, industry-funded studies were 20 times more positive than independent trials.' That would seem conclusive and almost damning of industry-funded research. But a 2014 study of statins conducted by one of the most prestigious schools in the world, the London School of Economics, concluded: 'Our analysis shows that the findings obtained from industry-sponsored statin trials seem similar in magnitude as those in non-industry sources.'[40]

At first glance, this would seem to disprove the 2007 study, and it's always so tempting to go straight to the conclusion of an article in a refereed journal and, using evidence-based medicine, quote the study and prove your point. In this case: that there is no difference between industry-funded and independent studies — but it depends.

It actually depends on the question asked. In the 2007 study, the question was: are there health benefits to taking statins? This showed conclusively that industry studies were 20 times more positive, raising possible doubts about why you might take the medication. The 2014 study asked a much simpler question: do statins reduce cholesterol? The answer in both industry-funded and independent research was conclusive. Statins do lower cholesterol. There's no argument there. On the more important question about whether there is a health benefit, there is disagreement, with the industry-funded studies clearly supporting the supposed health benefits. It's just a small example of the trouble with science and the difference between evidence-based medicine and 'evidence-based' marketing.

Another problem faced with medical research is reproducibility and reliability. As Stanford University professor John Ioannidis observes, 'In biomedical research, we are in the midst of a revolution with the generation of new data and scientific publications at a previously unprecedented rate. However, unfortunately, there is compelling evidence that the majority of these discoveries will not stand the test of time.'[41] This is another consequence of the race to market.

We are bombarded by health messages, and it can be difficult to work out who or what to believe. As I have explored in this chapter, the advice from pharmaceutical companies and corporations may not be in the best interests of our health and wellness. The desire for larger profits too often compromises health, and even costs lives.

Surely we can rely on other public health messages, like the Food Pyramid and dietary guidelines? Well, can we? Let's take a look …

CHAPTER 4

The Food Pyramid
and Other Myths

In 1930, there were 3,000 heart-attack deaths recorded in the United States; by 1960, this figure had skyrocketed to 500,000 deaths. Research in the 1930s showed no correlation between cholesterol and heart disease.[1] Most interestingly, if one were looking for why heart disease suddenly became such a problem, the rise in deaths coincided with the time when the use of seed oils such as sunflower, safflower, and canola became commercially and domestically available. The use of these oils that were cheap to produce and had a long shelf life, together with sugar and the newly invented high-fructose corn syrup, spawned a huge processed-food industry.

But in the 1950s and 1960s, there were two divergent views as to the reason for the rise in heart disease. One view was championed by a prominent British physiologist and nutritionist, John Yudkin, who identified added sugar as the primary agent for chronic heart disease (as well as diabetes and other killers);[2] he also showed that in most cases, weight could also be controlled by a low-carbohydrate diet.[3] His research and landmark 1972 book *Pure, White, and Deadly*[4] clearly did not receive the attention they should have. In fact, in a 2016 research article into the role of the sugar industry in funding research and formulating public health policy, the authors concluded:

The SRF [Sugar Research Foundation] sponsored its first CHD

[coronary heart disease] research project in 1965, a literature review
published in the New England Journal of Medicine, *which singled*
out fat and cholesterol as the dietary causes of CHD and downplayed
evidence that sucrose consumption was also a risk factor. The SRF set
the review's objective, contributed articles for inclusion, and received
drafts. The SRF's funding and role was not disclosed. Together with
other recent analyses of sugar industry documents, our findings suggest
the industry sponsored a research program in the 1960s and 1970s that
successfully cast doubt about the hazards of sucrose while promoting
fat as the dietary culprit in CHD. Policymaking committees should
consider giving less weight to food industry–funded studies ...[5]

The other view, that saturated fat was the main problem, was championed by Ancel Keys, a persuasive and charismatic physiologist at the University of Minnesota in the United States. He became interested in the causes of heart disease when he noticed business executives in the US had much higher rates than their counterparts in Europe. Keys believed high cholesterol levels in the blood were to blame, and that these were caused by eating certain types of fats — in particular, saturated animal fats. Keys wrote a paper in which fat consumption and heart-disease rates were mapped in six countries, and presented it to the World Health Organisation in 1955.[6]

Keys is often criticised for cherry-picking countries that fitted his hypothesis. It's claimed that he ignored other countries for which data was available (bringing the number of countries to 22) and that if these countries are included, there is no correlation between fat and heart disease — the 22-country graph doesn't show any particular trend.

The story is a little more complicated than that, but worth discussing. It's a good example of how poor science can still be used to build a public health policy — especially when supported by industry. At the time, academia was far from convinced about Keys' hypothesis. A review of his study was conducted in 1957, by Yerushalmy and Hilleboe — a Berkeley statistician and a New York State commissioner of health, respectively, who'd both attended the WHO meeting with Keys. They wrote a scathing critique of Keys' six-country graph. Even though they did in fact find a trend similar to Keys over the 22 countries, they warn of the limitations of this kind of observational study, reminding us that just because something occurs with something else doesn't mean it causes it — correlation does not imply causation.[7]

> *It is well known that the indirect method merely suggests that there is an association between the characteristics studied and mortality rates and, further, that no matter how plausible such an association may appear, it is not in itself proof of a cause–effect relationship. But quotation and repetition of the suggestive association soon creates the impression that the relationship is truly valid, and ultimately it acquires status as a supporting link in a chain of presumed proof.*

And indeed this was the case, as the 'lipid hypothesis', laying all blame on all fats, came to dominate the global approach to obesity. There is more to Keys' story, but this first set of claim, misunderstanding, and analysis is the prototypical exchange that would characterise how his subsequent work was received.[8]

Despite the warnings from academia, the low-fat dogma and demonisation of cholesterol was born nonetheless. The American Heart Association and US government, attracted by the simple cause-and-effect message, advised consumers to reduce their intake of butter, lard, eggs, and beef — despite the fact these foods had been consumed by humans for thousands of years before the epidemic of the last 50 years.

Another factor overlooked, but covered in undergraduate biochemistry and physiology, is that only 10 per cent of the body's cholesterol comes directly from our diet. Most cholesterol is produced by the liver — a point that even Keys conceded.

Given that heart disease remains the world's number one killer, it seems like it's time for a new hypothesis.

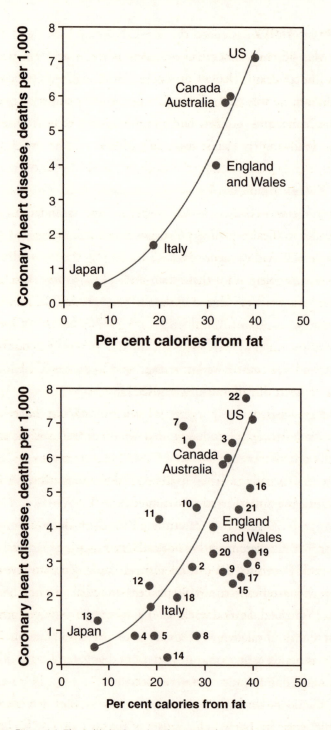

Above: Figure 4-1. The published results of Keys' paper.
Below: Figure 4-2. Results including 22 countries.

My father's story

When he was 56, my father had a minor heart attack. He wasn't overweight, never drank alcohol or smoked, and was physically very active. However, he was going through a particularly stressful time at work and at home, and certainly had a family history of heart disease. His doctor, following the 'latest research', advised that he switch to a low-fat diet, clearly influenced by the work of Ancel Keys and research funded by the sugar industry.

The message was clear — avoid cholesterol and saturated animal fat, and switch to 'health-giving' polyunsaturated margarine and seed and vegetable oils. As I've mentioned, it's interesting that heart disease was not such a problem until these man-made, highly processed, and unstable seed oils were introduced in the early part of the 20th century; but industry is a powerful influencer on public health. Without knowing it at the time, we were experiencing that influence in our own home, firsthand. Of course, we knew sugar was bad for teeth, but any connection to heart disease was never raised.

My father avoided eating eggs and butter, and our household switched to margarine, a product called Meadow-Lea, with a ratio of polyunsaturated to saturated fat of 2:1. In an effort to be even 'healthier', we eventually switched to Becel, another margarine, with an even 'healthier' polyunsaturated to saturated fat ratio of 4:1.

At the age of 75 and after carefully adhering to the low-fat, no-saturated-animal-fat diet, my father noticed he was getting progressively short of breath. He visited his cardiologist, and an angiogram revealed that his coronary arteries were now 90 per cent occluded. The new health regimen hadn't helped. Several weeks later, the heart surgeon performed a gruelling four-hour quadruple coronary-artery-bypass operation. The operation was hailed a 'success' — apart from one complication. Four hours is a long time for any operation, but for a 75-year-old it's even longer. While my father had displayed very early signs of dementia in the years preceding his bypass, the impact of the operation on his brain was soon obvious.

After a few months, we noticed my father's memory was badly affected and he was becoming forgetful about ordinary, everyday things. He was often frustrated and at times aggressive. Within two years, it became a serious problem, and my father was formally diagnosed with dementia. Eventually, at the age of 78, he had to be admitted to a medium-care dementia ward; he died three years later, unable to recognise anyone in our family. But dementia is like watching someone die very slowly, and sadly is a growing problem, even affecting people in their 60s (but that is another story).

The financial cost of the initial heart operation and for care in the dementia unit was more than AU$250,000. The emotional human cost to my father and our entire family was devastating.

Could my father's final years have been different? An integrative, holistic approach at the point of his minor heart attack at 56 — or at any time in the intervening years — might have advised him to eat more vegetables and avoid highly processed, unstable margarine and seed oils. What if he was told to eat moderate amounts of protein that was high in anti-inflammatory omega-3 fatty acids? What if he'd been advised to exercise and learn how to relax or meditate?

There is a whole range of simple interventions that could have been life-changing for my father, not to mention the rest of our family, and which I will outline in Part 3 of this book. If he had been given this information, I believe the financial and human cost of my father's final years would have been significantly different for all involved. It is an example of how health costs escalate and outcomes are compromised. It's a story that has been repeated millions of times in millions of ways.

And now for a word from our sponsor

Sponsorship of major health organisations by the food and pharmaceutical industries is also a problem. Take the effect of sugar on oral health as an example.

For over 50 years, I'm proud to say, the dental profession has warned about the dangers of sugar for oral health. In fact, Weston A. Price made the connection 80 years ago. Most people would agree that sugary drinks cause tooth decay. It's an example of a simple, common sense, widely accepted public health message. In 2003, the American Academy of Paediatric Dentistry reflected that clear message when it said, 'Frequent consumption of sugars in any beverage can be a significant factor in the child or adolescent diet that contributes to the initiation and progression of dental caries (cavities).' No one could possibly argue with that; sugar's effect is beyond doubt — or is it?

Just one year later, in 2004, Pepsi donated US$1 million to this same organisation, and its public health message changed to this: 'Scientific evidence is certainly not clear on the exact role that soft drinks play in terms of children's oral disease.' Despite the obvious and universally accepted evidence that soft drinks increase tooth decay, sponsorship created doubt — the greatest tool for industry interests. Creating doubt, uncertainty, and confusion is the best way of distracting attention from real health, and, for that matter, environmental issues.

How do other sponsorships and commercial interests affect messages that are not as clear-cut as this one?

Heart Foundation Ticks — health message or commercial interest?

In 1989, the Heart Foundation in Australia introduced a system known as the 'Heart Foundation Tick', in which foods that met its criteria could include a red tick on their packaging. The reality was that a product only needed to be low-fat and have had its producer pay a fee to the Heart Foundation for it to get the tick. 'The Heart Foundation tick is perceived by consumers to mean a product is healthy,' writes Sandra Jones, from the University of Wollongong.[9] 'But it's more complicated than that. The tick means a product is healthier than other options but it *doesn't mean it's healthy in its own right* [my emphasis]. A meat pie, for example, can get a tick if it's lower in fat and salt than other meat pies, but it doesn't mean this is a healthy food that should be chosen over a salad.'

Unilever, a global processed-food giant and the manufacturer of Flora margarine, received a Heart Foundation Tick, which was still in place as late as 2015. Like many global food and pharmaceutical giants, Unilever sponsors many professional dietitian associations around the globe. This a good example of the power of engaging healthcare professionals to promote a product. There will be many 'experts' and a great deal of research sponsored by manufacturers espousing the virtues of margarine over butter, and the decision may seem confusing.

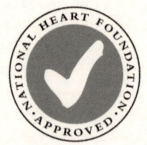

Figure 4-3. The National Heart Foundation Tick.

How is butter made? The sun shines; the grass grows; cows eat the grass and miraculously produce milk, the cream of which produces butter, which has been consumed in various forms for thousands of years.

Margarine on the other hand is the product of emulsifying, interesterification, hydrogenation, and more. This is clearly a complicated industrial process, so best summarised in Figure 4-4.

Reading the news and even the literature, it's easy to get confused. I will cover this in more detail in Chapter 12: Nutrition, but as a general guiding principle I would always choose a natural, minimally processed food over a highly processed one. I believe it's far better for healthcare professionals and their organisations to endorse simple health messages and products, or 'inform' the public that 'scientific evidence is certainly not clear on the exact role' of a particular food, rather than promoting foods that are 'proudly brought to you' by the sponsor.

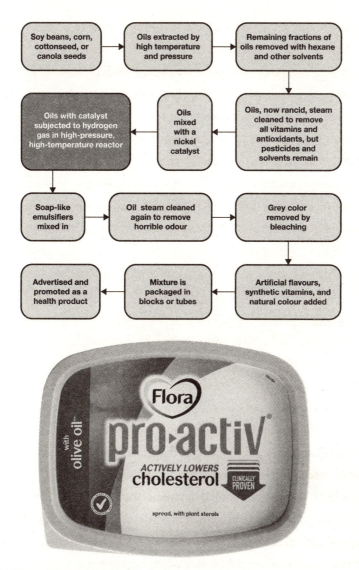

Above: Figure 4-4. The process of producing margarine.
Below: Figure 4-5. Heart Foundation tick-endorsed margarine in 2015.

People were often surprised to learn that companies paid to have their food assessed and then be allowed to carry the Heart Foundation's tick of approval. The fact is, if you didn't pay, your foods weren't assessed or allowed to use the Tick to market them. Again, a wonderful economic synergy bringing funding into health organisations while helping processed-food companies market their product with respected professional health endorsement. A great economic model, but a confusing one to say the least. A food item that was much healthier than another on a supermarket shelf simply couldn't have a Tick if the manufacturer hadn't paid the fee for assessment. I would have loved to have seen a Heart Foundation banner over the vegetable and fruit section of a supermarket, reminding shoppers that that's where the really healthy food was, but sadly the Ticks were restricted to the processed foods in the centre aisles.

To show just how far this can go, in February 2007, fast-food franchise McDonald's received nine Heart Foundation Ticks, including one for their Chicken McNuggets, at a cost of $330,000 Australian dollars.[10] On the day this was announced, Susan Anderson, national manager of the Heart Foundation's Tick program, told ABC radio reporter Jane Cowan that McDonald's had changed its recipes to earn the Tick and genuinely lifted its game. 'We've given them a tick of approval for meeting some very strict standards, because we know people are there, we know that they're not curbing their dietary patterns by not going to these sorts of places, so it is much better that they have a healthier choice when they're there.'[11] Cowan also was careful to make the point that the Tick didn't mean the item was healthy, just that it was healthier than other options in the category — in this case, other fast foods.

Ironically, one of the major changes McDonald's undertook was to stop frying their French fries in tallow, an unprocessed, traditional, and stable animal fat, and instead used a highly processed and unstable polyunsaturated, which when heated to high temperatures promotes inflammation. This is something I will cover in more detail in Chapter 6: Nutritional Stress and Chapter 12: Nutrition.

In 2011, after much community and health-professional pressure, the Heart Foundation reluctantly cut its relationship with McDonald's.[12] As an aside (and perhaps just coincidentally), I was fascinated to discover that six months after the removal of the Tick, the company reported a 5 per cent drop in profits.

The Tick program was belatedly, but thankfully, axed in December

2015. Ironically, removing the Tick from the supermarket shelves may be the Heart Foundation's greatest contribution to public health, particularly if it results in a significant drop in the sales of processed foods.

Health Star Rating

With the demise of the Tick, a new system has been introduced in Australia to help people make 'better choices'. As the Australian government describes it, the Health Star Rating is 'a front-of-pack labelling system that rates the overall nutritional profile of packaged food and assigns it a rating from ½ star to 5 stars. It provides a quick, easy, standard way to compare similar packaged foods. The more stars, the healthier the choice.'[13] The program rolled out in June 2014, funded by federal and state governments with the development and implementation overseen by various councils, groups, and multinational food and beverage companies.[14] I'm not reassured by this at all.

Once again, we are seeing corporations with the help of professional organisations 'educating' the public and influencing what we eat. They have created a complex nutritional calculation that breaks down the nutrients of a food product to arrive at the star rating. For example, many commercial breakfast cereals get 4 stars; Milo, a popular Australian chocolate and malt flavouring with a frightening list of ingredients, when consumed with skimmed milk gets 4.5 stars; while coconut oil, which *is* good for you, gets ½ star.

As independent consumer-advocacy group Choice put it, 'We're disappointed that food manufacturers are abusing the system to promote nutrient-poor foods as a healthier option.'[15] I'm disappointed, too, to say the least.

A rising epidemic despite dietary advice

A new epidemic has emerged in the last 20 years, one which does not discriminate by age. Type 2 diabetes used to be referred to as 'late-onset' diabetes but is now diagnosed among youth and even children.[16] Diabetes predisposes people to every degenerative disease, including cancer, heart disease, and dementia, and is at record levels in both the young and the old.

There are two widely accepted forms of diabetes:

- **Type 1 diabetes.** This is usually caused by an autoimmune destruction of the pancreatic beta cells that produce insulin. When the body's insulin production is impaired, the patient needs insulin injections or a continuous infusion through an insulin pump to survive. A paper published in 2010 revealed that the incidence of this autoimmune disease has increased globally by 2–5 per cent annually, and the prevalence of type 1 diabetes is approximately one in 300 in the US by 18 years of age.[17]
- **Type 2 diabetes.** This is when the body can't cope with the amount of glucose (a sugar) being ingested and produces too much insulin, to the point where cells become resistant to it. There is an excess of glucose in the body, which is then highly reactive and causes many health problems. Globally, approximately one in ten adults has type 2 diabetes, with the number of individuals more than doubling from 153 million in 1980 to 347 million in 2008.[18] The increased consumption of fructose, often in the form of high-fructose corn syrup (HFCS), found in many processed foods and drinks, contributes significantly to the problem.[19]

Dementia and type 3 diabetes

Today, some forms of dementia are being referred to as type 3 diabetes, where the brain cells become insulin-resistant and fail to adequately fuel brain cells for normal function and repair.[20] Given that we are seeing a dramatic increase in dementia occurring concurrently with the dramatic increase in type 2 diabetes, it's worth asking if nutritional factors are implicated in dementia more generally.

Dementia is another condition whose occurrence seems to be escalating each year, as our population ages. According to a recent global report: 'Today, over 46 million people live with dementia worldwide, more than the population of Spain. This number is estimated to increase to 131.5 million by 2050. Dementia also has a huge economic impact. Today, the total estimated worldwide cost of dementia is US$818 billion, and it will become a trillion dollar disease by 2018.'[21] The toll on carers and their families also places a huge emotional burden, which is impossible to quantify financially. Disturbingly, dementia is also affecting people at a younger age, even in their 50s and 60s.

The Food Pyramid — how much is too much?

Thirty years of dietary advice, the foundation of which has been the Food Pyramid and low-fat dogma, surely needs to be called into question.

We're all familiar with some form of the Food Pyramid. I've included the 1992 US Department of Agriculture (USDA) Food Pyramid here. It eventually morphed in 2011 into MyPlate, and in 2013 in Australia into the Australian Guide to Healthy Eating. Each is still built on grains and carbs, and each still demonises fats.

The American Food and Drug Administration (FDA) endorsed the USDA Food Pyramid as the foundation of an implied 'healthy eating' guide. It's worth pointing out that the USDA's primary role is to support US agriculture (in this case, growers of corn, wheat, and soy), not to promote a healthy way of eating. Those grain industries also receive massive government subsidies. While we are often reminded of the importance of an 'evidence-based approach to healthcare', I think it's worth asking, how did the evidence stack up?

Soon after its introduction, all major health organisations and professional associations, such as the American Diabetics Association and the American Heart Foundation, joined the FDA in endorsing the Food Pyramid. The graph in Figure 4-7 reveals what happened to the incidence of diabetes in the US from 1980–2011 and specifically once the Food Pyramid was introduced and so enthusiastically endorsed. Perhaps this is a coincidence and the Food Pyramid didn't lead to an increase in diabetes — but it certainly didn't help hold or reduce the rate.

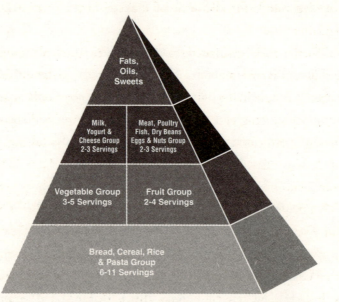

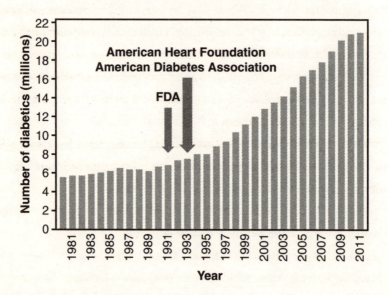

Above: Figure 4-6. The 1992 USDA Food Pyramid.
Below: Figure 4-7. Number of people with diabetes each year from 1980 to 2011, showing when the FDA introduced the Food Pyramid and when American Heart Foundation and the American Diabetes Association also endorsed it.

In 1980, fewer than six million Americans had diabetes. By 2011, just over 20 million Americans had diabetes. In 2014, the number increased to 29.1 million or 9.3 per cent of the US population.[22] The expected trends for all forms of diabetes over the next 20 years are alarming.

Then there is pre-diabetes, a 'condition' in which blood-glucose levels are higher than normal but are not high enough to definitively diagnose diabetes. People living with pre-diabetes are supposedly at an increased risk of developing type 2 diabetes, heart disease, and stroke. It's also known as impaired glucose tolerance or impaired fasting glucose. In 2012, 86 million Americans aged 20 and older had pre-diabetes — up from 79 million in 2010. There is, however, some doubt as to the value of such a diagnosis as pre-diabetes. A recent study found that between 90 and 95 per cent of those 'diagnosed' as pre-diabetics were not actually progressing to diabetes.[23] The scientific literature on nutrition is also often confusing and contradictory. For example, what actually qualifies as 'low-carbohydrate'? To some, this is defined as 70 grams per day. Others put it at 150 grams per day, and the official recommendation is 310 grams per day. The issue of high fat is also often poorly defined. It can vary from unhealthy saturated fats in hamburgers, pizzas, and French fries to healthy saturated fats such as those in butter, coconut oil, grass-fed animal fats, olive oil, or avocados. I'll cover this in more detail in Part 2 and Part 3 of this book.

Why is carbohydrate intake so relevant? Here is some basic scientific knowledge, known to all students of health studying biochemistry at undergraduate level:

- diet is a strong cause of type 2 diabetes
- insulin levels are affected when you consume too many carbohydrates that are quickly broken down into glucose
- healthy fats are an excellent way to stabilise hunger and blood sugar
- the lower your insulin levels, the healthier you will be.

Independent research now shows that a diet low in carbohydrates and high in healthy fat is more effective at controlling weight and blood sugar, and reducing the risk of heart disease.[24] Not surprisingly, this is a diet similar to that eaten by our grandparents before heart disease, diabetes, or obesity could ever have been described as epidemics; before food and healthcare became the major commodities they are today.

Despite the evidence, professional organisations (often financially supported by the food and pharmaceutical industries) persist in giving health advice that promotes a diet that clearly predisposes the population to an ever-increasing incidence of diabetes, obesity, and other chronic diseases. Diet and lifestyle is the common theme that runs through all degenerative diseases.

Each year, the International Diabetes Federation (IDF) organises a World Diabetes Day. On this day, the IDF acknowledges that it 'is particularly grateful to the following corporations and foundations for their *support towards helping promote diabetes care, prevention and a cure worldwide*' (my emphasis). Figure 4-8 shows a list of those corporate sponsors/supporters, which includes most major pharmaceutical companies in the world.

It's worth noting that for all those people with diabetes, 85 per cent have type 2 diabetes, for which the 'cure' is already well known: diet and exercise. And yet 70–80 per cent of people with diabetes in the US today take some form of medication. Addressing the cause with proper dietary advice and actually curing the condition is achievable, but it needs the correct advice. This would lead to you avoiding not only the wide-ranging side effects of type 2 diabetes, but also the medications — a huge win for individuals and public health.

But 'living with diabetes' and lifetime management seems to be the accepted norm. An example is the 2015 Australian Diabetes Council's '10 Steps to Good Health *with* Diabetes' (my emphasis). One only needs to look at step one of their ten-step program to be assured of a continued life *with* diabetes: 'Follow a healthy eating plan which is low in fat, particularly saturated fat, high in fibre and includes carbohydrates in every meal.'

MEET OUR PARTNERS

IDF is particularly grateful to the following corporations and foundations for their support towards helping promote diabetes care, prevention and a cure worldwide:

IDF Global Partners are engaged in long-term multi-faceted partnerships with the Federation. They support IDF's core activities and specific tailored programmes focusing on diabetes awareness, prevention, education and more.

IDF Corporate Supporters actively contribute to IDF's work and activities to promote diabetes care, prevention and a cure worldwide. They also participate in joint efforts to strengthen global awareness and advocacy.

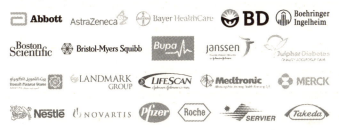

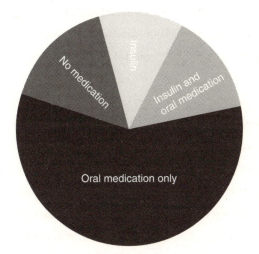

Above: Figure 4-8. International Diabetes Federation's corporate partners, as listed in 2013.
Below: Figure 4-9. People with diabetes in the US receiving conventional treatment.

According to research by the American Diabetes Association, the cost of diabetes has risen from $174 billion in 2007 to $245 billion in 2012 — a 41 per cent increase.[25] One starts to wonder … who are the main stakeholders for these professional health bodies? Is it the public

— or the organisations themselves and the corporations that support them in the search for a 'cure'?

Independent advice?

There is reason to be concerned about the independence of advice from organisations such as the Academy of Nutrition and Dietetics (formerly the American Dietetic Association — the world's largest organisation of food and nutrition professionals) when you look at their list of corporate partners (Figure 4-10).

Another major professional organisation is the American Society of Nutrition, established 1928, 'a not-for-profit organisation dedicated to bringing together the world's top researchers, clinical nutritionists and industry. Its corporate partners and sponsors support the Society in its pursuit of excellence in nutrition, research and practice' (Figure 4-11).

The Dietitians Association of Australia is similarly sponsored by corporations that, presumably, also assist in educational programs, research, and promoting important public health messages (Figure 4-12).

In recent years, the 'Paleo' diet has become popular, and with good reason. Foundations for this diet include fresh vegetables, ethically grown pasture-fed meats eaten in moderation, good fats, and the avoidance of grains and dairy products. The Dietitians Association of Australia has repeatedly branded it a 'dangerous diet', particularly because it avoids grains and dairy. Coincidentally, these industries have been two of the association's major sponsors for many years.

The growing impact of corporate advice

When determining which food is healthy, many consumers rightly, and yet perhaps naively, rely on advice from government authorities. From 1992 to 2005, the USDA Food Pyramid supposedly represented the ideal health diet. The method by which these recommendations were arrived at reveals more about the power of economics than of health.

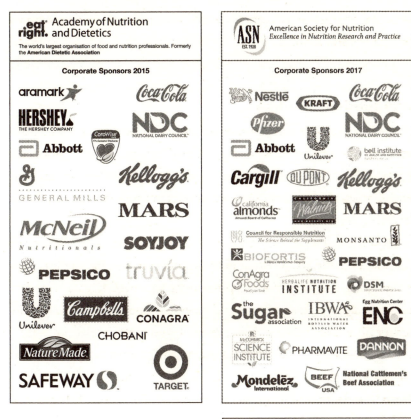

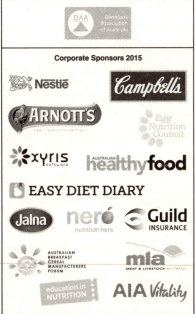

Above left: Figure 4-10.
Above right: Figure 4-11. 'The American Society for Nutrition is pleased to acknowledge the support by these organizations for educational programs of the society.'

Below right: Figure 4-12.

Dietitians initially recommended three to five servings of whole grains a day. But, after lobbying from the grain industry for between nine and 12 servings per day, the final recommendation was set at six to 11 serves of grains a day. This significant difference was based not on health, but on economics.

The US Centres for Disease Control and Prevention (CDC) has mapped the distribution of obesity across the states as the disease has spread. The percentage of obese Americans has grown despite the introduction of the Food Pyramid and its eventual replacement with MyPlate.

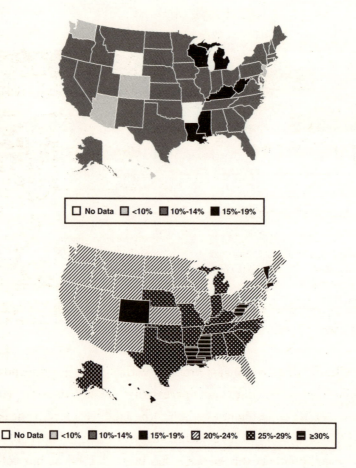

Above: Figure 4-13. The distribution of obesity across America in 1992, the year USDA Food Pyramid was introduced.
Below: Figure 4-14. The distribution of obesity across America in 2005.

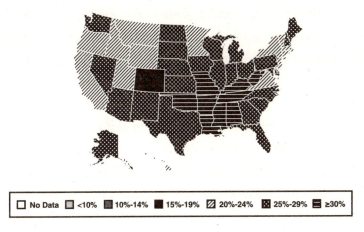

Figure 4-15. The distribution of obesity across America in 2009.

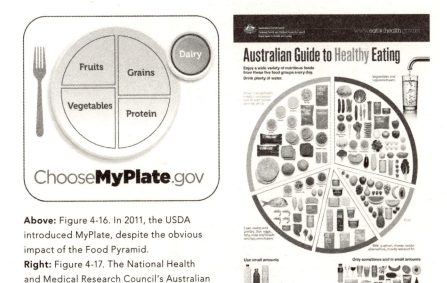

Above: Figure 4-16. In 2011, the USDA introduced MyPlate, despite the obvious impact of the Food Pyramid.
Right: Figure 4-17. The National Health and Medical Research Council's Australian Guide to Healthy Eating.

Clearly, there is a major problem with dietary recommendations. While correlation does not necessarily mean causation (and as I will outline throughout the book, the issues we face in health are multifactorial), the strong evidence suggests that the impact of official advice and public health messages has been harmful on our collective health. Since these various guidelines were released, diabetes and obesity have climbed to record levels. Childhood diseases are escalating, with even babies now suffering from obesity.[26] The increase in mental-health disorders, setting aside the impact of the *DSM-5*, may also be closely linked to nutritional issues.

The Harvard School of Public Health concludes: 'The US pyramid blueprint was based on shaky scientific evidence, and it barely changed over the years to reflect major advances in our understanding of the connection between diet and health.'[27]

The overriding message from official government sources, starting in the 1970s and 1980s and formalised in the 1992 Food Pyramid, is essentially: high carbohydrate (largely based on grains), low saturated fat, and low cholesterol. The effect of this nutritional advice is all around us. Surely the advice has changed by now?

Fast-forward to 2017, and the USDA has launched a new Interactive Dietary Reference Intake Calculator for Healthcare Professionals.[28] The dietary reference intakes have been developed by the Institute of Medicine and 'represent the *most current scientific knowledge* on nutrient needs' (my emphasis).

I entered my own age, weight, height, and activity levels, and the advice I received was essentially high carbohydrate (320–462 grams per day), low saturated fat ('As low as possible'), and low cholesterol ('As low as possible'). I will discuss the levels of macronutrients (carbohydrate, fat, and protein) in more detail in Chapter 12: Nutrition.

It's interesting to note in the daily-intake recommendations how fluoride has also found its way into the list of 'essential minerals', with a daily minimum requirement. As I will discuss in Chapter 8: Dental Stress and Chapter 12: Nutrition, of the 70 elements required for all of the biological functions to maintain good health in the human body, fluoride is not one of them.

My message to you

I believe government health authorities and professional health organisations are letting us down. They are too influenced by industries, slow to change, often more protective of their own reputations than public health, and often just seem to lack common sense.

When you become aware of these influences on confusing and contradictory public health messages, it allows you to put them into a broader perspective. For me, this knowledge has empowered me to take control of my own health, reflect on lessons from the past, and use some common sense. Hopefully, it will empower you to do the same. You are the major stakeholder of your health, and you and those who you care about are the major beneficiaries. Your health is too important to entrust to someone else.

You now understand public health messages. But to take control of your health, you must understand stress.

PART 2

Redefining
Stress

CHAPTER 5

Emotional Stress

Most of us understand that emotional stress can have an impact on our health, but you may be surprised at just how far-reaching its impacts can be. Emotional stress can affect your ability to sleep, your ability to breathe, your ability to eat, your ability to get up and move, and your ability to think. In Part 3 of this book, I will look at the five pillars of health and find ways to miminise the negative impacts that emotional stress can have on your wellbeing. The purpose of this book is to build physical and mental resilience into your life so you can better cope with past, present, and future emotional challenges. But first, let's take a closer look at emotional stress.

We all respond differently

During a visit to a fun park with our families, my friend Trevor convinced me to ride a roller-coaster with him. We climbed into the carriage, strapped ourselves in, and made our vertiginous ascent. As the roller-coaster teetered on the top of the track and then fell and swerved, I felt sick — I hate roller-coasters. Trevor, in sharp contrast, loved every minute of it.

At the end of the ride, he was smiling and flushed with excitement — presumably, the endorphins were pumping through his body — and he was ready for another ride. I, on the other hand, was pale and clammy; my cortisol and adrenaline levels must have been through the roof. We were two men of a similar age having just had exactly the same experience but with completely different responses, both mentally and physically. It's the same with emotional stress. We are often faced with stressful situations, which we may not have any control over. But we do have control over how we respond.

I was taught this very lesson by, of all things, a bird. The common koel is a migratory bird that arrives in Sydney each September. You know when it has hit our shores by the male's annoying whistle: a 'koo-eel' sound in an ascending tone — endlessly repeated. For most of my adult life, my bedtime was around midnight; I thought this worked well for most of the year, but, in September and October, I would be woken at 5.30 a.m. by that interminable 'koo-eel, koo-eel'. It was driving me crazy! But what could I do about it? The bird was there for the spring, but I needed more sleep. Clearly, I couldn't change the bird's desire to sing, so I decided instead to change my bedtime to 9.00 p.m. and use the bird as my wake-up call. Not only did this new routine work, it changed my life. Each day, I woke with the bird, and I started going to the gym in time for a 6.00 a.m. start. I ended up getting more sleep and improving my fitness simply because I changed my attitude to something I couldn't physically control.

I realise life is not as simple as that.

Avoiding stressful situations or relationships is one possibility. Taking a step back and looking at them in a different light is another possibility.

Stress is a growing problem

While everyone responds differently, we live in a world where there is a myriad of stressful stimuli, and an ever-growing number of us clearly feel the impact of that emotional stress. Research confirms what many of us suspect: that living with ongoing stress affects our health and can contribute to chronic illness. The *Stress and Wellbeing in Australia Survey 2014*, conducted by the Australian Psychological Society, found that 72 per cent of Australians reported their current stress levels had an impact on their physical health.[1]

Women reported a greater impact of stress on their health: 21 per cent, compared to 13 per cent of men, said that stress was strongly affecting their physical health — and 23 per cent of women compared to 14 per cent of the men studied reported that stress was strongly affecting their mental health. As a man, my experience tells me these results don't truly reflect the impact of stress on both the mental and physical wellbeing of males. My guess is that males are just not as introspective, analytical, or communicative about things that may have a negative impact on their health. It may be one explanation for why women, on the average, live five years longer than men. As with many other things, particularly when it comes to our health, we males have much to learn.

In that same 2014 study, almost six million people reported moderate to severe levels of distress in 2013, and lower levels of wellbeing compared with 2012 and 2011. Clearly, emotional stress plays a huge part in mental and physical health and wellbeing; the mind and body are intimately connected.

THE NERVOUS SYSTEM DEFINED

The nervous system coordinates its actions by transmitting signals to and from different parts of its body. It consists of two main parts:

- The central nervous system, which consists of the brain and spinal cord.
- The peripheral nervous system, which consists mainly of nerves that connect the central nervous system to every other part of the body.

The peripheral nervous system is further divided into three parts:

- Somatic nerves are associated with control of body

movements. These comprise both sensory nerves and motor nerves. Sensory nerves are responsible for relaying sensation from the body to the central nervous system; motor nerves are responsible for sending out commands from the central nervous system to the body, stimulating muscle contraction.

- The enteric nervous system controls the gastrointestinal tract. It has been referred as the 'second brain' because it can operate independently, but also because the brain and the gut are connected by an extensive network of neurons and a vast array of chemicals and hormones that provide a feedback loop, letting us know when we're hungry, whether we're stressed or not, and if we've ingested a potentially harmful microbe. The intricate and plentiful connections between gut and brain give a new meaning to the old expressions of having a 'gut feeling' or 'gut instinct'.

- The autonomic nervous system influences smooth muscle, glands, and internal organs. It acts mostly unconsciously, and regulates bodily functions such as heart rate, breathing, digestion, urination, and sexual arousal.

The autonomic nervous system is further divided into two parts:

- The sympathetic nervous system, which is activated in cases of emergencies or stress. This is called the 'fight or flight' response. Blood is diverted from the digestive system to skeletal muscles, immune system activity is minimised, and the reflexive, primitive part of the brain becomes dominant. From an evolutionary perspective, sympathetic activity should be over quickly. The problem is that in our world, this is not the case, and we are too often in 'sympathetic overload'.

- The parasympathetic nervous system is a much slower system. When we are breathing in a relaxed way, the parasympathetic nervous system is dominant and allows our body to function optimally. It helps to digest food properly, keeps our heartbeat regular, allows us to think more clearly, and allows the immune system to work optimally — facilitating 'rest and digest'. The vast majority of our time should be spent in the parasympathetic mode, to maintain a healthy balance in our body.

How does stress affect us?

Fight or flight. For our ancestors, this meant running away from a sabre-toothed tiger — or moving in for the kill.

Today, it means responding to a driver who pulls in front of you while on the road, pushing yourself to meet a deadline at work, trying to manage a hectic work-life balance, or constantly maintaining the 'lifestyle' or being the 'good consumers' we are all encouraged to aspire to. In contrast to the length of time the fight-or-flight response was active in our ancestors (only several minutes at any one time), this stress response may be constant, lasting for hours, days, months, or even years. Of particular interest is what happens when the adrenal glands produce stress hormones such as cortisol and adrenaline — and how these hormones affect all aspects of wellbeing, from the optimal operation of digestion and the immune system, right through to our ability to think clearly and make rational decisions.

Part of the physiological effect of the stress response is that blood is diverted from the digestive tract to the muscles in your arms and legs so you can run away from 'danger'. This explains why even if you eat the most nutritious diet and take all the supplements you feel you need, you may not be able to digest effectively and, most importantly, absorb those nutrients. Naturally, this interferes with not only how well you feel, but also the daily growth and regeneration of cells throughout your body that keep you healthy.

The gut is the location of at least 80 per cent of your immune system and, as such, is compromised by a prolonged stress response — making you more susceptible to disease. Stress hormones also affect other components that make up a well-functioning immune system. When faced with an actual or perceived danger, your body has to decide how to allocate its energy. The priority moves from dealing with bacteria, viruses, or even environmental toxins to addressing the immediate perceived 'danger' or stress. The outcome leaves you susceptible to infection, inflammation, and chronic disease.

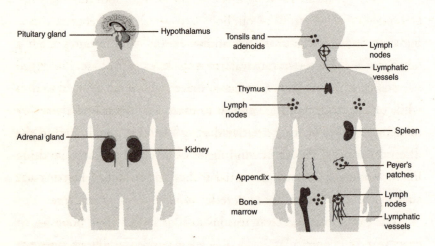

Left: Figure 5-1. Adrenal glands and hormones are affected by stress levels.
Right: Figure 5-2. Other components of the immune system.

But the impact doesn't stop there — our stress response also affects our ability to think clearly and logically. Adrenal hormones divert blood flow from the front of the brain (the part that helps process information and promote reason and logic), reducing its ability to function optimally and make well-considered, rational decisions. This can have far-reaching effects and may account for decisions about what to eat or drink when stressed — often things that you know aren't good for your health, but you buy them anyway. When stressed, you operate on reflex.

Hans Selye, who coined the term 'stress', referred to three phases of the stress response, which he termed 'general adaption syndrome':[2]

1. **Alarm phase.** Adrenaline and cortisol prepare the body for fight or flight.
2. **Resistance phase.** This varies in length according to the severity of the stress, and the resilience or adaptive capacity of the individual.
3. **Exhaustion phase.** If the stress is prolonged, the response enters this phase. The increased activity of the sympathetic nervous system starts to wear the stressed individual down, leading to health problems.

Essentially, we are running 21st century software (our modern lives) on pre-agricultural hardware (our body and mind). In Palaeolithic times, our stress response was protective and would last a few minutes or a few hours, somewhere between the 'alarm' and 'resistance' phase. Prolonged stress affects us in ways our bodies and minds have not evolved to deal with, exhausting the body's ability to maintain a healthy balance, or homeostasis; chronic degenerative diseases then take hold. And in the 21st century, it is worth reminding ourselves that stress is anything in the world that has the potential to knock you out of homeostatic balance. What we are faced with today is a multitude of stresses.

This is one of the main reasons I have written this book — to provide a broadened definition of what stress is, to discuss how the various stresses can affect your health, and to show you how to build resilience into your life.

HOMEOSTASIS DEFINED

The word 'homeostasis' refers to any process that living beings use to actively maintain the fairly stable conditions necessary for survival. The term was coined in the 1930s by Walter Cannon, a Harvard professor of physiology. Homeostasis is the tendency of a system (nervous, circulatory, lymphatic, immune, etc.) to maintain internal stability, owing to the coordinated response of its parts to any situation or stimulus or stress that would tend to disturb its normal condition or function.

More recently the term 'allostasis' has been introduced to recognise the importance of the brain, which activates internal homeostatic responses to bring the body back into balance. This is a recognition of the fact that the mind and body are inseparable. Throughout the book, I refer to the importance of factors that may compromise our health (stresses) and ways of achieving and maintaining an optimal balance (pillars). I will refer to 'homeostasis', which for our purposes encompasses the integrated role both brain and body systems play.

What causes emotional stress?

Emotional stress has many causes, from worries about money and work, to relationships and traumatic events, as well as caring for or giving support to others. It may also involve worrying about something that hasn't even happened.

A new source of emotional stress in our daily lives is technology. Don't get me wrong — I use technology as much as anyone. Technology has in many ways revolutionised our lives and provided us with enormous benefits.

Thanks to technology, I can talk with anybody, anywhere in the world, and even choose to see him or her via video. Tasks like banking, which used to take more time and people-power to complete, can now be done literally in the palm of my hand. The computing power of my mobile phone is greater than the computing power that helped send the first men to the moon!

Computers give us access to enormous amounts of information, with the ability to search the cumulative knowledge of the world. This 'democratisation' of knowledge and our ability to connect and communicate with one another is unprecedented in history and provides great potential for us as individuals and as communities. I believe that once we learn to harness and effectively share that power, the world will be a better place.

In my own dental practice, technology has revolutionised everyday tasks. Digital X-rays and photos improve our ability to communicate with patients; filling material is hardened by a light, literally with the flick of a switch; and ceramic fillings and crowns can be designed on a computer, milled to exact dimensions, and fitted at the same appointment.

Yet, while undoubtedly exciting, convenient, and stimulating, there are consequences of this 'switched on' and globally connected way of life — consequences to our health and wellbeing. For a start, the increased speed at which we live our lives is also making us feel more stressed than ever before. There's pressure to complete tasks more quickly, to respond immediately. Instead of waiting a few days for a letter to arrive in the mail and then consider its content and our response, it's delivered immediately through email or another networked message service, and with that delivery is the expectation that you will respond to it right away.

Social media is also a potential source of emotional stress. While it's wonderful that we are connected with the world, how often do you sit on a train or in a restaurant and notice that everyone is looking at his or her phone? They connect with the world but not with the person sitting right next to them. This paradox of connection and disconnection is another potential stress in our lives. On the one hand, we are more connected than ever, with hundreds of 'friends' and 'liked' by many, often globally; on the other hand, it is easy for people to feel isolated and lonely in a crowded city surrounded by people.

This is in total contrast to how we lived even a century ago — surrounded by the extended family unit, where we all knew our neighbours and, born out of necessity, tended to be engaged members of our local communities. Go back a short time, and belonging to a community was critical for survival — it meant food, warmth, and, yes, health and wellbeing. Our world has changed enormously, particularly in the last 40 years, but our responses to feeling isolated or connected, it would seem, have not.

Five revolutions that have shaped our world

In his exceptional book *Sapiens: a brief history of humankind*, Yuval Noah Harari describes the experience of our ancestors.[3] *Homo sapiens* appeared over 200,000 years ago, and Harari makes the point that, genetically and physiologically, we are not that different to our hunter-gather ancestors, who, for thousands of years, roamed in small tribes of up to 150 people. He outlines several revolutions since the appearance of *Homo sapiens* that have dramatically changed our physical and emotional environment.

The first, 70–80,000 years ago, was a cognitive revolution, which distinguished us from other *Homo* species, like *Homo erectus* or *Homo neanderthalensis*. It gave us what he refers to as a 'shared belief in an imagined reality' and our ability to communicate with one another, not just from one individual to another but from generation to generation or from tribe to tribe, in a way that is unique among life forms. This allowed much larger groups to interact and combine without personally knowing individuals, as people moved from small wandering groups of 150 to larger tribes — and eventually into villages, towns, cities, and countries. The shared belief would grow to include things like superstitions, religions, tribal leaders, governments, laws, and an agreement on the value of money.

Humans are unique in the animal kingdom in many ways, but our ability to organise ourselves into complex social structures and share knowledge has propelled us to the top of the tree with an unprecedented ability to alter and control our environment. In the process, we have developed complex societies and allowed millions of people to connect and live together in a civilised and orderly way.

The second revolution was 12,000 years ago. This was the agricultural revolution, which dramatically changed us as we made the move from nomadic tribal living. After many ice ages, the climate became warmer and more stable. This allowed us to domesticate grains and animals to provide a reliable food source, yet this revolution also made us 'slaves' to the weather, the seasons, and adequate yields to feed ever-increasing populations. Harari raises the intriguing question of whether we domesticated the grains and animals or they domesticated us. Whichever way you look at it, we are inextricably linked to the production of our food.

During this time, we worked harder tending our crops and animals, but our diet actually became more restricted, offering far less variety. Sanitation and infectious diseases never troubled us when we roamed in small groups and relied purely on untamed nature for our food, but in villages, towns, and cities they confronted us and became major challenges. Populations increased, and the production of food and the care of animals required constant attention, with physically demanding and repetitive work. As hunter-gatherers, our access to a wide variety of seasonal foods within our known environment, along with our mobility, became restricted by the limitations of a static place of residence dependant on our own agricultural potential. Trading filled the gaps. Commerce was born.

The third revolution occurred 500 years ago. Harari describes it as a scientific revolution, heralded by what he refers to as 'the discovery of ignorance'. People were willing to acknowledge that religious dogma or long-held superstition didn't accurately explain the world in which we lived, and so we embarked on an era of unprecedented scientific discovery. It raises an important, timely, and exciting point for us today as we balance our desire and need for certainty against our ability to say, 'We don't know or understand something or someone.' Acknowledging ignorance provides us with the impetus to find out, learn, change, and develop as individuals and as a society.

A fourth revolution, the industrial revolution, began some 250 years ago, when we harnessed energy, enabling machines to produce goods at unprecedented rates. This prompted the movement of huge numbers of the population into cities, disconnecting us further from the land than at any time in human history. The exodus from the countryside placed enormous strains on the cities — strains that still challenge us today.

While we may have solved the problems of clean water and sanitation that earlier communities faced, the size and demands of ever-larger cities pose new challenges. Our dependence on fossil fuels, generation of enormous amounts of waste, greater disconnection from our food sources, and increasing reliance on industrialised farming techniques are affecting human health as well as the health of our soils and, ultimately, our planet.

Today, we exist in what Harari describes as the fifth revolution, a globalised technological revolution. Our greatest strength as a species has always been our ability to communicate and adapt, to think in abstract and creative ways — and this is certainly the case in our technological age.

As part of this revolution, we have also entered the era of the 'individual', which has seen great strides forward in human rights, such as rights for women and children, and racial equality — but on the flip side, we may well have too many choices. A sense of individual entitlement with too many individual expectations and demands tends to place strains on us socially and environmentally. For millennia, family and 'village' structures met all our needs from cradle to grave. They provided us with childcare, education, health, jobs, aged care, a social life, and even helped with the construction of our homes. Of equal importance, the 'village' existence supplied us with moral, physical, and emotional support through times of celebration, as well as through times of grief, difficulty, or stress.

Today, our 'village' life has disappeared. In our globalised, individual-focused world, families and supportive social structures have become fragmented, and so we seek that support from governments, the private sector, or an online world for services that were once part of community life. Adding to the conundrum is the fact that as we have privatised what were previously government-run services, we have created a market-driven economy. It is this that now fulfils the needs of housing, healthcare, education, child care, aged care, and many other services, but it can only do so at an ever-increasing cost to the individual — and this means ever-increasing hard work and an emotional disconnect from those we seek support from.

We are at a point in history where the gap between rich and poor, haves and have-nots, has never been greater. While there have clearly been enormous technical advances in our world, we still require the same emotional support from family and community that we needed a thousand or thousands of years ago. The age of the individual and the sense of personal entitlement is often detrimental to our own health and wellbeing: physically, mentally, and emotionally. Chronic degenerative diseases, both physical and mental, are at epidemic proportions, just as the health of our planet is also suffering. Things have to change.

Will this technological age leave our planet in better health for future generations than the state in which we found it? The discussion on environmental issues (specifically climate change and waste) seems to be a conflict between evidence-based science on the one hand and a market-driven economy on the other. I will discuss this more in Chapter 7: Environmental Stress.

I am an optimist. I believe we are still learning to use this unprecedented access to and democratisation of information, together with our ability to communicate via social media, to effect change globally, to improve our own health and the health of the planet. It's another reason why I decided to write this book.

Does the news stress you out?

My parents lived through world wars, a global depression, racism, and the Holocaust. They left their war-torn, racist-fuelled countries of birth to escape to a nearby country, which they found was also consumed by conflict. From there, and with a young family, they eventually moved and resettled yet again, seeking a better and more peaceful life in

Australia. Millions of people share similar or even more traumatic and challenging stories. Over the last century, wars and conflicts have led to millions of deaths and displacements.

Yet in the 21st century — where we are bombarded daily with horrific stories of violence, conflict, murder, and terrorism as they occur in every corner of the world — it is surprising to learn that we actually live in the safest and most peaceful period in human history. You are more likely to die in a car accident than be killed in a conflict, and yet we still drive in our cars mostly without fear — depending, of course, on who is driving!

Nevertheless, the daily and relentless focus on negative news contributes to our emotional stress. Often, we get that news from our mobile devices, so we literally carry the news source and burden of that news with us. After seeing these shocking stories, we are often then encouraged (by advertising) to 'relieve' our stress by using our unprecedented access to credit to engage in a little retail therapy, which in turn adds its own financial, and eventually emotional, stress — a unique form of economic irrationalism.

The news rarely covers anything positive, such as acts of kindness or goodwill; instead, it reports when a bus crashes or a train derails in a remote corner of the world. There is a paradox here that, on the one hand, these stories often report on devastating human suffering, adding to our stress; yet on the other hand, because of the frequency and way this information is presented, it's easier for us to disassociate from the reality of the human aspects of such tragedies and suffering. Desensitised to that suffering of others, particularly those from different cultural backgrounds, we then continue our own lives in the pursuit of our own personal happiness.

There's less coverage of the complex stories and issues we face that require our careful consideration; this contributes to our ever-shortening attention spans. Sometimes, news stories are shorter than the commercial breaks that accompany them. Perhaps that's what the purpose of the news has become — a break from the advertisements.

When 140 characters per message, as occurs on Twitter, is the main form of communication for the leader of the free world, we know things have taken a turn for the worse at the highest levels — and we are justifiably stressed. Yet this reinforces the need for change to come from the ground up.

In his thought-provoking book *The News: a user's manual*, philosopher Alain de Botton argues that news should be the greatest friend of democracy.[4] It should cover issues that affect our community and be an ongoing forum to discuss the complexities of modern society — a springboard from which to think globally and act locally. However, rather than a friend of democracy, 'the news' has become a friend of the free-market economy, feeding consumerism, debt creation, a manic preoccupation with celebrity culture, and our disassociation from real issues. The news of today is fragmented, disconnected, and sensationalised. Ultimately, this sort of news creates even more stress.

A PATIENT'S STORY — PETER

Peter provides a simple yet perfect example of the potential impact of being connected with the world 24/7. At the age of 21, Peter complained of daily headaches, and neck and jaw pain in the morning on waking. He was sleeping poorly, depressed, and anxious. Teeth-grinding often causes this type of pain on waking, and a custom-made mouth splint (a much thinner version of a mouth guard) usually resolves 90 per cent of these headache problems. But on this occasion, after using the splint for several weeks, Peter told me that the dental appliance only made a marginal difference to his pain.

After further questioning, he revealed that he slept with his phone by his side in order to check Facebook during the night. It wasn't until I convinced him to leave his phone and computer out of his bedroom that his headaches disappeared, he slept well, and his depression and anxiety disappeared. It's obviously not always as simple as that, but it was a timely reminder that removing this obsession with technology can have a hugely positive impact. For me, it highlighted what a powerful source of stress technology and being 'connected' can be.

The deep impact of emotional stress on your body

I want you to imagine you are the mother of a chronically ill child. There are many hospital visits and your child requires constant care. You feel resentful for the time and effort the care takes, and guilty for feeling this resentment. Can you imagine living with the constant stress?

This is something Nobel Prize–winning molecular biologist Elizabeth Blackburn and psychologist Elissa Epel looked at in their groundbreaking research.[5] They evaluated the experiences of 58 women: 19 who had healthy children and 39 who had to take care of chronically ill children. Not surprisingly, the mothers of chronically ill children reported feeling more stressed, but here's the groundbreaking part: Blackburn tested what happened to these women's cells, in particular to their telomeres, which are located on the ends of chromosomes. The length of telomeres (and production of the enzyme telomerase, which repairs and lengthens telomeres) influences the amount of cellular ageing in our body — the shorter our telomeres, the greater our cellular ageing.

This study found a link between low telomerase and stress-related diseases. It was the first proof of the influence of the mind on the body's cells. As Blackburn explained to *The New York Times*: 'This was the first time you could clearly see cause and effect from a non-genetic influence. Genes play a role in telomerase levels, but this was not genes. This was something impacting the body that came from the outside [emotional stress] and affecting its ability to repair itself.'[6]

When she was asked if this was scientific proof of the mind–body connection, Blackburn answered, 'Researchers have found that the brain definitely sends nerves directly to organs of the immune system and not just to the heart and the lower gut. In that way, too, the brain is influencing the body.' The take-home message is that psychological stress affects gene expression and, in this case, ages your cells.

Does this process work in reverse? Can you reduce stress and improve cell function? In 2013, *Lancet Oncology* published a study by Elizabeth Blackburn and other researchers that looked at the experience of 35 men with early-stage prostate cancer.[7] Ten men made lifestyle changes including a plant-based diet, moderate exercise, and stress reduction such as yoga-based stretching and meditation. They also participated in a weekly support group. The other 25 men didn't make any changes to their lifestyle. The results are fascinating. When the five-year study ended, the men who made lifestyle changes showed a 'significant' increase in telomere length (approximately 10 per cent). The men in the control group who didn't change their lifestyle had shorter telomeres (nearly 3 per cent shorter). Even though the study was small, the results strongly suggest that managing stress and maintaining a healthy lifestyle can reduce susceptibility to chronic disease.

Needless to say, this study of 'early stage' prostate cancer was of particular interest to me, although my cancer was at a different stage. It again highlighted for me how complex decisions can be. Ultimately the lessons learned from the study, and I hope this book, are as relevant irrespective of the 'stage' of the disease. In my case, I combined all of those lessons with what modern medicine is best at: dealing with a crisis. It's not all or none; it's taking the best of both, or, even better, doing everything you can to stay out of the system altogether.

The key to health is the way in which we respond to stress — and realising that we do, in fact, have a choice in how we respond. It's also worth reminding ourselves at this stage of the book that it is never just one thing that makes the difference. There are a combination of things (stresses) that challenge our health and a combination of things (pillars of health) that have the potential to restore our health and maintain it. Read on!

The wonderful new science of epigenetics — take control of how your genes are expressed

The link between mind and body is further revealed in the exciting new field of epigenetics.[8] When you have a thought, your body produces small proteins called neurotransmitters, which include dopamine (pleasure), adrenaline (fight-or-flight), and serotonin (mood). These proteins travel through your body, attach to cell membranes, and cause genes within those cells to be expressed in a particular way. The outcomes can be positive or negative. And what's even more interesting is that the particular gene expression may be inherited in the next one or two generations.

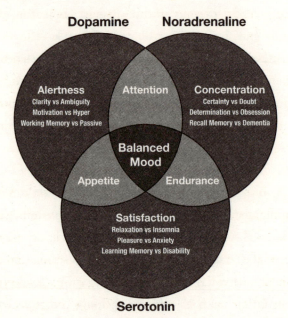

Figure 5-3. Examples of neurotransmitters and their effects.

This information is both frightening and empowering — again, it depends how you think about it. And how you think about it is very much the issue. Here is the mechanism by which your actual thoughts can affect your health. By controlling your genetic expression, neurotransmitters have an impact on your immune system as well as growth and development, and the impact can be positive or negative.

Negative effects include the promotion of cancer, heart disease, mental illness, and many other conditions.

Cellular biologist Bruce Lipton, in his enlightening book *The Biology of Belief*, discusses the moment he realised cells weren't just influenced by genes but also by the physical and emotional environment.[9] This includes thoughts, attitudes, and perceptions. He writes: 'I was exhilarated by the new realisation that I could change the character of my life by changing my *beliefs*. I was instantly energised because I realised there was a science-based path that would take me from perennial "victim" to my new position as "co-creator" of my destiny.'

While genes are clearly important, you are not beholden to your genes. Taking control of your health is such a powerful tool, on so many levels.

If biochemical components such as neurotransmitters can have this effect on gene expression, then it is only logical that this also applies to biochemical components that we commonly find in our nutrition and environment — as I will explore further in later chapters.

Emotional stress as a positive — the upside of stress

Stress is usually seen as having a negative impact on our health, but, according to health psychologist Kelly McGonigal, exciting new research suggests that stress can actually be a positive, and may even contribute to longevity.[10] This is because going through stress can make you better at dealing with it in future, helping you to face each new challenge. Again, your mindset is the key. For instance, in one study, 29,000 people were asked to rate their level of stress over the past year and how much they believed this stress influenced their health.[11] People who reported high levels of stress and who believed stress had a large negative impact on their health died in greater numbers in the following eight years: it was calculated that such people had a 43 per cent increased risk of death. Those who don't experience significant stress or who experience significant stress but don't perceive it as negative — that is, people who are less stressed by stress — are less likely to die.

Other studies support the finding that your own perception of stress is the most significant determining factor of health and longevity.[12] McGonigal suggests the harmful effects of emotional stress may be a consequence of your perception that the stress you are experiencing is bad for health, and argues for a paradigm shift that could be lifesaving.

Kelly Turner's book *Radical Remission* outlines the stories of people who made surprise recoveries or remissions from cancer.[13] It outlines the 'nine key factors that can make a real difference to surviving cancer against all odds'. Interestingly, seven of the nine factors focus on internal emotional factors: taking control of your health, following your intuition, releasing suppressed emotions, increasing positive emotions, embracing social support, deepening your spiritual connections, and having strong reasons for living. The other two are to change your diet and use herbs and supplements. In the cases studied by Turner, she shows that although the diagnosis of cancer was stressful, it prompted a major shift in the health of these people's lives.

While you may not have control over events in the world or the actions of people around you, you do have control of your attitude to those events and people — and that is a powerful tool to harness.

Conclusion

What should you do now? Keep reading! The next four chapters will continue to broaden the definition of what stresses our body and mind. These stresses affect our mental and emotional health, too. Building resilience by focusing on the pillars of health in Part 3 will help give you the physical and mental strength to deal with the emotional stresses of your world, past and present.

Today, emotional stress is difficult to avoid, but you have control over your attitude to traumas and stressful situations in your life or the world in general, and this can make the biggest difference of all. While building resilience is important, sharing your experiences, thoughts, and feelings through counselling can also be an important part of the picture. Just verbalising your feelings literally gives voice to past events and your reactions to them, which in itself can have dramatic and positive therapeutic effects.

Identifying the things that can stress your body and mind, while building on the pillars of health can influence your health in many positive ways — but the change has to come from you.

CHAPTER 6

Nutritional Stress

It's staggering to realise that 72 per cent of the global health burden is caused by largely preventable, lifestyle-related chronic disease.[1] For the World Health Organisation, this equates to 'billions of dollars of potentially avoidable healthcare spending and untold personal cost'.[2] Those lifestyle-related influences include nutritional and environmental choices we make each day, from what we eat and drink to our choice of homecare products, clothes, furnishing, or cosmetics as well as how much we choose to move our bodies.

Most of us are aware that the food and drink that passes our lips has a direct impact on our health and wellbeing. As the saying goes, 'You are what you eat.' If you eat too many French fries, you'll put on weight, clog your arteries, and increase your chances of contracting heart disease, cancer, or autoimmune diseases. But working out which foods are good for you isn't always straightforward.

In this chapter, I'll help you choose and explain exactly why healthy food choices are important not only for your body, but also for your mind.

Gut — brain — immune system

As I mentioned, the gut is where approximately 80 per cent of our immune system is located.[3] It has the largest accumulation of lymphoid tissue in the body, which is important for immune response and helps protect from infection and foreign bodies. But there is a whole new area of health called psychoneuroimmunology (PNI), which examines how the mind, immune system (including the gut), hormone balance, and nervous system interact — revealing a strong connection between gut health, mental health, and emotional wellbeing. People often associate food with mood, but they don't always make the leap to the influence food has on mental-health conditions.

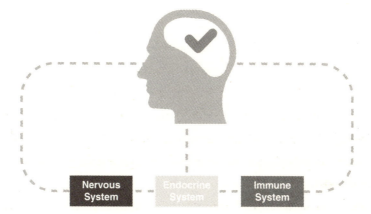

Figure 6-1. What is psychoneuroimmunology? Research has repeatedly demonstrated the profound influence the mind has on health and disease through the interactions between the nervous system, hormonal (endocrine) system, and immune system.

In his book *Grain Brain*, neurologist David Perlmutter outlines how grains and carbohydrates can have adverse effects on mental health, including: ADHD, anxiety, autism, depression, chronic headaches, and dementia.[4] The key message throughout the book is the importance of healthy fats for optimal physical and mental health, and the avoidance of grains and man-made seed oils, all of which can and often do promote chronic inflammation.

The other key point supported by many researchers is that while we expect the digestive problems with the food we eat to be reflected by symptoms in the digestive tract itself (such as indigestion, reflux, constipation, bloating, gas, or diarrhoea), surprisingly this is not always the case. Often, the only symptoms that appear are in the nervous system.[5]

The food we eat affects every cell in our body, which includes the skin, immune system, hormonal (endocrine) system, nervous system, and brain. While we are made up of almost 40 trillion human cells, we share our bodies with ten times that number of bacteria. Friendly bacteria promote health, while pathogenic (or 'unfriendly') bacteria promote disease, both physical and mental. When it comes to the bacteria in our gut, referred to as the 'gut biome', the key question is — do you choose to feed your friends or your foes?

The type and diversity of microbes in the gut biome are implicated in a wide range of diseases, from irritable bowel, Crohn's disease, ulcerative colitis, skin conditions, and cancer to obesity, depression, anxiety, and autism, and no doubt there will be many other connections made. The health of your gut biome is central to a healthy immune system and to both your physical and mental wellbeing. With all of the processed food, sugar, grains, preservatives, additives, and alcohol that is consumed today in our western diet, it is easy for the gut biome to be out of balance.

The good news is this can often be corrected, sometimes within a period of weeks or months. If the condition is a longstanding one, it may take many months or even years to 'rebuild' a healthy gut — but it's important not to become discouraged. The effort is well worth it, and you may even start to feel improvements in your health straightaway!

Is your digestive system telling you something?

Your digestive system gives you feedback each and every day and is an excellent indicator of overall health. Symptoms such as gas, bloating, indigestion, bad breath, burping, constipation, diarrhoea, intense sugar cravings, and brain fog are signs that the digestive system isn't working properly. Unfortunately, the way our modern world deals with these issues — looking at the obvious symptom and looking for a short-term fix — often exacerbates the underlying problem or creates another one. Let's explore further by looking at some common problems: indigestion, constipation, and diarrhoea.

If you have heartburn, reflux, and indigestion, this suggests a problem with acidity. The western medical solution is to neutralise this 'acidity' by prescribing over-the-counter 'remedies' such as Alka-Seltzer, Gaviscon, and Mylanta, or prescription medications including Nexium and Zantac. The latter are two of the world's bestselling drugs — Nexium sales alone are worth over US$6 billion annually — and therefore belong to the growing category of medications referred to as 'blockbuster drugs'. If only the patient saw as much benefit as the drug companies' shareholders.

Prescribing a pill is a short-sighted, symptom-based, linear way of approaching the problem because stomach acid is essential to effective food digestion. We need stomach acid to break down and absorb proteins, which are essential for every system in our body. Stomach acidity is also a built-in barrier to infection. Some of the side effects that come from prolonged use of these medications include an increased susceptibility to infections such as pneumonia and colitis (an inflammation in the intestinal lining). They also affect the body's ability to absorb minerals, particularly calcium, and so increase the risk of osteoporosis — another growing problem in our society. Prolonged use of these medications may also cause a vitamin B12 deficiency with resulting anaemia, tiredness, and weakness.

The ideal approach when treating heartburn is to look at the patient as a whole and find out why the reflux is happening in the first place. An integrative, holistic, and patient-centred approach identifies problem foods and eliminates them, or corrects deficiencies or imbalances in essential vitamins and minerals, while maintaining healthy stomach acidity to encourage good digestion and absorption of nutrients. Not only would rising acidity be dealt with, but also many seemingly unrelated overlying health conditions may also improve as a result.

The quality, frequency, and shape of your stools offer daily clues and important messages about the state of your digestive health. The ideal time it takes food to pass through the digestive tract is 18–24 hours, with between one and two bowel movements a day. In our western diet, this is rarely achieved; for many, the transit time for food to pass through the digestive tract can be up to 60 hours or more. Constipation, which is defined as two or fewer bowel movements a week, reflects an underlying disorder. This problem can stem from inadequate water intake or from not eating enough fibre, particularly vegetables. Other causes of constipation include an underactive thyroid, irritable bowel, colon cancer, or neurological conditions such as Parkinson's disease or multiple sclerosis. Constipation can also be the result of emotional stress as the blood supply to the gut is reduced, affecting its normal function. There are also over 150 medications that can cause constipation, including some antacids, antidepressants, and painkillers.

If you are on the other end of the spectrum, and regularly have diarrhoea or stools that are watery and loose, it may be a reflection of an underlying bacterial or viral infection. It could also be a response to a food intolerance or a chronic condition such as irritable bowel, inflammatory bowel disease, coeliac disease, non-coeliac gluten sensitivity, or diabetes, to name but a few. Medications can also cause diarrhoea, including chemotherapy medications to treat cancer as well as some common prescription medications for heartburn such as Nexium or Zantac. Take the trouble to 'read' the message your body is sending you.

So what does healthy stool look like? Ideally, your stool should be log-like and walnut in colour; it should not contain any undigested food particles or be overly smelly. When 'launched', it should initially float and then subside. It is important to spend some time looking at your stools. If they aren't normal, take action, not necessarily medication — keep reading, identify some of the causes, and change your diet. Your stool is one of the best barometers of gut health; don't ignore it.

What does your poo say about you?

Every day your body sends you a report card giving you a 'tick' or a 'cry for help'. You don't need a prescription or a lab test, and it doesn't cost a cent. Your body is sending you a message, so listen. Use your brain to help your body; it's a win-win for both!

Okay, you've got it — it's important not to ignore that message. But what does your poo say about you? The Bristol Stool Chart is a medical aid that classifies human faeces into seven categories.[6] After you pass faeces, what you see in the toilet bowl is the result of your diet, fluids, medications, gut health, and lifestyle. Everyone has different bowel habits, but it's important that stools are soft and easy to pass.

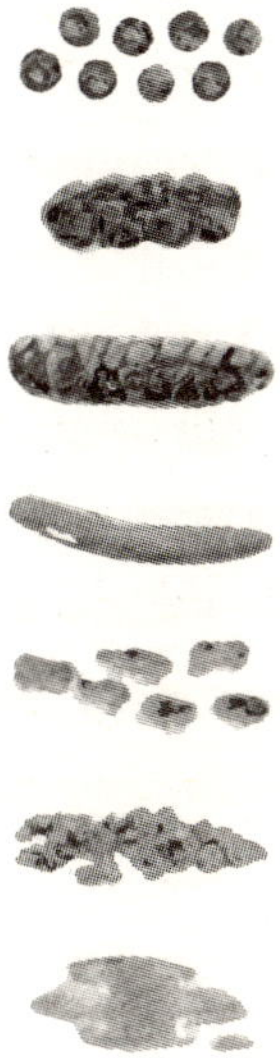

	Type 1	Separate hard lumps	Very constipated
	Type 2	Lumpy and sausage like	Slightly constipated
	Type 3	A sausage shape with cracks in the surface	Normal
	Type 4	Like a smooth, soft sausage or snake	Normal
	Type 5	Soft blobs with clear-cut edges	Lacking fibre
	Type 6	Mushy consistency with ragged edges	Inflammation
	Type 7	Liquid consistency with no solid pieces	Inflammation

Figure 6-2. The Bristol Stool Chart.

Eight problems with today's food

Many of the issues surrounding digestion and the health of our gut come down to what we eat and, of equal importance, how our food is grown, processed, prepared — and, ultimately, absorbed. As we have evolved from hunting and gathering to domesticating plants and animals, we have had to adapt. I will give examples of what constitutes a nutrient-dense diet in Chapter 12: Nutrition, but, suffice to say, food production changed radically during the agricultural revolution — but never more so than in the last 50 years. During this more-recent period, our food production has become industrialised in an unprecedented way, and if the evidence of rising chronic diseases is anything to go by, that change has been harmful to human health and the health of our planet.

Problem 1 — the demonisation of saturated fat and cholesterol

For the last 50 years, saturated fat, particularly animal fat, has been demonised. While it's true that not all saturated fats are good for you, it's worth noting that over 60 per cent of our brain and half of the cell membranes surrounding the 37 trillion cells in our body are made up of saturated fat. Good saturated fats, which have been traditionally used for thousands of years, are today found in meat from pasture-fed, free-range animals, lard (pork fat), tallow (beef or mutton fat), butter, ghee (clarified butter), and coconut oil. As for bad saturated fats, they are contained in French fries, pizzas, potato crisps, and other processed foods, which are also often high in carbohydrates, hydrogenated fats, and vegetable oils. Somehow, whenever saturated fats are vilified, there are usually photos of these fast-food products to accompany them, further adding to the confusion. Yes, those foods are bad for many reasons, but healthy saturated fats are good.

Another important compound that's been much maligned is cholesterol, which also happens to be an integral part of every cell in our body. Quite simply: without it, we wouldn't function properly. One of cholesterol's most important jobs is hormone production. Cholesterol is stored in the body, and converts to steroid hormones that help the body function optimally; the adrenal glands produce cortisol, the ovaries produce oestrogen, and the testes produce testosterone. Without these steroid hormones, there are malfunctions in weight, sex, digestion, bone health, and mental health. Cholesterol also plays an important role in the production of vitamin D, which can be considered both a vitamin and a hormone, and is central to the function of all cells throughout the body.

The demonisation of these traditional animal fats along with warnings to stay out of the sun — both of which provide us with excellent sources of essential vitamin D — has seen a huge jump in the number of people with deficiencies in this vital fat-soluble, anticancer hormone/vitamin. Research confirms that vitamin D deficiency has reached pandemic proportions, affecting between 30–50 per cent of the global population.[7] To give you an idea of how important vitamin D is: its deficiency is implicated in cancer, heart disease, type 2 diabetes, dementia, depression, rheumatoid arthritis, high blood pressure, and osteoporosis — to name just a few.

Cholesterol also plays an important role in repair and damage. Disparaging cholesterol is like blaming the firefighter for the fire, just because they both happen to be at the same place at the same time. What makes demonising, measuring, and targeting cholesterol so appealing for health practitioners, however, is that 'cholesterol causes heart disease' can be so simply explained and then cholesterol in all its forms can be easily measured and monitored by blood tests, opening the market to the blockbuster profits of statins.

Despite decades of the Food Pyramid, low-fat dogma, and demonisation of cholesterol, heart disease is still the number one killer in the world. But 'cholesterol' is good for business. John Ioannidis from Stanford University estimated that the total sales of statins may approach $1 trillion worldwide by 2020; the most commercially successful drug in history, atorvastatin (Lipitor®), alone had sales exceeding $120 billion between 1996 and 2011.[8]

While I covered this in Part 1, I think that as statins are so widespread and cause so much confusion, it's worth reminding you what Pfizer (the manufacturer of the world's bestselling statin, Lipitor®) warns:

LIPITOR has not been shown to prevent heart disease or heart attacks.

As I've also mentioned, with so many reputations built on this saturated fat/cholesterol/statin dogma and with the billions of dollars of profits involved, you can be sure this approach will not be surrendered lightly.

Problem 2 — seed oils and trans fats

Seed oils were developed and marketed for the first time in human history by the food industry in the early part of the 20th century. They were developed to extend the shelf life of processed food and provide a source of inexpensive fat. Examples of commonly used seed oils include cottonseed, canola, soybean, safflower, and sunflower oil. Margarines are an even more highly processed by-product of the already highly processed seed oils. It's important to reiterate that as seed oils became a part of the human diet, there was also a sudden and dramatic increase in the incidence of heart disease.

Cancer levels have also skyrocketed in the 20th century. One in two men and one in three women will contract cancer by the age of 60. According to Samuel Epstein, professor of environmental and occupational health at the University of Illinois, even allowing for the increase in life expectancy, there has been a 25–30 per cent increase in cancer rates since 1975; childhood cancer rates have also increased by 36 per cent since 1975.[9] Foods that humans have never eaten before may be implicated in these disease levels. Again, it's never just one factor or stress that causes these medical issues, but as you read on you will see it's probably a combination of nutritional and environmental factors, poor sleep, and lack of exercise that are impacting our health.

We now know seed oils are harmful to health — they are highly processed and unstable, particularly when heated. Despite this, they are widely used in processed food. Ironically, even as saturated animal fat was demonised, health authorities (often sponsored by the food companies that manufacture seed oils and margarines) promoted these foods as a 'healthy alternative' — and many still do.

In addition, these seed oils are often hydrogenated to avoid rancidity, but hydrogenated seed oils produce trans-unsaturated fatty acids when they are heated to high temperatures — and these trans fats have been implicated in cancer and other degenerative diseases. Better fats are natural ones that have been used throughout human history, which are produced from pasture-fed, free-range animals. They include lard; tallow; chicken, duck, or goose fat; butter; and ghee. From plants, coconut oil is another. They all contain some vitamin D and are stable at high temperatures.

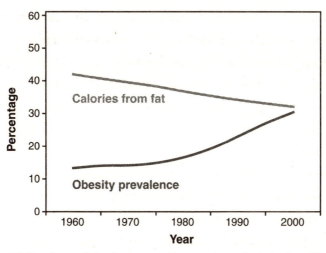

Figure 6-3. Prevalence of obesity compared to percentage of calories from US adults 1950–2000. The low-fat dogma of public health messages has resulted in a reduction in the consumption of fats, which has gone hand-in-hand with the increase in obesity.

Problem 3 — too much sugar

CARBOHYDRATES DEFINED

A carbohydrate is a biological molecule consisting of carbon (C), hydrogen (H), and oxygen (O) atoms, usually with a hydrogen–oxygen atom ratio of 2:1.

Monosaccharides are the simplest forms of carbohydrates. Examples include glucose (also known as dextrose), fructose, and galactose, found in many fruits and dairy. The chemical formula for all three is $C_6H_{12}O_6$, but the arrangement of atoms is different.

Two monosaccharides can combine to form a disaccharide, such as sucrose (common table sugar, derived from sugarcane), maltose (derived from grain), and lactose (found in milk).

Monosaccharides and disaccharides are referred to as simple carbohydrates or sugars.

Monosaccharides can also combine into larger molecules, called complex carbohydrates. These fall into two classes: oligosaccharides (comprising three to nine monosaccharides), such as maltodextrin; and polysaccharides (comprising ten or more mono-saccharides), such as starch and cellulose.

When it comes to carbohydrates, there a few things to consider. First, how many molecules are present that can be quickly broken down into simple sugars, the excess of which is stored as fat. Second, do the carbohydrates you are eating (such as those in many grains) irritate the digestive system or increase the likelihood of leaky gut. Finally, does the food contain dietary fibre (such as cellulose) to promote a healthy gut microbiome with the many accompanying health benefits and bowel movements you can be proud of.

Ideally, we want low-carb, low-irritant, nutrient-dense, high-fibre vegetables and some fruits.

Our relationship with sugar has changed over the years. Growing up, I often sprinkled white sugar (sucrose) over my already sugar-laden breakfast cereal. I would also add two teaspoons of sugar to my morning cup of tea, and even two spoons of Chocolate Quik or Milo to a glass of milk! Sugar, sugar, and more sugar. What was I thinking? It certainly kept my dentist busy, but, back then, oral hygiene, tooth brushing, and flossing weren't promoted in the same way they are today; it wasn't part of people's daily routine in avoiding dental decay. I brushed my teeth as a child but not as diligently as I do today, and I've had my time in the dental chair as a result. But the even bigger difference between then and now is that, back then, adding sugar was optional.

Today, sugar is an embedded ingredient in most processed food and many drinks. A recent study in Australia has shown that at least 70 per cent of packaged foods contain added sugar.[10] The average American consumes 60–70 kilograms (130–150 pounds) of sugar a year. That's the equivalent of 40 teaspoons of sugar every day. Australians consume an average of 45 kilograms per year, or 32 teaspoons of sugar daily.[11] I hardly consume any today, so a lot of other people must be having more than their share.

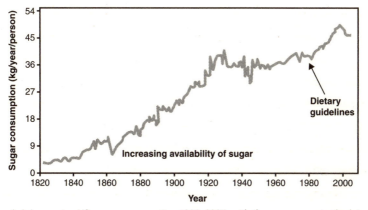

Figure 6-4. Increasing US sugar consumption 1822–2005, with the emergence in the late 1970s of the low-fat dietary guidelines.

Whether it is white, brown, organic, or raw, sugar should be thought of as empty calories that can actually strip the body of vital nutrients, particularly when consumed in excess. Sugar affects key hormones in the body, specifically insulin and leptin levels, both of which help regulate how we store and metabolise carbohydrates and fat.

Sugar is associated with an increased risk of heart disease and adverse changes in lipids (fats) and chronic inflammation. It's no wonder the dramatic increase in the consumption of soft drinks and fruit juices by children over the last 30 years is contributing to the huge increase in childhood type 2 diabetes, as well as the epidemic in childhood obesity.[12] Again, the government and health authorities have been focused on fats, while presiding over this epidemic in chronic disease.

Let's take a closer look at sugar and the hormones it affects in our bodies.

INSULIN

This hormone is made by cells in the pancreas. When you eat sugar — or, for that matter, excessive carbohydrates that are quickly converted to sugar — insulin is released into the bloodstream, where the hormone moves glucose from the food into cells to be used as energy or stored. In groundbreaking research on this subject, Cynthia Kenyon, a professor at the University of California, San Francisco, found a pathway involving insulin that extends lifespan and delays age-related disease in species throughout the animal kingdom.[13] Further research on humans confirmed that the less you use insulin, the lower your insulin levels are, and the healthier you are likely to be.

When you eat too much carbohydrate, the body can't produce enough insulin to deal with the higher levels, and the cells throughout the body become resistant to the effect of insulin. This is called insulin resistance and leads to elevated levels of glucose in the bloodstream, which ideally should contain no more than four to eight grams of glucose at any one time. Too much glucose leads to glycation, a highly reactive process in the body that damages tissues and organs. That's why diabetes, which is a problem of insulin resistance and the ability to metabolise sugar correctly, has such wide-ranging problems throughout the body.

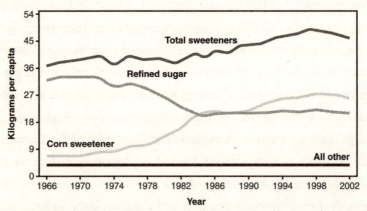

Figure 6-5. Estimated per capita sweetener consumption, total and by type of sweetener, 1966–2004 (source: USDA Economic Research Service).

LEPTIN

This hormone plays a crucial role in appetite and weight control. It's produced by adipose (fat) tissue and secreted when weight is gained to signal to the brain (specifically, the hypothalamus) that there are adequate energy stores. It crosses the blood–brain barrier and binds to receptors in the appetite centre of the brain, which signals how much to eat. The hypothalamus should then stimulate metabolic processes that result in weight loss, including a reduction in hunger, a full feeling, an increase in resting metabolism, and an increase in fat breakdown.

Many overweight people who have difficulty losing weight may also have leptin resistance; the brain understands this as a form of starvation. In this situation, several mechanisms are activated to increase, rather than burn, excess fat stores. Leptin resistance also stimulates the formation of reverse T3, a thyroid hormone that blocks the regulatory effects of leptin on the metabolism. Leptin resistance is a complex issue with no single cause. Factors affecting leptin levels include the presence of fructose (especially high-fructose corn syrup), high stress levels, lack of sleep (as we will cover in Chapter 10: Sleep), yo-yo dieting, high insulin levels, overeating, and grains (specifically, the lectin — not leptin — within grains like wheat, barley, and rye).

GLUCOSE AND FRUCTOSE

These are both forms of sugar, but they metabolise differently. Glucose is a very unstable molecule. There are between four and eight grams of glucose circulating in your body at any one time. Insulin makes glucose available to cells as they need energy, or stores excess glucose as glycogen — up to about 400 grams. Any remaining glucose — which would not be uncommon in a high-carbohydrate diet — is converted to fat and also stored. This stored fat tends to sit around the organs, including the liver.

While fructose isn't directly affected by insulin in the same way as glucose, it is nonetheless stored in the liver or converted to fat.

An excess of either fructose or glucose causes the body to go through glycation, which is, as I've mentioned, implicated in tissue damage and ageing. Fructose is far more potent in this process, which is what makes diabetes such a challenge to health on so many levels.[14]

HIGH-FRUCTOSE CORN SYRUP (HFCS)

First developed in Japan in the 1960s, it became ubiquitous in processed foods from the 1970s onwards. HFCS is much cheaper to produce than sucrose from sugar cane, and, again, as with seed oils, we see industry influence on our food taking precedence over the effect of those products on our health.

Like seeds oils, which are a 20th-century food, never before consumed by humans, HFCS is also a new invention. In his research, Barry Popkin, professor of nutrition at the University of Carolina, outlines that in the US, the consumption of HFCS increased by greater than 1,000 per cent between 1970 and 1990, and goes on to say 'that HFCS is absorbed more rapidly than regular sugar and that it doesn't stimulate insulin or leptin production. This prevents you from triggering the body's signals for being full and may lead to overconsumption of total calories.'[15] Clearly, this plays a role in the epidemic of type 2 diabetes we see occurring today, with all of its accompanying health implications, as well as the huge increase in obesity for young and old alike.

FRUIT

Another, possibly more surprising source of sugar in our modern diet is fruit, which contains both glucose and fructose in varying quantities depending on the type. Over the last 50 years, fruit has been bred to be sweeter than its ancient relatives — in other words, today it contains more sugar. Excess consumption of fruit, particularly in the form of fruit juices, dramatically raises blood-sugar levels, elevating insulin levels. This insulin then takes the sugar and stores it within the body's fat cells. Similarly, excessive glucose or fructose also affects leptin, lowering levels of this vital regulatory hormone. As I have discussed, this then affects the body's ability to metabolise fats, as well as affecting appetite — specifically, it distorts our ability to know when we have had enough to eat.

REDUCING SUGAR

In March 2015, the WHO issued guidelines recommending adults and children reduce their daily intake of added sugars to less than 10 per cent of their total energy intake,[16] going on to say a further reduction to below 5 per cent, or roughly 25 grams, per day would provide additional health benefits.

Eliminating all added sugar and HFCS, which are commonly associated with processed foods and drinks, is the ideal. When eating fresh seasonal fruit, we do also ingest vitamins and fibre, which are beneficial to health, but, due to its high fructose level, fruit should be consumed in moderation. Any benefits that go with 'freshly squeezed' juice, such as vitamins, are minimal unless the fruit has been literally squeezed and consumed within five to ten minutes. Fruit juices contain little fibre and a great deal of sugar, so it's best to avoid drinking them altogether.

OTHER CARBOHYDRATES, PROTEIN, AND FAT

Apart from sugar, other carbohydrates, particularly starchy grains or tuber vegetables, can also be a problem because the body rapidly breaks them down into glucose, which then gets stored as fat and affects insulin levels, adding to the total sugar load. Going back to undergraduate biochemistry, it is worth mentioning that glucose, which is the primary fuel the body uses for energy, can also be derived from both protein and fat. There may be many reasons for eating carbohydrates — such as vitamins, minerals, phytonutrients, and fibre for gut health — but it's important to realise that we are not completely dependent on carbohydrates for energy. I'll deal with this in more detail in Chapter 12: Nutrition.

Independent scientific studies suggest that diets low in carbohydrates and higher in good saturated fats are better for you. Lydia A. Bazzano, of the Tulane University School of Public Health and Tropical Medicine, led a year-long trial in which people were placed on either a low-carbohydrate or a low-fat diet.[17] The low-carbohydrate group lost about 3.6 kilograms more on average than those in the low-fat group. Even more interestingly, the low-carb group had significantly greater reductions in body fat than the low-fat group, had lower insulin levels, and saw improvements in lean muscle mass — even though neither group changed their levels of physical activity. The important message is that fat doesn't make you fat, carbohydrates (and sugar) make you fat.

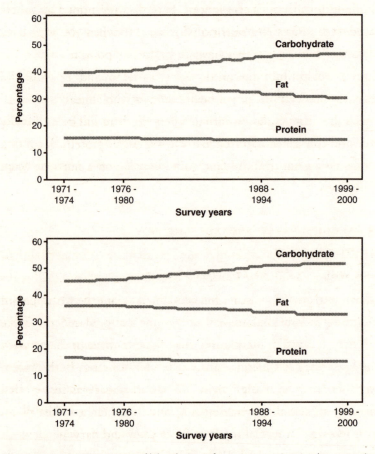

Above: Figure 6-6. Percentage of kilocalories is from macronutrient intake among American men aged 20–74 years (source: National Health and Examination Surveys).
Below: Figure 6-7. Percentage of kilocalories is from macronutrient intake among American women aged 20–74 years.

I wrote this section because I wanted to include some basics beyond the fact that sugar, when eaten in excess, will be converted to fat and affect insulin levels predisposing to diabetes. Too much carbohydrate in the form of grains or starchy vegetables also break down quickly into glucose and follow the same pathway to fat production, insulin and leptin resistance, diabetes, and obesity.

As US president John F. Kennedy once said, 'Too often … we enjoy the comfort of opinion without the discomfort of thought.' Around the same time, Martin Luther King said, 'Nothing in all the world is more dangerous than sincere ignorance and conscientious stupidity.' They weren't talking about nutritional stress, but when you look back on public health messages, they have an important point to make.

Many people think they can do both 'low-carb' and 'low-fat', and that way take 'full advantage' of both pieces of public health advice. I don't agree. If you go both low-carb and low-fat, there will be a problem; you will probably get hungry or just eat too much protein. Lowering your carbs and eating healthy fats while focusing on a nutrient-dense diet is the answer.

Problem 4 — grains
MODERN WHEAT ISN'T WHAT IT USED TO BE

Wheat has been part of our diet for 10,000 years, but the wheat grown today is very different from that grown by our predecessors. Since biblical times, emmer and einkorn wheat varieties have been the main wheat grown; they have literally 'given us our daily bread'. In the 1960s, however, a new variety of high-yield semi-dwarf wheat was created that dramatically increased the yield and lowered the height of the plant, requiring less water and making it easier to grow and harvest.

But this new variety also had much higher proportions of gluten and fewer nutrients such as zinc, copper, iron, and magnesium. In addition, industrialised agriculture, with its high dependency on fertilisers, has depleted soils of selenium and many other trace elements that are essential for good health. More about that later.

While I understand that correlation does not necessarily mean causation, and it's never just one thing that causes all problems, it is interesting to note that since the introduction of this wheat variant (ably supported by governments, 'health authorities', and public health messages promoting 'pyramids' and 'plates'), there's been a dramatic increase in chronic degenerative diseases, which includes a multitude of digestive disorders. As the population followed those government-endorsed, industry-sponsored eating guidelines, assuming them to be good for health, it seems instead to have created a perfect storm.

Cardiologist William Davis, in his book *Wheat Belly*, outlines the ways in which modern wheat has been modified.[18] These include:

- **Changes to the gliadin protein.** This makes wheat a more potent opiate and encourages *addictive eating behaviour*. Yes, wheat is an opiate; gliadin binds to the opiate receptors of the brain. But instead of making you high, gliadin makes you hungry: this may explain why demolishing a loaf of fresh crusty hot bread has always been so appealing; wheat eaters consume, on average, 440 more calories per day.

- **Enrichment of glia-alpha-9.** This genetic sequence was mostly absent in wheat grown prior to the 1960s, but is found in most modern semi-dwarf wheat and could explain why coeliac disease has quadrupled in the last 30–40 years. It stimulates the production of a unique protein in the gut called zonulin, which increases gut permeability (leaky gut) as well as intestinal inflammation.

- **Changes in wheat-germ agglutinin.** This toxin protects wheat from insects, yeast, and bacteria and could also be responsible for intestinal permeability by causing direct intestinal damage, allowing foreign substances to get into the bloodstream, resulting in autoimmune conditions.

- **Changes in wheat lectin.** This may also block the hormone leptin, contributing to the obesity epidemic we are faced with today.

- **Changes in alpha-amylase inhibitors.** These are the enzymes that help break down carbohydrates into glucose. Inhibitors slow this process but may also be a source of wheat allergies and obesity.

PROCESSING OF WHEAT ISN'T WHAT IT USED TO BE

Modern food-processing techniques also affect the nature of reactive components in today's wheat products. Some processing practices over the last 50 years may have increased exposure to components of wheat implicated in sensitivity, such as gluten and lectin. Modern processing differs from traditional methods in three major ways: First, today's mass production means wheat has become highly refined, using harsh chemical processes. Second, the fermentation of yeast — which helps break down gluten — used to take up to 18 hours; today, it takes only two hours, thanks to the use of fast-acting baker's yeast. And third, the addition of wheat proteins and inulin (a starchy, soluble fibre considered a prebiotic and important in nurturing healthy gut bacteria; unfortunately, it also nurtures harmful bacteria).[19]

A LEAKY GUT PREDISPOSES YOU TO AUTOIMMUNE CONDITIONS

The problem for many of us is that our digestive systems are being compromised, meaning these high-gluten, highly-processed grains are passing more easily from our gut and into the bloodstream. Put simply, our gut linings are becoming more permeable, or 'leaky'. Our bodies then attack these 'leaked' undigested proteins and, depending on your genetic predisposition, you may develop an autoimmune response. Autoimmune diseases are on the increase and responsible for a wide variety of health problems.

The digestive system is lined with billions of cells with finger-like projections called villi. When functioning well, those cells are tightly joined. Ideally, food passes along the gut and is broken down, and the resulting nutrients are then absorbed by these finger-like projections attached to the cells of the gut wall. When working effectively, they also keep the food in the gut while it is being broken down. If you eat grains, particularly modern varieties of wheat, containing the glia-alpha-9 genetic sequence and higher gluten content, the body itself may produce a unique protein called zonulin, which causes the tightly joined cells to become loose.

Zonulin and its effects were discovered in 2000 by Harvard Medical School professor Alessio Fasano and his team.[20] As Fasano explains in his groundbreaking work on gluten and zonulin and their relation to autoimmune diseases: 'We, as a species, are not engineered to eat wheat because for the 2.5 million years of evolution, 99.9% of that time our species has been gluten-free. Gluten came into the picture only 10,000 years ago, with the advent of agriculture.' Modern wheat and its processing has further exacerbated the problem. For many years, the impact of zonulin was referred to as 'leaky gut', but, more recently, as the medical profession has become more aware and accepting of this phenomenon, it has taken on the more-impressive, scientific-sounding term 'intestinal permeability'. They are essentially the same thing.

Depending on your genetic predisposition, leaky gut can manifest through:

- skin, e.g. psoriasis or lupus
- gut, e.g. Crohn's disease, ulcerative colitis, or Coeliac disease
- joints, e.g. rheumatoid arthritis
- nervous system, e.g. Parkinson's or multiple sclerosis
- endocrine glands, e.g. overactive thyroid (Graves' disease) or underactive thyroid (Hashimoto's disease).

Research suggests that leaky gut is implicated in a wide range of diseases by contributing to chronic inflammation, autoimmunity, and even cancer.[21] It has also been linked to diseases like endometriosis and polycystic ovarian syndrome, and, while these are not strictly autoimmune diseases, they do affect many women, and numbers are on the rise.

Autoimmune responses are rarely a direct result of eating non-processed foods, such as vegetables. But once you have sensitivity, the body often becomes cross-reactive and sensitive to more than just one food group, chemical, or protein, resulting in multiple sensitivities. So if you develop one sensitivity, you may also begin to react to a much wider range of foods, such as dairy or even certain types of fruits and vegetables. You could also become more sensitive or reactive to environmental chemicals in household and personal-care products, physical stress, neurotransmitters released by emotional stress, as well as other infections and some medications. It can work both ways.

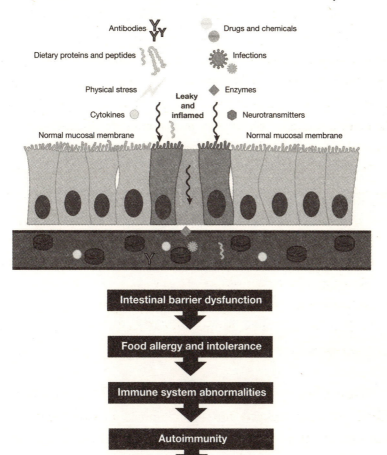

Figure 6-8. The many stresses assaulting our gut, resulting in leaks into the bloodstream.

The first step in rectifying these issues is eliminating the foods to which you are reactive, followed by rebuilding the gut lining and gut biome — that is, rebuilding the resilience of your digestive system. Consulting a knowledgeable integrative medical practitioner, nutritionist, or naturopath gives structure and meaning to what can be a complex problem. As I've mentioned, depending on how long this has been a problem, it can take many months or years, but, seen in the long term, the health benefits far outweigh any effort required.

Acute disseminated encephalomyelitis	Lupus
Addison's disease	Mixed connective-tissue disease
Alopecia areata	Morphea
Ankylosing spondylitis	Multiple sclerosis (MS)
Antiphospholipid antibody syndrome (Hughes syndrome)	Myasthenia gravis
	Narcolepsy
Autoimmune haemolytic anemia	Neuromyotonia
Autoimmune hepatitis	Opsoclonus myoclonus syndrome
Autoimmune inner-ear disease	Pemphigus vulgaris
Bullous pemphigoid	Pernicious anemia
Chagas disease	Polymyositis
Coeliac disease	Primary biliary cirrhosis
Crohn's disease	Psoriasis
Dermatomyositis	Psoriatic arthritis
Endometriosis	Rheumatoid arthritis
Goodpasture syndrome	Schizophrenia
Graves' disease	Scleroderma
Guillain-Barre syndrome	Sjogren's syndrome
Hashimoto's thyroiditis	Stiff-person syndrome
Hidradenitis suppurativa	Temporal arteritis
Idiopathic thrombocytopenic purpura	Ulcerative colitis
IgA nephropathy	Vasculitis
Interstitial cystitis	Vitiligo
Kawasaki disease	Wegener's granulomatosis

Figure 6-9. A sample of the wide range of autoimmune and autoimmune-like conditions.

Problem 5 — industrialised meat production

The industrialised production of meat is not just an ethical and environmental issue (which I will deal with in Chapter 7: Environmental Stress); there are health implications for us, too. These health issues include the over-consumption of meat, which has become a relatively cheap source of protein. But, even more importantly, we must consider the type of fat we consume thanks to industrialised farming practices, which produce the vast majority of our meat.

When essential fatty acids, which are vital to our health, are in balance, they help regulate or reduce chronic inflammation. A healthy diet needs a healthy balance of these essential fatty acids, called omega-3 and omega-6 fatty acids. When animals eat grass, as they have in nature for millions of years, the proportion of omega-3 (anti-inflammatory) and omega-6 (pro-inflammatory) is usually in the ratio of between 1:1 and 1:3.

Today, this healthy balance of essential fatty acids in our meat can be hard to find. Instead of eating grass, many animals are reared in feedlots where they are fed grains to literally fatten them up. From an economic perspective, this is great — it can increase an animal's weight by 100–150 kilograms in the space of four to six weeks. But it does little to promote healthy fatty-acid ratios, in fact quite the opposite — from a health perspective, this is not so great.

The problem is that apart from grain-fed meat being higher in fat, the proportion of the type of fats has also changed dramatically and, again, not in your best health interests. After just six weeks, the fat from grain-fed animals has minimal amounts of anti-inflammatory omega-3 and up to 20 times the amount of omega-6. This makes the meat higher in fat, and, more importantly, these fats also promote inflammation. Now, it is well accepted that the common denominator running through almost every chronic degenerative disease is chronic inflammation, so it's logical that anything that promotes inflammation, such as grain-fed meat, is best avoided.

When you are told that red meat is linked to heart disease and cancer, the question must be: 'What was that meat fed throughout its entire life, including the last four to six weeks of its life — grass or grains?' The issue of how animals are treated in our industrialised meat production is another issue of great concern.

Remember, our goal is to achieve good health for our families and our wider community not just ourselves as individuals. To me, the 'wider community' includes the animals that help feed us, so we must examine the ethics of how we treat these animals as we 'grow' this food. Questions need to be asked about the use of antibiotics to control infection in the confined housing of factory-farmed animals, along with the use of hormones and other additives to promote growth. Not to mention the stress we place these animals under in this confined industrialised environment. These are animals with feelings, and those feelings have an impact on their health, and that needs to be respected. I have no problem eating healthy animals that have led healthy and happy lives, but I think we should honour the animals we eat, from nose to tail.

Problem 6 — not enough fibre to nurture your healthy gut bacteria and good bowel movements

Non-starch polysaccharides occur naturally in many foods and are also referred to as dietary fibre, roughage, or bulk. They have many unique and important properties. One of the most important features is that they can be fermented by the gut microbiome in the large intestine into short-chain fatty acids, which in turn have important health benefits, including reducing the risk of coronary heart disease, colorectal cancer, inflammatory bowel disease, and breast cancer.[22]

Dietary fibre includes cellulose and other indigestible parts of food derived from plants. Unlike other macronutrients, such as fats, proteins, or other carbohydrates, which your body breaks down and absorbs, fibre isn't digested by your body itself but rather the trillions of microbes that make up the gut microbiome.

Dietary fibre is commonly classified as soluble, which dissolves in water, or insoluble, which doesn't.

- **Soluble fibre.** This type of fibre dissolves in water to form a gel-like material. By slowing digestion, it slows the absorption of glucose, which is helpful to people with diabetes. Soluble fibre is good for both diarrhoea and constipation. Soluble fibre is found in most fruit, asparagus, beans, beetroot, broccoli, Brussels sprouts, carrots, peas, sweet potato, zucchini, barley, lentils, nuts, oats, and seeds.

- **Insoluble fibre.** This type of fibre promotes the movement of material through your digestive system and increases stool bulk, so it can be of benefit to those who struggle with constipation or irregular stools (together with drinking enough water). Insoluble fibre is also found in bananas, Brussels sprouts, figs, nuts, okra, parsnips, pears, raspberries, spinach, strawberries, sweet potato, and many above-ground vegetables such as asparagus, broccoli, cauliflower, green beans, and zucchini.

There are many benefits in dietary fibre, but there are some potential problems, particularly if you have an imbalance of gut microbes or just too many, as is the case in small-intestinal bacterial overgrowth (SIBO), which often causes irritable-bowel symptoms or food intolerances. With more longstanding and complex digestive issues, it's best to work with integrative medical practitioners, nutritionists, or naturopaths, who are familiar with some of the issues I've covered.

I will discuss some basic guiding principles further in Chapter 12: Nutrition. Suffice to say, a wide variety of fresh foods contain a diverse range of nutrients, including both soluble and insoluble fibre. While grains are often presented as an excellent source of dietary fibre, this overlooks their potential for irritating the gut.

Not surprisingly, processed and most fast foods contain less fibre. 'Fibre added' to processed foods is (I believe) a great marketing tool, but eating whole fresh foods is just so much better for your health. After millions of years of 'research', nature seems to have got the 'ingredients' just right.

Feeding your gut biome and creating your own healthy team of friendly bacteria is central to a healthy digestive and immune system. Healthy microbes in your gut are an essential part of a long, harmonious, and healthy life. Bad bacteria have the potential to compromise your immune system and contribute to both physical and mental illness. Good bacteria support the immune system and help maintain homeostasis, health, and wellbeing. What you eat determines which bacteria are dominant — good or bad. Feed your friends, not your foes.

Problem 7 — additives, preservatives, and pesticides — and a reduction in micronutrients

We are potentially exposed to thousands of chemicals every day, through our clothes, furniture, and household and personal-care products, but mainly through our food. In particular, chemical additives and processed foods go together — you rarely have one without the other. The more processed foods you eat, the more additives you'll eat, too. The easiest way to avoid additives is to eat fresh food and, if necessary, 'lightly' processed foods such as canned tomatoes and frozen vegetables. But as a general rule, fresh is best.

Food Additives to Avoid

Artificial food colours 100s 102, 104, 110, 122, 123, 124, 127, 129, 132, 133, 142, 143, 151, 155: Cordials, lollies, soft drinks, chips, Natural colour Annotto 160b	**Synthetic Antioxidants** **Gallates** 310-312 **TBHQ, BHA, BHT** 319-321: Vegetable oils, chips, chewing gum	Sodium/Cal. Cyclamate 952 Saccharin 954 Any diet product **Other additives** **Brominated Vegetable Oil:** Sport drinks
Preservatives 200s **Sorbates** 200-203: Cheese, jams, soft drinks, dips **Benzoates** 210-213: Fruit juices, soft drinks **Sulphites** 220-228: Dried fruit, wine, vinegar **Nitrates/Nitrites** 249-252: Cured meats, ham, salami, bacon **Propionates** 280-283: Bread, pizza, cheese	**Flavour Enhancers** **Glutamates** 620-625 **MSG** 621 **Ribonucleotides:** Disodium guanylate 627 Disodium inosinate 631 Sodium Ribonucleotide 635 **Hydrolysed Vegetable Protein:** Stocks, fast foods, instant noodles, flavoured chips **Artificial Sweeteners** Acesulfame potassium 950 Aspartame 951	**Potassium bromate 924:** Sport drinks **Brominated Vegetable Oil:** Breads **Trans/Hydrogenated fats:** Margarine, chips, crackers, baked goods, fast foods **Olestra (Olean):** Synthetic fat **High Fructose Corn Syrup:** Soft and sport drinks, cereals, lollies

Figure 6-10. Food additives to know about and avoid.

The connection between soil and plate is an important one, but much of the soil we use today to grow our food is out of balance. Magnesium, selenium, zinc, and other trace elements are essential for many biochemical processes throughout body, but are deficient in Australian soils and most soils used in industrial agriculture. Fertilisers, pesticides, herbicides, and fungicides all adversely affect the balance of the bacteria and fungi that are so important for healthy soils, just as antibiotics affect the gut biome so vital for our health (I examine these connections in more detail in Chapter 7: Environmental Stress).

Our need for a wide range of essential elements are also relevant to any discussion about salt. The components of conventional table salt are sodium, chloride, and sometimes iodine. More recently, potassium chloride has been substituted because of concerns about higher sodium intake on supposedly causing elevated blood pressure. It's another example of reductionist thinking and looking for the one answer resulting in a simple public health message: 'salt causes high blood pressure and heart attacks, therefore avoid salt'.

There is certainly disagreement with this message, with much research pointing out that salt doesn't increase blood pressure or lead to heart attacks.[23] What there hopefully is universal agreement on is that the processed foods these salts, be they sodium chloride or potassium chloride, are found in are the real problem. I believe the main point is that both simple salts miss an important opportunity to consume a nutrient-dense food with many important elements.

So when you read that 'salt is bad', the question you have to once again ask yourself is *which* salt? I agree that conventional table salt, which also finds its way into most processed food, is bad. On the other hand, Celtic sea salt and Himalayan rock salt contain over 50–60 micronutrients, which our bodies cannot produce themselves and are essential to our health.

Finally, there has also been a significant loss of biodiversity in the actual food we consume. The greater the diversity of foods and colours, the greater the number of vitamins, minerals, and other nutrients we have available. Figures 6-11 and 6-12 outline how things have changed over the last 100 years. Looking beyond 1983, chemical companies such as Syngenta, BASF, Dow AgroSciences, Bayer Crop Science,

DuPont Pioneer, and Monsanto have dominated the agricultural seed world — 90 per cent of the food we eat sprouts from seeds owned by chemical companies.

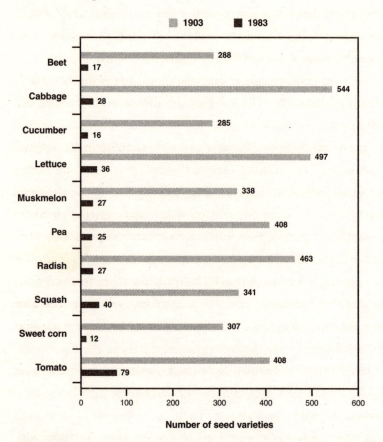

Figure 6-11. In 1903, commercial seed houses offered hundreds of varieties, as shown in a sampling of ten crops above the line; 80 years later in 1983, few of those varieties were found in the National Seed Storage Laboratory.

Seed	1983	2016
Artichoke	34	2
Beetroot	288	17
Cabbage	544	28
Cauliflower	158	9

Figure 6-12. US mail-order seed listings.

Problem 8 — overconsumption of alcohol

Alcohol has become ubiquitous with almost every social engagement or celebration. I would describe myself as a 'social drinker', but there have been times in my life when I have been too 'social'. Like many people today, I have a job that can be stressful and demanding — it's easy to feel you need to 'reward' yourself after a hard day's work.

Alcohol is not good for our health, and drinking too much alcohol, as we all know, is actually really bad for us. But how much is too much? Let's take a look.

The part of the body most affected by the consumption of alcohol is the liver. Our liver performs many essential functions, including clearing toxins from the body, processing food nutrients, and regulating the metabolism. With greater chemical exposure in our modern environment, it's even more important that our liver functions optimally.

In addition to its impact on liver function, chronic alcohol use also changes the way in which the central nervous system regulates inflammation and the delicate balance of hormones and neurotransmitters. This can lead to persistent, systemic chronic inflammation and, ultimately, organ damage.[24]

But the effects of alcohol don't stop there — alcohol also makes you gain weight, affects heart health, predisposes you to type 2 diabetes, and promotes depression and cancer.

When the liver breaks down alcohol, it creates acetaldehyde, which is a known carcinogen. Normally, the liver uses the antioxidant glutathione to neutralise acetaldehyde. Drinking too much alcohol means the liver can't keep up. This isn't just a problem because of the excess acetaldehyde; glutathione detoxifies many other chemicals, including those that your body creates naturally, as well as thousands of chemicals and pollutants we are exposed to on a daily basis.

Sleep is also disrupted when you drink alcohol. It might be easier to fall asleep, but the quality of your sleep is reduced. Poor sleep has far-reaching effects on many physical and mental-health conditions, which I will cover in detail in Chapter 10: Sleep.

However, we live in the real world and finding the right balance for yourself is important. It's easy to fall into the habit of one or two glasses of wine each night — before you know it, a whole bottle is gone, all in the name of 'unwinding and relaxing' or just 'being sociable'.

Going alcohol-free for a few weeks is a worthwhile experience for so many reasons. So many things (bowel movements, indigestion, exercise, tiredness, depression, and so on) are affected by alcohol — after a while, we tend to just accept it, and it can become your 'normal'. A short period of going alcohol-free will at least give you a benchmark against which to compare how good you can feel.

There are many countries in the world where alcohol is consumed regularly and in moderation, and appears to enhance health. It's always interesting to look at the whole picture rather than just one thing in isolation. Often these countries have a lifestyle (emotionally, nutritionally, environmentally, and posturally) conducive to health and longevity.

If you are healthy and free of chronic degenerative diseases, you should still aim for a few alcohol-free days per week. And when you do drink, do so in moderation. Once you realise how well you can feel, you will at least start to realise the real effects of alcohol.

If, on the other hand, you have health challenges, eliminating alcohol is an important part of the healing process, quite apart from it also being an interesting social experiment.

Conclusion

Diet has a dramatic impact on wellbeing for both body and mind. If we don't consume a healthy and balanced diet, we are at huge risk of suffering from nutritional stress. Slowly, western medicine is starting to accept the message that alternative, complementary, or integrative health practitioners have championed for the last 80 years, one that Hippocrates highlighted over 2,000 years ago: that in food we may find excellent medicine or terrible poison. We are beginning to embrace that self-evident 'revelation' — that what you eat has the potential to stress your system and promote the chronic degenerative diseases that plague our modern world. Or, for a more positive way to look at it, we are coming to understand that what you eat can extend your life by years or even decades.

The choice is yours. Nutritionally stress your system or nourish it? What you eat has the potential to control chronic inflammation, restore healthy gut bacteria, and affect your physical, mental, and emotional health. It is central to building resilience and is more important than ever in today's toxic, chemical world.

CHAPTER 7

Environmental Stress

Our environment is under stress: melting glaciers and icecaps, rising sea levels, bleaching of coral reefs, clearing of rain forests, increasing desertification, extinctions, and unprecedented floods, fires, heat waves, and other 'unseasonal', 'once-in-a-century' weather events. In addition, an alarmingly under-regulated range of chemicals and electromagnetic radiation we are exposed to on a daily basis.

It would seem 'progress' and our human footprint is having a significant impact on our fragile environment, both for us as individuals and our planet. We do not stand alone; we are not separate from the environment — all these things are connected. As we degrade the environment, we degrade ourselves. Seeing this is what I mean by 'taking a holistic view'. I want to show you the interdependence of our world.

How the health of our soils is directly linked to the quality of our food, our own health, and the health of our planet. How decisions we make about the foods we eat and how they are grown directly affect those health outcomes. How the choices we make, and a little caution, can dramatically reduce our exposure to thousands of chemicals and poorly understood levels of radiation.

While environmental stress may seem beyond our control, by being informed and aware we can make a big difference. But the change has to start with you and me.

It starts with soil

This may sound obvious, but we need healthy soil in order to grow healthy plants and rear healthy animals. It takes 500 years for two centimetres of soil to form, so it is a precious resource. A crucial part of healthy soil is the life within it. Just as we are learning the crucial role that healthy microbes play in human health, healthy microbes play an equally important part in the health of soil, and, ultimately, all that it nurtures.

An extraordinary example of this is a group of microorganisms known as mycorrhizal fungi. These fungi form a symbiotic relationship with many plants, increasing their resistance to drought and disease while forming a network around a plant's roots to extend its range and resilience. In exchange for this favour, the plant feeds the fungi liquid carbon (the only energy source it can use), some of which is used by the fungi and some of which is used by soil bacteria to generate other nutrients, including many of the trace elements and minerals so essential for our health. This system also allows plants to store up to 15 times more carbon in the soil than they could without mycorrhizal fungi — and storing, or 'sequestering', carbon, as we are often reminded, is an important goal in combating our biggest current environmental challenge, climate change.

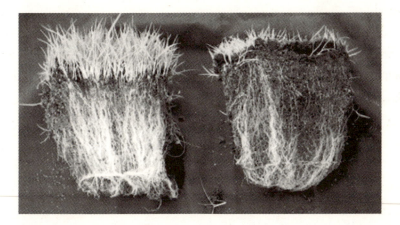

Figure 7-1. The plant on the left has an intricate and deep network of mycorrhizal fungi and its associated root structure, while the one on the right does not.

This group of microorganisms is very rare in conventional industrialised agriculture. The networks of mycorrhizal fungi are very delicate, so tilling easily destroys them. And since the fungi rely on plant roots as their only source of food, the bare ground left after a harvest quickly starves them. Worst of all, the widespread use of fertilisers (largely consisting of nitrogen, potassium, and phosphate) together with the use of herbicides and fungicides seems almost purposefully designed to kill these soil-enriching fungi. As plants monitor the level of nitrogen in the soil to determine how well-fed the mycorrhizal fungi are, many fertilisers cause the plants to shut down their supply of food, starving the fungi because — to the plants and the farmers, at least — crops appear to be thriving. But we need more than just nitrogen, potassium, and phosphate to thrive as humans. We need over 60 elements, which have to come from healthy soils, healthy plants, and healthy animals. Microorganisms such as mycorrhizal fungi that occur in healthy soils provide us with many of the vital trace elements we require.

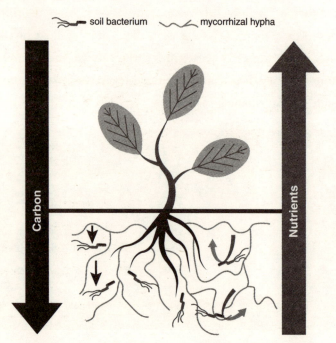

Figure 7-2. A symbiosis between plant and soil microbes (both bacteria and mycorrhizal fungi) involves a two-way exchange.

Unhealthy soil = unhealthy plants = unhealthy animals = unhealthy humans = unhealthy planet

The vast majority of microbes in our body help us maintain a healthy immune system, just as the vast majority of microbes in soils ensure the soils and plants that grow in them are healthy and resilient to disease. Over the last 100 years, the chemical and pharmaceutical companies have been instrumental in promoting an adversarial approach to both.

The overuse of antibiotics, for humans *and* animals, and our obsession with antibacterial products have been now been recognised as major contributors to many human health challenges, specifically antibiotic resistance, both now and, more worryingly, in the future. Similarly, the widespread use of fertilisers, herbicides, fungicides, together with lack of diversity in crop planting and poor grazing practices deprive the soil of those enriching, supportive soil microbes and have contributed to an unsustainable level of soil degradation and the widespread creation of deserts.

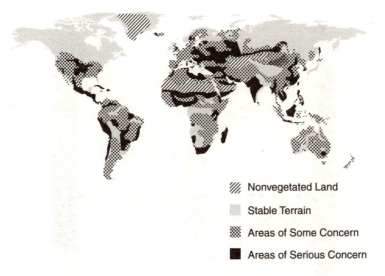

Nonvegetated Land

Stable Terrain

Areas of Some Concern

Areas of Serious Concern

Figure 7-3. 1.2 billion hectares of the world with moderate to severe soil degradation.

Over the past 40 years, the world has lost a third of its arable land due to overgrazing, erosion, or pollution. The loss of this finite resource, arable fertile land on which to grow nutrient-dense food, could see potentially disastrous consequences, with catastrophic effects on world food production and both human and planetary health.

Researchers at the Grantham Centre for Sustainable Futures at the University of Sheffield in the UK have identified some specific issues of serious concern when looking at soil degradation.[1] Duncan Cameron, professor of plant and soil biology at the university, has said:

Soil is lost rapidly but replaced over millennia and this represents one of the greatest global threats for agriculture. Erosion rates from ploughed fields averages 10–100 times greater than rates of soil formation and nearly 33% of the world's arable land has been lost to erosion or pollution in the last 40 years. This is catastrophic when you think that it takes about 500 years to form 2.5 cm of topsoil under normal agricultural conditions. A sustainable model for intensive agriculture could combine the lessons of history with the benefits of modern biotechnology.

Cameron goes on to explain:

Enhancing the biological functionality of soils allows them to store more water and nutrients, and support microbial communities that can boost plant health through direct suppression of soil-borne diseases and priming plant immune systems. A sustainable soil-centric re-engineering of the agricultural system would reduce the need for fertiliser inputs and pesticide application, and require less irrigation, thus contributing towards safeguarding finite natural resources.

In North America, industrialised agriculture alone has been responsible for 66 per cent of soil loss, while, in Africa, poor grazing practices are responsible for about half of the soil degradation. The economic reasons for these processes are linked to characteristics specific to each region — a holistic view of soil degradation accepts there is a complex interplay of cultural, political, and economic issues.[2] Solutions need to extend beyond the next quarterly corporate reporting cycle or half-yearly dividend to shareholders. Given that the earth's resources are finite, the answer certainly does not lie in the continual clearing of forests and the degradation of our soil.

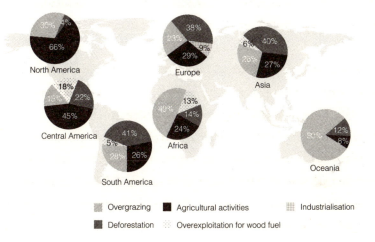

Figure 7-4. Causes of soil degradation globally include deforestation, over-exploitation for fuel wood, overgrazing, agricultural activities, and industrialisation.

Industrialised meat production is an assault on many levels

For 10,000 years, we have domesticated animals as a food source, and these animals have throughout human history and to this day played a critical role in human health. But for the last 40 years in particular, the treatment of these animals through industrialised farming has become another assault on the natural world, affecting not just the health and welfare of those animals, but our own health and again the health of our planet.

When humans first inhabited North America, more bison roamed and grazed on grasslands than the number of cattle present today, and had been doing so in harmony with the environment for thousands of years. A cycle of eating, defecating, urinating, trampling, and moving to new grasslands occurred in a sustainable cycle that continually enriched the soils on which they grazed.

Today, millions of acres of forests and grasslands are cleared to grow grains to feed animals held in massive enclosures, feedlots, cages, or pens. Their excrement is regarded as a problem, a waste product challenging their health and requiring chemical or antibiotic management, rather than as an enriching organic resource that is so valuable in replenishing the earth.

We are looking for ways to take carbon out of the atmosphere and if possible sequester it into the soils. When excrement becomes waste instead of the valuable resource it has been for millions of years, an important natural cycle is broken. That process, the breaking down of nutrients from animal waste into the soil, has the potential to significantly sequester carbon into the earth, where it also helps create and maintain nutrient-rich soil. This has the potential to help control climate change rather than contribute to its acceleration. Nurturing the soils for future generations while feeding the planet and treating animals humanely — surely this is our goal?

Unfortunately, modern industrialised livestock farming is a growing problem as we try to satisfy our insatiable and unhealthy appetite for more meat, oblivious to its quality, its impact on our health, or the environmental price. According to the United Nations Food and Agriculture Organisation, the second half of the 20th century saw global meat consumption increase five-fold.[3] In 1950, 45 million tonnes of meat was consumed; today, the figure is 250 million tonnes. The amount is set to double by 2050, particularly if China and India follow the lifestyles of western industrialised countries.

Land isn't the only resource that livestock farming affects. Animals reared for food need to be fed and watered in order to grow. In industrialised farming, animals consume far more resources than they produce in meat, milk, and eggs. For instance, to produce one kilogram of grain-fed beef requires around 15,500 litres of water and seven kilograms of plant-based food. The meat and dairy industries alone use one-third of the earth's fresh water. In the US, 5 per cent of fresh water is used in homes and 55 per cent on animal agriculture. Clearly, things are out of balance — and given that we tend to eat far more meat than we require for nutrition purposes, this is something we could readily address with our consumer choices.

Is there an alternative?

There is a view that industrial farming is the only way to feed the planet. Another view is that animals, and specifically meat production, has no place in a sustainable global food production. But it is not a view held by everyone. Environmentalist, farmer, and ecologist Allan Savory proposes alternatives to land management and food production that use large herds of grazing animals.[4] His approach — which involves mimicking the behaviour of wild grazing animals such as bison — is designed to regenerate soils, grow food ethically and sustainably, and sequester carbon from the atmosphere while addressing the reality of human needs and sustainable, ethical animal agriculture. His TED Talk in 2013 on reversing climate change has had over four-and-a-half million views and challenges accepted wisdom. It's worth a look.[5]

While you may not be able to organise animal agriculture, there are simple everyday decisions that you can make that can influence its direction. Animals that are free-range and pasture-fed are happier and healthier animals, maintaining a balanced cycle of carbon consumption (grasses, seeds, etc.) and returning carbon to the soil in excrement. Their products for our consumption are also healthier, particularly if we consume only what we need. A win-win for animals, planet, and us.

Global food waste and efficient land use

Each year, one-third of food produced globally for human consumption (or approximately 1.2 billion tonnes) is wasted.[6] This situation is further exacerbated by a system that sees inefficient subsidies paid by governments, at huge costs to taxpayers, to the food industry. Take, for instance, the corn industry in the US.[7] A tiny fraction of corn grown in the US directly feeds the nation's people, and much of that is in the form of high-fructose corn syrup (HFCS). Ironically, this government-subsidised product finds its way into most processed food, even though it's now almost universally accepted as a significant nutritional stress on our health.

In 1997, the US produced enough grains for animals that could instead have been used to feed 800 million people.[8] A report in 2013 suggested that an additional four billion people could be fed if agricultural production was focused on feeding people — not feeding animals or providing biofuel for cars.[9]

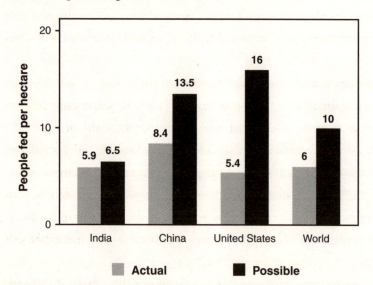

Figure 7-5. The purpose of agriculture is to feed humans — clearly there is scope for improvement.

I'm not suggesting we feed all that grain to people, but, with a holistic approach to land management and food production, vast amounts of land, water, and fossil fuel could be used far more efficiently, in addition to a reduction in the billions of kilograms of chemicals used to sustain the system.

There are many factors involved in food waste, including the food's production, handling, storage, processing, distribution, marketing, and, of course, actual consumption. The greater a geographical area's access is to refrigeration and transport, the greater the proportion of waste is attributable to consumption, particularly in our western society. The seemingly insatiable appetite of industrialised countries is environmentally unsustainable in its current form; its effect on our individual health is another important matter to consider.

It is rather sobering to observe that over 800 million people in the world do not have enough food to lead a healthy, active life. That's about one in nine people on earth (or 11 per cent). On the other hand, according to the WHO in 2014, more than 1.9 billion adults aged 18 years and older were overweight. Of these, over 600 million adults were obese. The number of overweight or obese infants and young children (aged zero to five years) increased from 32 million globally in 1990 to 42 million in 2013.

Once again, things are clearly out of balance.

In addition to the environmental and nutritional stresses in play here, we should also consider the emotional stress of the situation. As I've discussed, there is a strong link between mood and food. Poor nutrition is inseparable from physical, mental, and emotional health. It's no coincidence that industrialised food production has led to environmental degradation, over-consumption of nutrient-poor food, and an epidemic in chronic degenerative diseases and mental-health problems.

Something has to change. A more integrative, holistic, ethical, sustainable, and socially and environmentally conscious approach to how we grow our food, what we eat, and how much we eat is a worthwhile goal for our own health and the health of our planet.

The human impact on our environment

While there is rightly a focus on the impact of highly subsidised fossil fuels on the environment, we often ignore the fact that industrialised animal agriculture in its current form accounts for 51 per cent of global greenhouse gases. This compares with 13 per cent of emissions from road, rail, air, and sea transport. Animal agriculture is also the reason that 91 per cent of the Amazon rainforest was cleared, one-third of which has already gone on to be lost forever to desertification.

It's ironic that we should even be arguing (let alone be surprised) that human activity is the main driver in global warming.

But no matter which side of the argument you are on, there can be little doubt the scale and speed of detrimental change in the last 40–50 years could have catastrophic effects. The world is littered with thousands of examples, and the world's climate scientists are almost unanimous in their assessment.

> *Earth's climate has changed over the past century. The atmosphere and oceans have warmed, sea levels have risen and glaciers and ice sheets have decreased in size. The best available evidence indicates that greenhouse gas emissions from human activities are the main cause. Continuing increases in greenhouse gases will produce further warming and other changes in Earth's physical environmental ecosystems.*
>
> *Source:* The Science of Climate Change: questions and answers
> *Australian Academy of Science*
> *February 2015*[10]

The suggestion that human activity hasn't affected carbon emissions (and thus climate change) conveniently turns a blind eye to the last 70,000 years of human history. As the dominant species, we *Homo sapiens* have either survived or wiped out all other human species, including *Homo erectus* (which inhabited the world from 1.9 million to 143,000 years ago) and *Homo neanderthalensis* (600,000 to 40,000 years ago), along with tens of thousands of animals on land, in the sea, and in the air.[11] These mass extinctions include entire megafauna species (animals over 50 kilograms), great forests, and vast grasslands.

In our march to dominate planet earth, humans destroyed ecosystem after ecosystem.

Evidence-based medicine is held up as the gold standard of healthcare, but, sadly, evidence is not so valued for our environment. When it comes to the health of our planet, an evidence-based approach is too often manipulated or ignored in favour of an economic imperative, where the market and profit take priority. The way we view and even care for our environment has fallen prey to the Tobacco Playbook, which I mentioned in Chapter 3: Big Pharma, Big Profits.

This is a worrying situation: when it came to tobacco, even in the 1950s, the science was clear — smoking was harmful and addictive — but government action and important public health messages were hindered, frustrated, and delayed. It's sobering to consider that the USA FDA only declared smoking an addictive substance in 2009, almost 50 years after scientific evidence had clearly shown the health risks!

When it comes to our planet's climate, the same delay tactics and political manipulation are being employed, but today the stakes are much higher. Irreversible harm is being done to our world, multiplying the health risks to present and future generations. Why then is there such confusion in public health and also environmental messages, so much inertia in government policies? Put simply, though the stakes are higher, the potential industry profits are also much higher.

News services deal with this critical issue in the interests of providing a 'balanced' report. The same news emphasis, publicity, or airtime is often given to a report put together by 3,000 highly qualified climate scientists as is given to a climate-change denier with absolutely no climate-science credentials and, more often than not, links to the fossil-fuel industry. Often, the denier may even get more coverage, as their claims of 'poor science' make for better quotes and higher ratings. Important issues are lost as the 'news' is reduced to short, attention-seeking headlines rather than informed analysis and discussion.

A surprising fact for many of us is the depth of resources at the disposal of this 'fossil-fuel industry', reaching deep into the media, regulatory bodies, and governments themselves. Mining and other resource extraction are sacrosanct. Just as in the food and pharmaceutical industries, the fossil fuel industries lobby elected government representatives. Media campaigns result in proposed mining taxes and regulations being withdrawn, and arguably even in changes of government. Renewable energy is another favourite for industry and media to meddle with. It's interesting to see how little exposure in the media, or consideration in government debate and policy, is given to what must be one of the most significant areas of reform in energy and environment.

Limited media or government attention has been given to a highly significant International Monetary Fund (IMF) report which reveals that the fossil-fuel industry receives US$5.3 trillion in annual subsidies worldwide, which equates to a staggering US$10 million every minute.[12] This subsidy is a far greater amount than the annual health spending of all world governments combined. Clearly, if we are expecting the change to come from above, from governments or media being influenced by industry, we will be disappointed. In Australia, the change is coming from the ground up, from people individually embracing renewable energy — despite government inaction, for instance, more than 1.5 million households have already installed solar power.

This official response to climate change in particular, and our health in general, is, I believe, a sad legacy of a free-market economy. In the same way climate change has altered our external environment, adding environmental stress to the health of our planet, this stress has serious implications on our individual and community health as well, not to mention what our legacy will be for future generations. The market has successfully globalised stress. We are all connected, so we are all affected.

The external environment affecting the internal environment — our modern human experiment

There is another way we're connected, one we hear about all the time these days — through technology. The paradox here is that almost everyone carries a mobile phone, connecting us all to information, people, and the world. Yet technology also has the potential to harm us all.

Advances over the last half-century have seen us all become part of a modern 'human experiment' unprecedented in the history of our world: our exposure to electromagnetic radiation (EMR). This exposure comes from a multitude of sources: electrical appliances, microwaves, wi-fi, Bluetooth, X-rays, CAT scans, MRI, even air travel, and, most importantly, mobile phones. I say, 'most importantly' because we all carry them on our bodies and put them next to our brains. These technologies are recent innovations, and it's difficult to not be swept up in the excitement of change. Even though industry often provides the assurances of 'safety' when faced with questions on EMR and our wellbeing, the actual long-term effects on health are not yet known.

What we do know for sure is that our bodies are walking electricity. As Albert Einstein noted in his theory of relativity, every atom in the universe, which includes every atom in our bodies, is both energy and matter. Every cell in the human body functions through small electrical currents. We know that EMR has the potential to affect our body by interfering with the billions of finely tuned processes that allow us to live, function well, and stay healthy. It would be naive to assume that we are not affected by the EMR from our modern devices, and those effects are unlikely to be positive. Sometimes, common sense and caution should prevail.

Countries such as Switzerland, Italy, France, Austria, Luxembourg, Bulgaria, Poland, Hungary, Israel, Russia, and China have set exposure limits between 100 to *one million* times less than Australia, the United States, and the United Kingdom. Do they know something we don't, or is this something we conveniently just choose to ignore?

These countries recognise there is more to the safety of electronic devices than just how hot they get, and are increasingly recognising that non-thermal biological effects from EMR are potential problems. More than a dozen countries restrict, or advise precautions regarding, the use of mobile phones by children. Growing numbers of authorities from around the world are banning or warning against wi-fi use in schools.[13] Two new studies, which looked at the effects of wi-fi on brain function, have found that electromagnetic fields from wi-fi transmitters can alter electrical brain activity and decrease a measure of attention in young adults when performing a memory task.[14]

It's worth reading the fine print tucked away deep within the instructions on your mobile phone. If, like me, you use an iPhone, you can tap Settings > General > About > Legal > RF Exposure to read: 'Carry iPhone at least 5mm away from your body to ensure exposure levels remain at or below the as-tested levels. Cases with metal parts may change the RF [radio frequency, i.e. EMR] performance of the device, including the compliance with RF exposure guidelines, in a manner that has not been tested or certified.' In fact, while I was writing this book, Apple removed the instruction to carry the phone 'at least 5mm away from your body'. Now, they blandly assert that testing for EMR exposure was carried out 'with 5mm separation' — that is, they make no claims about what happens if the phone is carried closer to your body. Suddenly, texting and using the speaker phone seems more appealing than I ever thought.

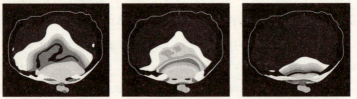

5 yr old child   10 yr old child   Adult

Figure 7-6. The younger the child, the deeper radiation penetrates their skull. This is because their skulls are thinner and still developing. Unfortunately, bone marrow in a child's skull absorbs ten times more microwave radiation than does an adult.

Our daily chemical environment

Our daily exposure to chemicals is another issue we should be paying more attention to. Today, there are over 140,000 chemicals in our environment, with 2,000 new chemicals added each year;[15] once again, we're part of a huge and unprecedented human experiment. We rather naively assume that if it is sold, it has been tested. When it comes to chemical exposure in our food, personal-care products, or home environment, it's sobering to realise only a small percentage of those thousands of chemicals have been tested for links to health — and many of them are toxic.[16]

To add to this, the testing of these materials is fraught with problems: How do you test it? What is the health status and age of the person tested? How long do you test for? What happens if one chemical is combined with another?

Just read the label on any product and you will understand that each day we are exposed to a cocktail of chemicals — it's never just one chemical at a time. Even more alarmingly, most tests on the harmful effects of a particular chemical are only conducted on a single chemical exposure, over a period of just weeks or months — and often on a young, healthy subject. The synergistic interaction of several chemicals over a lifetime on people of various ages and degrees of health is rarely, if ever, considered. So my advice is: it's better to be cautious than cavalier.

For an example of how cavalier health authorities and regulatory bodies can be when it comes to the dangers of chemical exposure, you need only look at the example of dental mercury, which I discussed in Chapter 2. Mercury is universally accepted as one of the most toxic elements — see Chapter 8: Dental Stress for even more details — yet the International Dental Federation, while acknowledging it as an environmental hazard, still endorses its use in humans? It's crazy but true. I haven't used mercury in my clinical practice for over 30 years, so I can assure you there are alternatives.

My point here again is that if you are expecting governments, health authorities, or regulatory bodies to deal with toxicological concerns that are less obvious or more nuanced than the problem of highly toxic mercury, you may be waiting a long time. When it comes to environmental stress, taking control of your own exposure and exercising the precautionary principle is the best alternative.

In the United States, legislators are more inclined to argue that if a consumer is harmed, they should pursue compensation in law courts, and that is how harm from toxins is determined. The burden of responsibility is on the public to make the claim and the court to decide. The problem with this approach is that the damage has already been done, not only to the claimant, but also possibly to millions of other people. It also assumes that individuals have the financial resources to pursue legal action against major corporations. It's hard to put a price on good health — even if you 'win' in court, you're still left with health problems.

If something has the potential to cause you harm, and you can avoid it or minimise your exposure to it, it's probably best to do so. Use your consumer dollars to choose wisely and reduce chemical loads. By making informed choices you can reduce your chemical load by 80–90 per cent. That's empowering.

THE PRECAUTIONARY PRINCIPLE DEFINED

The precautionary principle has four central components:

- take preventive, cautious action in the face of uncertainty
- shift the burden of proof to the proponents of an activity or product
- explore a wide range of alternatives to possibly harmful actions
- increase public participation in decision-making.

In other words, if something has the potential to harm either the health of the public or the environment, it is best avoided unless there is *independent* scientific consensus that the action is not harmful. The burden of proof rests with the promoter — often an entire industry — not the public.

Ten toxic truths about environmental toxins

Much of what I have discussed in this chapter was clearly and cleverly articulated by Professor Marc Cohen on *The Good Doctors* podcast. I want to highlight the points he talked about — encapsulating for you just how ubiquitous environmental stress can be for us all.

Professor Cohen leads the Wellness Discipline in the School of Health Sciences at RMIT, Melbourne. He's a pioneer in integrative and holistic medicine in Australia, and is passionate about informing the public on the dangers of toxins in our environment. Cohen created a list of '10 Toxic Truths',[17] and, while he admitted they could sound depressing, he also argued that awareness and knowledge of these truths could encourage people to make informed choices. I have covered some of the points he makes, but it's worth going over them and taking a closer look at some of the other issues he raises:

1. **Everything is connected, and everyone is affected.** Whether we like it or not, whether we believe in it or not, we're all connected and so we are all affected by toxins in the environment.

2. **We don't know the full extent.** As Cohen outlines, 'There's an estimated 140,000 commercially produced chemicals in our environment, and probably another 500,000 produced inadvertently. These chemicals weren't in the environment 200 years ago.' There is also often a long lag-time before a disease becomes clinically apparent or diagnosed.

3. **Very small doses can cause very large effects.** In 2014, the World Health Organisation released a document on endocrine-disrupting chemicals.[18] Cohen says, 'We previously thought it was the dose that made the poison and, below a certain dose, everything was okay. And if you had a small amount of the toxin, it didn't really matter. Now, we're realising that very, very small amounts can affect our endocrine system, which matters because it's the endocrine system that [by producing hormones] controls the regulation of our organs and their growth and development. Another document released by the World

Health Organisation recognised that these chemicals are in our water, our soil, and our air.[19] They're in consumer goods, furniture, personal care products, our food, and they have a huge effect on chronic diseases, diabetes, depression, neurological problems, human reproduction and fertility, and childhood development.'

4. **Chemical cocktails are synergistic.** How toxic is mercury? What if we combine it with lead? If a small dose makes a difference and these chemicals are combined, that becomes a bigger problem. For example, if we give mercury a toxic value of 1 and we give lead a toxic value of 1, adding both together doesn't necessarily make 2. The toxicity of two or more chemicals could equal 10 or 100; the combined effect could be exponential.

5. **Timing is important.** It's not just the dose or mixture of toxic chemicals, but the timing of the exposure. This was seen in the 1970s when pregnant women were prescribed thalidomide for morning sickness. The timing of the chemical exposure meant thousands of children were born without limb buds.

6. **Foetuses, children, and the young are at greatest risk.** Children have much higher chemical exposure than adults because they literally live closer to the ground, where many toxins are located. They have much more hand-to-mouth behaviour and eat, drink, and breathe more per kilogram than adults. Children also have a faster metabolism and so extract more toxins when exposed to them. While they have a higher exposure, they have less ability to process the toxins, because of immature detoxification and immune systems. And because they are exposed so early in life, they also have a longer period to develop latent diseases — it can often take 20–30 years to develop a disease, and it will be much more obvious in a child than in an older adult. Recent data suggests organophosphate pesticides, commonly used as water-soluble pesticides, and phthalates found in plastics and personal-care products can have cumulative, synergistic, and adverse health effects, and again children are most vulnerable.

7. **Biomagnification happens up the food chain.** This occurs when

large organisms consume smaller organisms — big fish eat little fish — magnifying the toxic chemical consumption. There could be a tiny amount of mercury in plankton, for example; but when shrimp eat plankton, it's aggregated. Then when little fish eat shrimp, it's aggregated again. Then bigger fish eat little fish and it is aggregated again. Then predatory fish or seabirds eat the other fish. In this way, the amount can be magnified by up to ten million times. When it reaches the top of the food chain — humans — there are much higher concentrations. Another good reason to eat plant-based, organically grown food.

8. **Bioaccumulation.** Persistent organic pollutants (POPs) are chemical substances that persist in the environment, bioaccumulate through the food web, and pose adverse effects to human health and the environment. They are stored in fatty tissue. When a male blue whale was killed in 2013, Baylor University scientist Stephen Trumble and his colleagues extracted the whale's 25-centimetre-long earwax. When this wax was tested, it had traces of environmental contaminants such as DDT and its breakdown products, and mercury. These substances were deposited in the layers of wax from the bloodstream, enabling the scientists to assemble a profile for each of these chemicals over the lifetime of the whale.[20] Certain fruits and vegetables are also more likely to be contaminated by pesticides and herbicides than others. See the 'Dirty Dozen' and 'Clean Fifteen' in Chapter 12: Nutrition.

9. **Effects are epigenetic and transgenerational.** As I discussed in Chapter 5: Emotional Stress, when you have a thought, it produces a protein called a neurotransmitter that causes a gene to be expressed. This is the epigenetic effect. When a pregnant woman is exposed to a nutrient, a toxin, or a thought, it affects how her genes express themselves. That gene expression, the epigenetic effect, can then be passed on to the foetus and even to genes in the following generation. You don't start life with a clean slate, but inherit your parents' or grandparents' exposure. With knowledge comes power, and the science of epigenetics is empowering because it suggests that by taking a precautionary approach, you can influence the way in which genes are

expressed; admittedly, it can also frightening when you consider the number and amount of environmental toxins we're exposed to — it's a double-edged sword.

10. **Injustice and accidents happen.** Catastrophic accidents expose populations to chemicals — this is something beyond their control. Examples include the 1984 Bhopal toxic gas leak in India, the 1986 Chernobyl nuclear-reactor disaster in Ukraine, and the 2010 BP oil spill in the Gulf of Mexico. There are justifiable concerns when local disasters can have global effects. In March 2011, an earthquake and subsequent tsunami in Japan led to the Fukushima nuclear-reactor disaster, when nuclear waste and toxins from the stricken factory flowed into the sea, and currents carried them around the north Pacific and down the American west coast. Following the events in Japan, marine scientists from Stony Brook University and Stanford University tested 15 Pacific bluefin tuna caught off the coast of southern California and found small amounts of radioactive elements from the Fukushima nuclear power plant in their bodies.[21] According to the research, the migratory tuna were one to two years old, and swam in radioactive waters between Japan and California.

This reinforces the number one 'toxic truth' — that we are all connected and so we are all affected. Globalisation in the modern world offers us many opportunities, but it also offers us many challenges. Government regulations (or lack thereof) in one part of the world, far removed from you, may still have an impact on your health.

Oceans and seafood — danger, humans present! — planet earth beware!

As you can see, another natural environment suffering from degeneration is our oceans. Humans are also damaging our marine ecosystems at an unprecedented rate from overfishing, polluting, fertiliser run-off from farming, and acidification from increased carbon-dioxide emissions.

Our oceans are reaching a critical point: fish, sharks, whales, and other marine species are in danger of extinction, and are disappearing more quickly than originally predicted.[22]

Clearly, this problem flies in the face of advice that we should be eating more seafood — advice I have two major concerns with. The first is that it's unsustainable. Seafood consumption is reaching record levels; the world's per capita fish supply has increased from an average of 9.9 kilograms in the 1960s to 18.4 kilograms in 2009.[23] Global fish stocks are exploited or depleted to such an extent that without urgent measures, we may be the last generation to catch food from the ocean.

My second concern centres on the toxicity of seafood. As I mentioned, many chemicals are stored and passed up the food chain. Seafood is affected by runoff from human effluent laced with pharmaceuticals, fertilisers, industrial waste, toxins, pesticides, insecticides, and herbicides, as well as chemical breakdowns from the disposal of plastics and other rubbish. A 2015 report estimates that around eight billion kilograms of plastic waste enters the ocean each year.[24] Plastics are not biodegradable (harmless), but they *are* degradable, breaking down into smaller and smaller but equally toxic components, ingested by organisms large and small.

Today, most fish that we are sold is farmed, and this only compounds the environmental and health challenges. Farmed fish is often fed from ocean stock that's been indiscriminately trawled in vast ocean nets and turned into fishmeal. According to *National Geographic*, 'Across the world's oceans, large commercial fishing boats haul aboard huge nets and 60-mile (97-kilometer) lines teeming with unwanted creatures — bycatch, sometimes referred to as "bykill" or "dirty fishing." Bycatch is a mix of young or low-value fish, seabirds, marine mammals, and sea turtles, often considered worthless and tossed overboard — dead or dying.' In effect this is like 'vacuuming' the ocean, and it destroys the delicate balance of sea life, large and small, old and young — it is a process that has resulted in areas of ocean literally stripped of life.

In fact, if we look at how efficient it is, as Matthew Evans points out in his excellent book *The Real Food Companion*, 'According to the sustainable fisheries advocate, The Australian Marine Conservation Society (AMCS), it can take up to 4 kg of wild fish turned into feed to produce 1 kg of farmed salmon and up to 12 kg to produce 1 kg of tuna.'[25] I would also recommend watching his excellent three-part TV series *What's the Catch*, which reviews the environmental and health issues surrounding today's seafood consumption.[26]

Unlike wild fish that has been caught in the ocean, farmed seafood does not eat krill or plankton, or other smaller fish that have themselves also eaten the krill or plankton. Though this means no biomagnification, it also means that farmed seafood lacks the health-giving fat content of ocean-caught seafood that makes it supposedly such a healthy food.

Fish farms also need to use chemicals and antibiotics to maintain the 'health' of the fish that are confined in an unnatural, unhealthy, stressful, and often small enclosure. The farmed fish also produce significant waste, and, as with land animal in feedlots, farmed fish are stuck in confined spaces where their faeces and urine are a challenge rather than a resource. These conditions have the potential to cause algal growth, reducing the water's oxygen content and making it harder to support life.

Building sustainability, resilience, and health into our cities — is 'the triple bottom line' enough?

'In 2008, the world became more urbanised for the first time in human history, with more people in cities than living in rural environments,' explains Geoffrey Roberts. He's one of Australia's leading environmental scientists and urban planners, and a good friend of mine.

'This trend is exponential, not linear, and this century is often called the century of the city. By 2050, around another billion people will live in cities. This meta-trend has shifted the environmental debate to a very large degree, pushing it from the "green debates" of the 1960s in rural areas to the "brown debates" of cities today.

'And the terminology being used has also changed. For the last 20 years, the word "environment" was very much used as a part of a greater problem, that of sustainability. This period has been dominated by thinking around what is referred to as the triple bottom line, which includes environmental, social, and economic factors as a way of measuring the health of a city.'

There is also the issue of equity and its effect on individual health. Geoffrey observes: 'We know that socio-economic advantage or disadvantage is a direct determinant of community health. In other words, lower education levels, poor access to transit-based transport systems, lower average family income, increased family size — all present higher determinants of poor community health: obesity levels, type 2 diabetes, heart disease, etc.

'So, if we as a society believe in equity of opportunity, then cities also need to become more equitable. We can't subject new residents of cities to lack of access to services like transit services, green infrastructure, schools, and health systems or we will get poor individual health outcomes. In effect, cities become the scaffolding for individuals to take control of their own health.'

How we live in our cities affects our health. How much time we spend travelling to and from work is a key predictor of a person's physical and mental health. Proximity and access to infrastructure and support is also vital to individual and community health. Perhaps the triple bottom line that guides urban planners should be expanded to the quadruple bottom line, with the 'health and wellbeing of the individuals that inhabit the cities' as the fourth and key component added to the environmental, social, and economic measures. Building resilience on a personal level is what this book is about, but as we are all connected and everything is connected to us, the resilience of an individual is intrinsically linked to the resilience of a city and vice versa. The same goes for countries and the planet.

In our modern world, there appears to be two types of people: those who want more and those who need more. If current levels of growth

159

are maintained, and if people living in third-world countries are to enjoy the 'spoils' of industrialisation and urbanisation, things need to change. 'Economic rationalism' has to give way to a period of 'planning rationalism'.

Building sustainability, resilience, and health into our rural environment — the bottom line

While we may be in the century of the city, that doesn't mean we can forget about the rural environment — it's important to build resilience here, too. As in cities, there are major health, environmental, social, and economic factors to consider in building a sustainable rural environment.

I have had the pleasure of meeting many farmers through a venture I cofounded with Vicki and Tim Poulter in 2006 called Nourishing Australia, a not-for-profit organisation dedicated to educating and inspiring people about the critical importance of nourishing our soils, plants, animals, people, communities, and planet. It is humbling when you realise the effort that goes into producing a seemingly simple item of food. You very quickly become aware that when you compare what we spend on discretionary items in our urban environment, it's clear we are paying very little for our most essential items, the nutrient-dense food we need to be healthy. But that 'cheap' food is all too often at the expense of the farmer and the planet.

In the emerging age of 'planning rationalism', I'd like to think that we will get our priorities right and elevate farmers to be the most revered and highly paid people in our society. Perhaps the coming century will also be known as 'the century of the revered farmer'. Particularly those who make every effort to nurture the soils, plants, and animals in their care. After all, not only do they grow the food we need to survive, they are at the frontline of nurturing the earth in which that food is grown and protecting the very environment that sustains us.

If money talks, and clearly it does, our greatest power to bring about change individually and collectively is to make choices about how we spend that money. Sadly, it's more powerful than our votes, but, through it, we have an opportunity to say something each and every day, to industry and therefore government — a message that goes beyond convenience and immediate gratification.

Conclusion

Environmental stress may seem overwhelming and at times depressing, but I believe the first step in dealing with a problem is to become aware of it. With knowledge comes the power to take control, and the precautionary principle should be our guiding light. If something has the potential to cause harm, it is best avoided — particularly if you are exposed to that 'something' on a daily basis.

As Julian Cribb points out in his excellent book *Poisoned Planet*:[27] we should demand a right not to be poisoned; eliminate fossil fuels; encourage clean, renewable, sustainable energy; eliminate toxins from the food chain; test all chemicals for safety; train scientists to 'first, do no harm'; reward industry by buying 'green'; and practise zero waste.

Remember: we are all connected, so we are all affected.

The heartening news is that if you make informed choices, you can dramatically reduce your chemical and radiation exposure; you can encourage and support those farmers that truly sustain the soil and nurture the animals. You have the ability to change your own life and also what is available in the marketplace. Choosing well to be well, not only for your own sake, but also for all that you are connected with.

CHAPTER 8

Dental Stress

Did you know that problems with your mouth and teeth can stress your body? In fact, they contribute to a vast range of problems from heart disease and tension headaches to poor sleep and a compromised immune system. If the eyes are the windows to the soul, the mouth is the gateway to the body.

Here are the facts:

1. The mouth and face are the most sensitive parts of the body, with huge neurological input to both the central and autonomic nervous systems. Imbalances in individual teeth or the way teeth meet, referred to as your 'bite' or 'occlusion', can contribute to facial pain, tension headaches, neck aches, jaw pain, and more.
2. The mouth is the site of the two most common infections that affect humans: gum disease and tooth decay.
3. Because of these two common infections, it is also the site of chronic inflammation, which is linked to all degenerative diseases, including cardiovascular disease and cancer.
4. Because of tooth decay and the need to repair and restore holes or defects in teeth, or replace missing teeth, there are many foreign materials implanted in the body, in the form of fillings, crowns, implants, or dentures.
5. The mouth is the gateway to the respiratory tract and so the shape and size of the upper and lower jaws, and the position of the lower jaw and the tongue, affects your ability to breathe and sleep well.

6.   The mouth is also the first part of the digestive tract, so imbalances
     in the occlusion or the jaw joints can affect your ability to chew food
     effectively — and this is the first stage in digestion.

But here's the problem: the mouth has become a sort of 'black hole' of health, with many medical and health practitioners, not to mention patients, failing to even consider oral health when making a diagnosis, or trying to get well. Too often, oral health is simply equated with the absence of pain — nothing could be further from the truth.

But even for specialists, there can be challenges to thinking holistically. Dentists are often caught up in the minutiae of the everyday challenges and complications of restoring broken-down teeth, making it easy to forget the connections with the rest of the body. This needs to change — we need to broaden our perspective.

To me, what defines a holistic dentist is that, as well as looking after the details of dental treatment, they also remember the person attached to the teeth and are mindful of the many connections between oral health and general health. Thankfully, by that definition, there are probably many more dentists who think holistically than dentists who actually call themselves 'holistic'. But the point is, oral health and general health are intimately connected, and in this chapter I am going to explore some of those connections.

Why the health of your gums matters

Most of us know that failing to take care of teeth and gums may well lead to gum disease — no big deal, you might think. Yet ongoing gum disease, the most common form of chronic inflammation in the body, may interfere with conception in women[1] and is also linked to preterm low birth weight[2] and osteoporosis.[3] Chronic inflammation often has no obvious symptoms, but it exacerbates other chronic health problems.[4] Once triggered, chronic inflammation can persist undetected for years or even decades without pain, causing imbalance and even cell death throughout the body.

Gum disease is often characterised by bleeding gums. Healthy gums look firm and pink, and shouldn't bleed when you brush or floss your teeth. When plaque builds up around the crevice where the gum meets the tooth, it causes inflammation in the gums (gingiva), resulting in gingivitis. The only sign may be the aforementioned bleeding, bad breath, or both. If the plaque persists, the crevice between the gum and tooth deepens to form a pocket. At this stage, the gingivitis has progressed to involve the attachment of the tooth to the underlying bone (periodontium), resulting in periodontitis. This undermines the periodontal ligament that connects the tooth to the jawbone, and the bone supporting the teeth is lost.

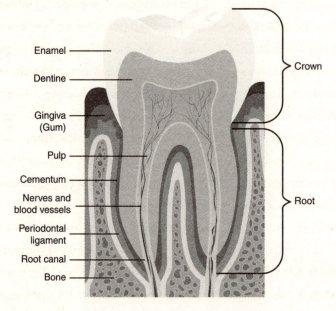

Figure 8-1. Healthy tooth anatomy and supporting structures.

According to the latest research there are up to 1,400 microbial components in the mouth.[5] The oral microbiome comprises many different species of microorganisms and sticky glycoproteins. Ideally, this microbiome should be stable and diverse, avoiding the build-up of destructive bacteria in what is called plaque or biofilm.

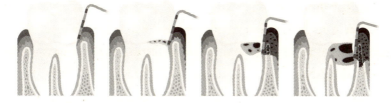

Figure 8-2. The stages of periodontal disease: a healthy tooth; gingivitis; periodontitis; severe periodontitis. The dentist investigates the tooth with a periodontal probe, which bears one-millimetre markings to measure the crevice or pocket.

If you eat a healthy diet and maintain good oral hygiene, the oral microbiome remains in balance; the healthy bacteria are dominant and don't cause chronic inflammation, bleeding gums, tissue damage, or tooth decay. A poor diet combined with poor oral hygiene allows the unhealthy bacteria to proliferate. Once a periodontal pocket has formed, these bacteria have a place to hide, becoming impossible to clean off with daily brushing or flossing. After 12–14 weeks, the more-destructive types of bacteria begin to multiply in the pocket and periodontium. This is why regular professional cleaning — every six months or, if a deep pocket has formed, every three to four months — by a dentist or dental hygienist is so important. Bleeding when you brush or floss should not be ignored.

If every time you washed your hands the cuticles of your nails bled, it is unlikely you would ignore it — and even more unlikely you would stop washing your hands altogether. Yet people do just that when it comes to the mouth. They dismiss or ignore the fact that their gums bleed when they brush or floss their teeth, and often say, 'The gums only bleed when I floss, so I stopped flossing.' This is not the answer.

So what actually happens when the gum is chronically inflamed and bleeds easily? It means that bacteria can enter the bloodstream in a process called bacteraemia. This is actually the reason blood donors are asked if they have visited a dentist or dental hygienist in the last 72 hours. Blood banks prefer to avoid harmful bacteria in the blood of their donors, and so should you. If your gums are inflamed, the body also produces C-reactive protein (CRP), which is an important indicator of chronic inflammation and can result in systemic effects in other parts of the body, such as the heart or the joints. This is the main mechanism that links the chronic inflammation in the gums to so many chronic health conditions.

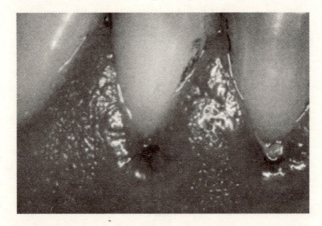

Figure 8-3. Gingivitis: gums are red and puffy, and bleed easily.

Gum disease is also the most common cause of tooth loss in adults, and is the main reason behind bad breath. In 70–80 per cent of cases, bad breath is caused from a build-up of plaque in the mouth, but it can also emanate from nasal passages, sinuses, the throat, or lungs. (Bad breath can also occasionally indicate an undiagnosed disease: a sweet smell may indicate diabetes, a fishy smell may indicate kidney disease, and a rotten egg smell suggests liver disease.)

As occurs with so many symptoms we are faced with in our modern world, bad breath is big business. The business of masking bad breath with chewing gum, mouth rinses, lozenges, or mints has spawned a $10-billion-a-year industry. It's another good example of a symptom-based approach to a health issue; but rather than masking the problem, like so many other symptoms in health, it's much better to discover the underlying causes and restore a healthy balance — in this case, in the oral microbiome. It would cost far less and achieve far more.

I'm often asked which toothpaste is best to remove plaque and promote healthy gums and good breath. Many commercial brands contain a list of chemicals, additives, detergents, and even sweeteners, while fluoride toothpaste even contains a warning not to swallow, as poisoning may occur. Personally, I use organic toothpaste: it contains herbal components, which are said to be good for the teeth, and I like the taste. Overall — despite the advertising claims — I don't believe there is a magic bullet toothpaste or mouth rinse.

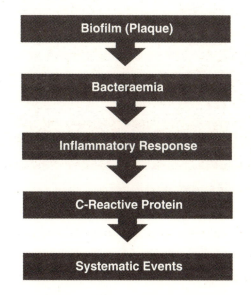

Figure 8-4. Inflamed gums leading to systemic chronic conditions in other parts of the body.

Yet it's so important to physically remove plaque by carefully brushing twice a day, and flossing each night. Promoting oral hygiene has been one of the greatest oral health initiatives over the past 50 years, and, while avoiding sugar has become part of our current health conversation, I am proud that the dental profession has been warning about the dangers of sugar for at least as long.

A regular check-up with a dentist or dental hygienist to carefully remove calcified biofilm, called calculus or tartar, which you can't get off with a brush, is also important. Don't wait for pain; by the time something becomes painful in the mouth from decay or gum disease, it is often quite advanced, and the solutions are more complicated and expensive than they need to or would otherwise be.

The mouth is the most sensitive part of the body

The orofacial region of the body includes the mouth, the jaws, and the face and is the most highly sensitive part of the body. Our senses of sight, smell, hearing, and taste are centred in this region, and touch is exquisitely present, too. Thirty to forty per cent of our body's sensory and motor nerves are found in the mouth and face.

Our ability to perceive the texture of what enters our mouth and then to effectively chew it or spit it out relies on our ability to detect tiny details. As I pointed out, the periodontal ligament attaches teeth to the jawbone — but it also does so much more. The periodontal ligament acts like a shock absorber, protecting our teeth from pain or excessive pressure. Embedded in the periodontal ligament of each tooth are nerve receptors so sensitive that they can detect displacements as small as 20 microns (0.02 millimetres). Fortunately, there is an adaptive range that makes discrepancies tolerable, but, when stressed, such pressures can become significant, causing teeth and fillings to become sensitive or even painful.

Sensory   **Motor**

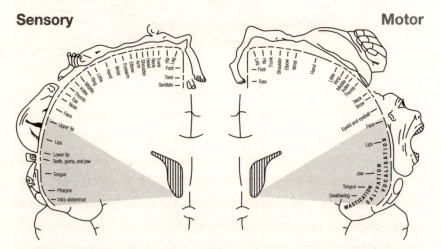

Figure 8-5. Homunculus — shaded areas show the proportional representation of sensory and motor nerves in the orafacial region.

Then there is the tongue, the most sensitive part of the body, not just to taste but also to touch. To make the point of just how many nerves there are in the mouth and thus how sensitive the area is, I often use the example of a hair. When you go to the hairdresser and talk too much while your hair is being cut, you may end up with a strand of hair in your mouth. You are immediately able to locate its position. A strand of hair is 20–100 microns (0.02–0.10 mm) thick. If the same hair were placed on any other part of your body, apart from your fingers, you wouldn't be able to detect it.

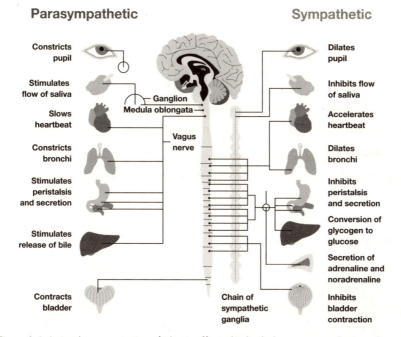

Figure 8-6. A visual representation of what is affected in both the parasympathetic and sympathetic nervous systems.

The processes of chewing and swallowing are a complex interplay of taste and touch, involving both voluntary and involuntary activation of more than 30 nerves and muscles, which must be coordinated with breathing.[6] Apart from preparing food for passage to the stomach, these processes protect the airway — the consequences of dysfunctional swallowing can be catastrophic. Yet thanks to the marvel of our mouths, we swallow 600 times throughout the day, even while we are asleep.

The nervous system is an important mediator of health and wellbeing, so, as the mouth is so richly innervated, chronic infections and inflammation as well as imbalances in the occlusion and the jaw joints also have an impact on the nervous system, sometimes with surprising results — affecting vision (blurred vision), balance (dizziness), mucous secretions (runny nose or sinusitis), and digestion.

Stress in the jaw is a two-way street. As stress is so common in modern life, the body often suffers fight-or-flight overload, disordered breathing while asleep, clenching, or grinding — all implicated in chronic musculoskeletal pain, tension headaches, neck aches, and jaw ache.

Gateway to the respiratory tract — breathing well and sleeping well

We know that breathing is important: while you can survive without water for a few days and without food for a few weeks, if you stop breathing for more than three minutes you die. But there is a difference between breathing to stay alive and breathing to be well. I will look at this, and how to achieve it, in more detail in Chapter 11: Breathing. But sub-optimal breathing is part of what I also include as a dental stress. The mouth is the gateway to the respiratory tract, and influences your ability to breathe well both during the day and, more importantly, during sleep, when the body and mind are meant to rebuild, reboot, and recover.

The actual shape and size of the jaws can impact on your ability to breathe well. The upper jaw should be a broad U-shape with a flat palate (roof of the mouth) and enough room for all of the 16 teeth in the upper jaw. There are also 16 teeth in the lower jaw. Over millions of years, we have evolved to have enough room in our upper and lower jaws to provide enough space for a total of 32 teeth. But today, in over 95 per cent of the population, that is not the case — the vast majority of us have a crowded jaw, with many of us having our third molars (wisdom teeth) removed because of inadequate space.

So why exactly is this a problem? If teeth are crowded or the jaws are narrow, it means there is less space in the upper airway, and less room for your tongue, which in turn can lead to upper-respiratory problems, such as recurring airway, nose, and throat infections; allergies; and asthma. It can even alter your posture in an attempt by the body to get more air — the head tilts back to open the airway and results in a head-forward position, which can also strain head, neck, and spinal muscles, something I will deal with in Chapter 9: Postural Stress.

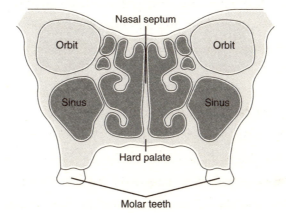

Figure 8-7. A cross-section through the front of the face showing a broad palate and resulting good spaces in the sinus and nasal passages.

Problems can also stem from how and where we breathe. Ideally, you should breathe through your nose to warm, humidify, and filter the air before it enters your lungs. If you breathe through your mouth, you bypass your built-in, comprehensive air-filtration system, making you more susceptible to respiratory problems. Breathing through your nose also helps regulate body chemistry and homeostasis, engaging the parasympathetic nervous system. Mouth breathing loses these advantages and predisposes you to the same posture problems as having a narrow jaw or crowded teeth.

The ideal breathing posture is through your nose, with lips lightly closed and the tongue at rest on the palate. If you breathe through your mouth, the tongue drops from the palate to rest on the floor of the mouth, and, over time, pressure from the lips and cheeks cause a narrowing of the upper and lower jaw, which can lead to a narrowing of the nasal passages and sinuses in the upper airway.

As I just mentioned, dental crowding or a narrow jaw also results in a lack of space for the tongue. The body has a few ways to accommodate this, but none of the options are ideal. One way to make more room for the tongue is to keep the mouth open — this certainly provides extra space. The problem with opening your mouth to make space is that you then also tend to breathe through your mouth, when really you should be breathing in through your nose. Another way for the tongue to get enough space is to retreat or fall to the back of the airway, restricting or blocking your breathing. A narrow jaw can therefore lead to sleep disorders, including snoring, upper-airway resistance syndrome (UARS), and obstructive sleep apnoea (OSA).

Jaw development and physical degeneration

I'm often asked why narrow jaws and crowded teeth are so common. Most people, even dentists, have come to accept that an overcrowded mouth is normal. Yet if we had insufficient room for all five fingers on our hands, I doubt we would be as accepting if it was suggested that the removal of the fourth finger was no big deal when we all reached the age of 20.

There is evidence to show crowded teeth and narrow jaws can also reflect physical degeneration that starts from the moment of conception, then continues in the womb and throughout life. This was suggested 80 years ago by dentist, researcher, and nutritional anthropologist Weston A. Price, who found the link between diet, dental decay, narrow crowded jaws, and physical degeneration — including many of the degenerative diseases of our modern world.[7]

Price was in search of the cause of tooth decay. He visited isolated communities all around the world and found that those villagers on traditional diets of nutrient-dense foods were not only free of tooth decay, they also had sufficient space for all 32 teeth, with broad, well-developed jaws and faces. Additionally, they were free of any chronic degenerative diseases.

When he visited the local towns, and viewed the same racial

groups who were consuming a western diet, high in sugar and refined carbohydrates, he found tooth decay was rampant. What was even more interesting was that after only one generation, the jaws were narrowed and the teeth were crowded. The populations on the western diet also displayed chronic degenerative diseases we commonly see today, such as heart disease, diabetes, and cancer.

Development of the craniofacial area, which includes the upper and lower jaws, sinuses, and nasal passages, is influenced by the parents' diet prior to conception, the mother's diet during pregnancy, and the baby's diet from birth throughout life into adulthood. As Price discovered, the best diet for oral and general health is one that focuses on nutrient-dense food (Chapter 12: Nutrition). As I discussed in Chapter 6: Nutritional Stress, avoiding the 'antinutrients' found in most processed food, as well as sugar, high-fructose corn syrup, and seed oils discussed, is also important.

Another factor influencing jaw formation is the position and function of the tongue, lip, and cheek muscles when breathing and swallowing. We swallow 600 times per day and breathe between 17,000 and 30,000 times per day — how we use those muscles is the subject of a relatively new specialty called 'oral myology' or 'myofunctional therapy'.[8] The tongue is your very own built-in, best-ever 'orthodontic appliance' and, when functioning properly, helps develop and maintain a wide, broad, flat palate, and well-balanced, well-spaced teeth and jaws.

An extensive study from the University of Washington over 40 years showed that irrespective of which orthodontic treatment was undertaken, whether teeth were extracted or not, or even whether wisdom teeth were present or not, jaws tended to narrow and teeth became more crowded over time.[9] Oral myology sheds some light on why this might be so. Unless breathing, posture, and muscle activity of lips, tongue, and cheeks are addressed, as well as addressing foods that might be promoting nasal and sinus congestion, teeth that are perfectly aligned at the end of orthodontic treatment, may after just a few years relapse to a crowded position.

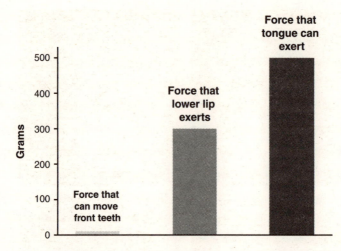

Figure 8-8. Tongue and lip function may be the cause of forcing the teeth into the crowded position they occupy. It only takes very light forces, of less than two grams, to move teeth. Lower lip can exert 300 grams and tongues up to 500 grams of force.

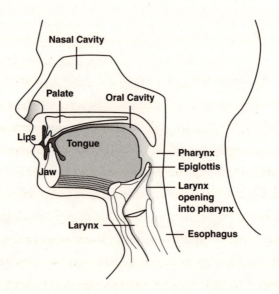

Figure 8-9. Side-on view showing ideal position of the tongue, which does not impinge on the pharynx (airway).

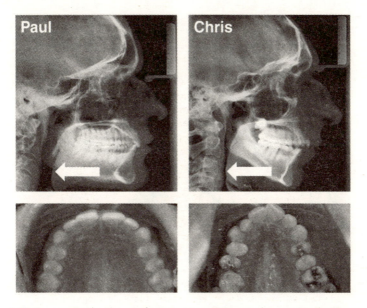

Figure 8-10. You can see the impact of a narrow jaw on tongue placement in the X-rays of two patients, both aged 38: Paul (left) has a broad upper jaw, adequate space for his tongue, and an open airway (see arrow). Chris (right) has a narrow jaw, restricted space for his tongue, and a restricted airway (see arrow).

Night-time clenching or grinding of teeth

When your teeth touch firmly in function (during chewing, talking, and swallowing), it is not only the jaw muscles that contract, but also the neck muscles. If you add up in a 24-hour period how much time your teeth touch in those instances, the duration would be less than half an hour per day. For the other 23 hours, the jaw should be at rest, with tongue resting on the roof of the mouth, lips lightly touching, and teeth either slightly apart or lightly touching. In this rest position, the neck muscles only need to balance out contracted jaw muscles for 15–30 minutes a day. The neck muscles' main function is to keep the head up and allow you to move your head in various directions.

But if you clench or grind your teeth, which most commonly occurs at night, the teeth could be contacting with considerable force for several hours. That means the neck muscles also need to contract for those extra hours. So if you have a neck problem with associated restrictions or pain, it may persist for years unless the jaw clenching is also addressed.

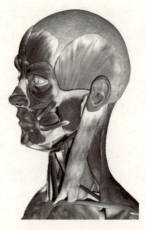

Figure 8-11. All of these muscles tighten when you clench your jaw.

Signs of nocturnal bruxism — the clenching and grinding during sleep — include worn or cracked teeth, hypersensitivity of teeth to air and cold, fractured dental restorations, indentations of the teeth in the tongue or cheek, exacerbation of gum disease (particularly when localised to one or two teeth), failures of dental implants, and waking in the morning with a headache, neck ache, or jaw pain.

In the majority of cases, wearing a well-fitted and correctly balanced occlusal splint to protect the teeth from wear while correctly balancing the muscles and jaw joints can resolve the bruxism and its effects. Another approach is using a mandibular-advancement splint (anti-snoring appliance) to maintain a more-open airway at night. This can boost energy levels by improving the quality of sleep, and dramatically improve mental and physical health. More about that in Chapter 10: Sleep.

OCCLUSAL SPLINTS DEFINED

An occlusal splint is a removable appliance, usually fabricated of resin, most often designed to cover all the surfaces of the teeth in the upper or lower jaw or both. Occlusal-splint therapy has been shown to be useful for the diagnosis and management of various musculoskeletal pain disorders and sleep-disordered breathing conditions. Other names for occlusal splints are: biteplates, night guards, occlusal orthotics, occlusal devices, stabilisation appliances, and mandibular-repositioning or -advancement splints.

There are several reasons for using occlusal splints:

- to determine the role clenching or grinding might play in a chronic musculoskeletal pain condition or jaw-joint issue
- to protect the teeth or restorations from excessive wear or mobility caused by the destructive forces of clenching and grinding
- to relieve tension in the muscles of the jaw, head, and neck
- to relieve pressure or tension in the jaw joint (TMJ) to address clicking or locking of that joint
- to reposition the lower jaw (mandible) in a more forward position to correct a clicking TMJ
- to reposition the lower jaw in a more forward position to improve airway clearance as a treatment for sleep-disordered breathing conditions such as snoring or OSA.

While various splints may look the same to a layperson, nothing could be further from the truth.

An occlusal splint is most effective if custom-made. This means that accurate impressions are taken for a patient's upper and lower teeth so that stone models of the teeth can be used to make an appliance specifically for that patient. This ensures accuracy of fit, better comfort, balance, and more stability.

Stabilising the spine

There are two structures that sit atop the spinal column and play a significant role in its stability: the skull and the lower jaw, or mandible.

The mandible pivots on two joints, called the temporomandibular joints (TMJs), just in front of the middle ear.

One of the things that makes the jaw joint unique is that it has a rigid endpoint, teeth, which position it when you bite together. Also, you can't move one joint without affecting the other. The jaw joints and occlusion help stabilise the cervical spine (neck), particularly the atlas (C1) and the axis (C2) vertebrae.

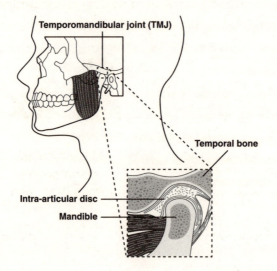

Figure 8-12. The temporomandibular joint (left), and the disc separating the jawbone from the skull (inset).

Within the jaw joints, there is a pressure-bearing disc (meniscus) separating the jawbone from the skull, allowing the two bones to move smoothly and quietly. The disc within each jaw joint is also important in absorbing the heavy load of chewing, clenching, or grinding, and doesn't contain nerves or blood vessels.

If, however, your jaw clicks when you open and close your mouth, this usually indicates the disc is out of place and the jaw joint is not as stable as it should be. TMJ clicking means the disc may have slipped forward (anteriorly displaced disc): the disc makes the sound as it moves back into place when you open your mouth; it then goes out of place again as you close. A clicking jaw may mean that when you chew, clench, or grind, the load is put on the ligaments that hold the disc in place rather than the disc itself, and those ligaments *do* contain nerves and blood vessels. You might compensate by eating too quickly because your jaw tires more easily, and this haste can affect digestion. You may also compensate by tightening muscles around the jaw and neck to protect the TMJs.

So a narrow, poorly aligned jaw, crowded teeth, or a clicking jaw may lead to instability in head posture and the spine, particularly if you also clench or grind your teeth. All of this can significantly contribute to headaches, neck aches, and ear and jaw ache.

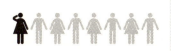

1 in 8
of the American population
is currently affected by TMJ.
This number may be low due
to undiagnosed cases.

TMJ is 4x more
common in
women than men.

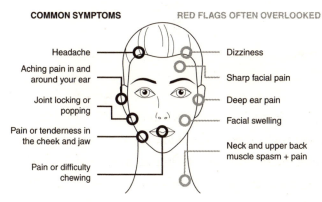

COMMON SYMPTOMS   RED FLAGS OFTEN OVERLOOKED

Headache

Aching pain in and
around your ear

Joint locking or
popping

Pain or tenderness in
the cheek and jaw

Pain or difficulty
chewing

Dizziness

Sharp facial pain

Deep ear pain

Facial swelling

Neck and upper back
muscle spasm + pain

Above: Figure 8-13. While at least one in eight Americans (and most probably a similar proportion of other westerners) is currently affected by TMJ dysfunction, the number may be much greater due to undiagnosed cases.[10] The fact that over 95 per cent of the population in western societies has some degree of narrow jaw or crowded teeth means it would be not unreasonable to assume the jaw joint is often compromised.

Below: Figure 8-14. TMJ disorders are always assessed by the degree of pain a person has, but one of the common symptoms that is often overlooked (particularly when there is no pain associated with it) is difficulty chewing effectively. This disorder is one reason that food is not chewed and broken down properly, an important first step in digestion.

Tooth decay and jawbone infections

Apart from determining our occlusion, teeth are also, of course, necessary for chewing (mastication), the process by which we tear, cut, and grind food in preparation for swallowing. Chewing allows enzymes and lubricants released in the mouth to begin the digestion of food. By chewing properly, you also increase the surface area of food as it enters the stomach, allowing stomach acid and other digestive enzymes to break down the food more thoroughly for its transit through the rest of the digestive tract. So what happens when these teeth, the hardest substances in our body, are compromised?

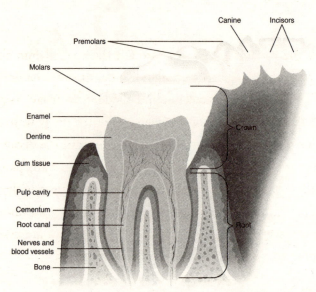

Figure 8-15. The structure of teeth. The hard enamel covers the softer dentine, both of which protect the nerve in the tooth.

The two most common infections in the mouth are gum disease and tooth decay. The main causes of tooth decay are sugar and acidity from drinks and foods, including starchy carbohydrates or processed food that quickly converts to sugars. Apart from weight gain, these sugars cause the destructive bacteria in the mouth to secrete acid that over time demineralises the tooth, starting with tiny pinholes that occur in the enamel.

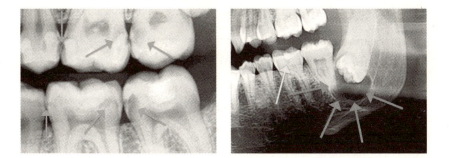

Above: Figure 8-16. Dental X-ray — arrows show shadows, which indicate the presence of pain-free tooth decay.
Below: Figure 8-17. Dental X-ray — white arrow shows shadow indicating decay under a filling; grey arrows indicate a very large (pain-free) cyst around an unerupted third molar (wisdom tooth) on a 40-year-old male.

Once the pinhole progresses through the enamel into the softer dentine beneath, decay can spread and undermine the harder enamel. Eventually, the enamel will collapse and 'suddenly' you have a significant hole — a 'cavity'— in the tooth, when in fact the decay wasn't sudden at all. This often occurs with little or no pain until the decay actually approaches the nerve; but even then, there may not be any pain at all.

It still surprises me how often decay can progress without pain. I've seen patients with teeth literally decayed to the gum line yet who say they've never had any pain at all. Dental X-rays are essential in determining the presence, extent, and depth of decay.

Are dental X-rays necessary and safe? Yes

To do a comprehensive dental examination, we need dental X-rays. They are invaluable diagnostic tools. Today, dental X-rays use digital sensors instead of X-ray films, delivering significantly less exposure to radiation than their old-fashioned counterparts. They are low-dose, involve no chemical developers, and are instant and easily reproducible.

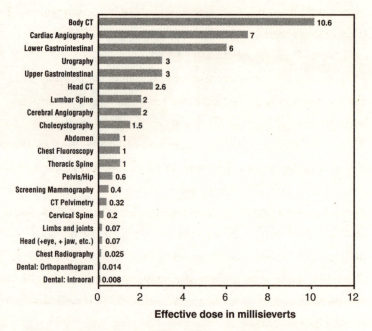

Effective dose in millisieverts

TYPICAL VALUES OF DOSE FOR VARIOUS MEDICAL AND DENTAL X-RAY PROCEDURES

Figure 8-18: Both panoramic X-rays of the jaw (called 'dental orthopantomogram') and the smaller intra-oral X-rays (called 'dental intra-oral') are an important diagnostic tool in doing a thorough dental examination, and give relatively little exposure to radiation.

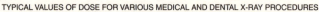

A PATIENT'S STORY — PATRICK

When Patrick, 62, came to my clinic, he described how he 'could barely walk from his bedroom to the bathroom'. His decline in mobility over two years was attributed to rheumatoid arthritis, and he had sought various traditional and alternative medical solutions, but his condition was only worsening. At this point, he had already lost 20 of his 32 teeth, so clearly oral health had not been a high priority for him throughout his life. Dental decay on four of the remaining 12 teeth had progressed through to the nerve of the tooth and into his jawbone. Patrick also had extensive plaque and calculus/tartar deposits around his teeth, causing both the more-superficial gingivitis and the deeper periodontitis.

Surprisingly (but as you will now appreciate, not uncommonly), despite these serious dental infections and chronic inflammations, he didn't feel any dental pain at all.

I removed the infected teeth; importantly, I thoroughly curetted the surrounding infected bone; and I cleaned the remaining teeth to restore gum health. I also constructed removable partial dentures to support and balance his bite and jaw, allowing him to effectively chew his food. Within a few weeks, his symptoms abated, and, within three months, Patrick resumed his active lifestyle — amazingly, he even cycled from Perth to Sydney via Melbourne, almost 4,500 kilometres! While I have no doubt his general debilitating health conditions improved because we addressed the source of his chronic infections and inflammation — namely his oral infections — I can't claim credit for his achievement of cycling across Australia.

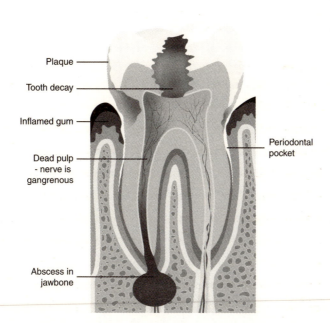

Figure 8-19. The progression of decay through a tooth from the pinhole cavity in the enamel, spreading to the softer underlying dentine, through to the nerve and into the jawbone.

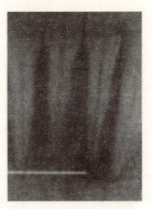

Abscess in jawbone

Figure 8-20. Once the nerve in the tooth dies infection will also spread into the jawbone resulting in bone loss around the tip of the tooth, which shows up as a shadow.

How mercury leaches into the body

A further source of dental stress is the restorative materials used in dental procedures. The use of foreign materials in dentistry is inescapable, but care needs to be taken when implanting anything into a patient's body, including the mouth. The best 'filling' material is your own natural tooth; everything else is a compromise to some degree.

As mentioned in Chapter 2, dental mercury amalgam fillings are 50 per cent mercury with the remainder comprising silver, tin, zinc, and copper. They have been used in dentistry for over 160 years as a cheap, durable, and relatively straightforward way to restore decayed teeth.

In 1991, a panel set up by the WHO to determine levels of mercury exposure included the advice of dentists, who were aware that mercury escaped from fillings. This was the first time that the daily exposure to mercury from dental mercury amalgam had even been considered. Previously, the panels without dentists assumed or did not consider 'silver' dental fillings to be a problem — they were apparently unaware that such fillings contained mercury or that any mercury escaped from these fillings. Not surprisingly, the results in 1991 showed that filling material, which is in the mouth 24/7, is the main source of mercury in the body.

Mercury source	Micrograms per day
Dental mercury amalgam	3–17
Fish and seafood	2.3
Other food	0.3
Air and water	Negligible

Figure 8-21. Sources of daily exposure to mercury according to the World Health Organisation.

Mercury is released from a filling as elemental mercury vapour, and the rate at which it is released increases with chewing, clenching, grinding, or drinking something hot.[11] In a more recent 2003 report by the WHO, the assessment of dental-mercury vapour is more concise, showing it to be by far the greatest contributor of mercury in the body.[12] This so-called 'harmless' form of mercury becomes a more-toxic form via a process called methylation, which can occur throughout the body.[13] The more-toxic form is then stored, mainly in the kidney, liver, and brain,[14] and is the greatest source of mercury load in the body.[15] It can cause tissue damage,[16] impaired kidney function,[17] neurological effects similar to Alzheimer's disease,[18] autoimmune conditions,[19] a compromised immune system,[20] and even an increase in antibiotic resistance.[21] Dental staff members who come into contact with mercury also (and not surprisingly) have adverse neurological effects.[22] Exposure is also a special concern for pregnant women, with research showing the quantity of mercury in a foetus is proportional to the number of mercury fillings in the mother.[23]

The Australasian Integrative Medicine Association (AIMA), of which I am proudly a member, has done an excellent position paper with extensive references on dental mercury amalgam.[24] Another comprehensive review, entitled 'The Scientific Case Against Amalgam' can be found in the 2016 report by the International Academy of Oral Medicine and Toxicology (IAOMT), identifying the many potential environmental, occupational, and health issues of using this material.[25]

Of course, dental authorities that support the use of dental mercury amalgam provide their own 'well-referenced evidence' for its safety.[26]

So where does this leave us? I encourage dentists and health professionals to consider the person attached to the tooth, and the impact of mercury on the body, not just the external environment. Mercury is toxic — and as we are trying to reduce the environmental exposure in our air, water, and food, it would seem logical to me that the human body is a good place to start. Stop using mercury fillings and exercise caution in their removal.

When removing dental mercury amalgam, several precautions should be taken, and this at the very least should include:[27]

- a dental rubber dam — a sheet of rubber that acts like a shield to prevent mercury from being swallowed or inhaled
- a separate air source that fits over the nose and prevents the inhalation of mercury vapour when the filling is removed
- cutting the filling out in manageable chunks
- copious amounts of water to dampen down any vapour produced — important for patient, dental assistant, and dentist alike
- high-speed suction to make sure the mercury and vapour are taken away as quickly and efficiently as possible.

Biocompatibility of dental materials

There are also concerns about other metal alloys used in prosthetic devices, joint replacements, and dental restorations. Recent studies suggest that metal-induced chronic inflammation might play a role both in chronic fatigue syndrome (CFS) and fibromyalgia, as well as in other autoimmune diseases.[28] Practitioners are now beginning to recognise this, with dentists moving away from the use of metal in the mouth in preference for ceramic, non-metallic dental restorations, although the changes are often driven by cosmetic concerns.

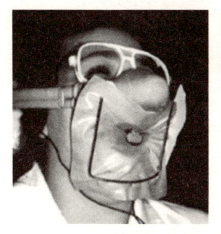
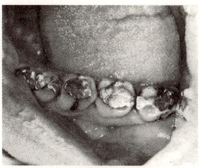
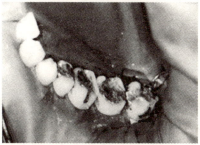

Figure 8-22. Left: rubber dam and nosepiece with separate air supply. Right, above: no rubber dam, exposing the mouth and airway to mercury when it is removed. Right, below: rubber dam in place, acting as a barrier.

ALLERGY AND HYPERSENSITIVITY DEFINED

Allergy is caused when the immune system reacts to a foreign material (or allergen) that may pose no threat to the body and yet the body mounts a violent immune response in the form of inflammation, which may lead to cell and tissue destruction. Because of this overreaction, allergy is also called hypersensitivity. Allergens include other organisms (pets, dust mites, pollen, moulds), foods, metals (nickel, gold, palladium, cobalt, chrome, titanium, mercury), and some medicines. There is a genetic (inherited) tendency to develop allergic diseases.

When susceptible people are exposed to allergens, they can develop an immune reaction that leads to allergic inflammation (redness and swelling). Some allergens produce obvious results, such as hay fever (allergic rhinitis/conjunctivitis), eczema, hives (urticaria), and asthma. But some reactions can occur over a longer period, making it easier to overlook the source of chronic inflammation.

There are essentially four types of allergies:

- **Anaphylactic hypersensitivity (Type I).** One of the most common allergic reactions, it is characterised by an immediate reaction to the offending allergen, usually within minutes, although it can take two to four hours. It is an immunoglobulin E (IgE) mediated response, resulting in the release of mediators of inflammation such as histamine. It triggers physiological responses such as smooth-muscle contraction, mucous secretion, and increased vascular permeability, and is potentially life-threatening. Symptoms include rashes, swelling, nausea, vomiting, and difficulty breathing. In Australia, more people die of anaphylactic shock from bee and ant stings each year than from our famously dangerous sharks, snakes, and spiders. For this reason, EpiPens, which deliver life-saving adrenaline (epinephrine), are a common sight in classrooms and childcare facilities.
- **Cytotoxic hypersensitivity (Type II).** This involves the destruction of entire cells, mediated through immunoglobulin M (IgM) and immunoglobulin G (IgG). Cytotoxic responses are immediate. They may occur when a patient is given the incorrect blood type during transfusion. Other examples are rheumatic fever, Goodpasture syndrome (affecting lungs and kidneys), and pemphigus (affecting skin).
- **Immune complex–mediated hypersensitivity (Type III).** Another IgG-mediated immune response, it occurs when an excessive amount of allergen is present and the body's normal mechanism for coping is overwhelmed, leading to undesirable inflammation and damage to surrounding tissue. Type III is subtle, and the immune response and inflammation may go on for years without the trigger being recognised and

diagnosed. It most commonly affects kidneys, blood vessels, joints, and skin, and is involved in lupus and rheumatoid arthritis. If a little bit of something was okay, but too much causes symptoms to appear, this may be the type of allergic hypersensitivity you are experiencing. Type III is implicated in food sensitivities, which are easy to overlook.

- **Cell-mediated (delayed) hypersensitivity (Type IV).** This is not mediated by immunoglobulins (with their more-immediate response) but rather by a type of white blood cell, the T lymphocyte cell, which typically only begins to appear after 24 hours. The maximum reaction may occur up to three days later. Type IV is implicated in many autoimmune diseases and metal-induced chronic inflammation.

A 1993 study reported that 3.9 per cent of healthy subjects tested positive for metal reactions.[29] If this figure were applied to the current world population, it would mean that dental-metal allergies potentially affect as many as 273 million people. Others studies suggest that the incidence of metal allergies is on the rise and may be linked to increased exposure to metals, infections, or environmental triggers, making our immune responses more sensitive and defensive to a multiple 'assault'.[30]

Just as dental mercury amalgam is an alloy of five or six different metals, materials commonly used for crowns, dentures, and orthodontic braces are also alloys of several metals. Metal alloys have been an important part of dentistry for over 150 years. Porcelain crowns with a metal base have been commonly used in dental restorations for the last 50–60 years, and the choice of alloy is an important one, especially bearing in mind the potential for biocompatibility issues.

Some dental alloys contain nickel, a very common allergen, and yet are still certified as biocompatible. It's estimated that up to 17 per cent of women and 3 per cent of men are allergic to nickel,[31] with the incidence in sensitivity to this material also on the increase.[32] It is cheaper to use nickel than metals such as gold or platinum, but there is clearly a high risk of nickel-allergic hypersensitivity in the patient. Even titanium — usually regarded as a highly biocompatible metal commonly used in dental implants — can cause sensitivity in 5 per cent of people.[33]

Example of Porcelain Bonded to Non-precious Metal Crowns

Nickel-Chromium ceramic alloy

Predominantly a base metal alloy with ideal mechanical and physical properties for both conventional feldspathic and newer generation ceramics.

Advantages

- Excellent melting and flow properties
- Easy to divest
- Reduced hardness
- Works with conventional feldspar ceramics
- Certified biocompatibility

Indications

- Single crowns
- Posts
- Short and long span bridges

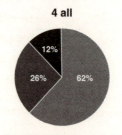

4 all

Nickel 62%, Chromium 26% and Molybdenum 12%

Figure 8-23. A non-precious alloy for porcelain bonded to metal-base crowns — 62 per cent nickel, 26 per cent chromium, and 12 per cent molybdenum.

The body's immune response to different metals can be tested using the Memory Lymphocyte Immuno-Stimulation Assay, or MELISA test, a blood test that detects hypersensitivity to metals, chemicals, environmental toxins, and moulds from a blood sample by looking at the reactivity of white blood cells called lymphocytes.[34] Swedish toxicologist Vera Stejskal developed this unique test, which is performed by labs in Europe and the US. Unfortunately, the test is not currently available in Australia, but information is available online.[35] Exposure to metals in dental fillings and implants, joint prostheses, pacemakers, environmental pollutants, and jewellery are easy to overlook yet can lead to significant health problems, caused by allergic responses leading to chronic inflammation.

Today, composite resins and ceramics are emerging as the materials of choice for dental materials. Some concerns have been reported about the potential for endocrine disruptors (which interfere with our hormonal system) in certain composite resins,[36] but there are newer, purely ceramic-based resins that are free of such material.

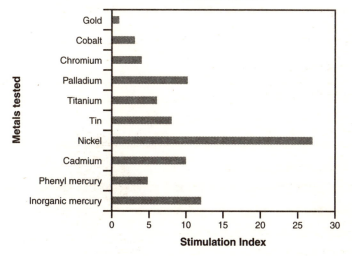

MELISA® results

Figure 8-24. The graph above shows percentage of the study group affected by different metals. As noted nickel sensitivity is high at over 25 per cent; titanium is just over 5 per cent; gold triggers little sensitivity relative to other metals.

Oral galvanism — creating batteries in your mouth

As I've mentioned, the body is a mass of bioelectrical reactions. Whether you look at how muscles and nerves work, or just look at how each cell membrane in the body moves nutrients and waste about, micro-currents play a vital role. A combination of metal in the body, as happens with metal alloys used in dental restorations, can produce their own micro-currents, which can interfere with our natural micro-currents and create problems of their own.

Dental mercury amalgam fillings are made up of at least five different metals. If you have a porcelain crown with a metal framework in your mouth, the metal used is an alloy made up of anywhere between four to ten different metals, and may include gold, platinum, palladium, copper, zinc, nickel, and iron. A metal denture framework may also contain several metals, including gold, cobalt, chromium, titanium, and molybdenum.

It's not unusual to find up to 15 different metals in one mouth.

Going back to high-school chemistry, you may remember that when two or more metals are placed in a moist environment, a galvanic reaction occurs. Combining metal dental restorations, saliva, and body heat, the mouth is the perfect environment to produce electrical currents — our own mini battery.

These micro-currents have a biological effect, of course. Some symptoms associated with oral galvanism include fatigue, loss of strength, lack of stamina, insomnia, unexplained painful conditions that resist treatments, gingivitis, inflammatory mouth disorders, burning-mouth syndrome, frozen shoulder (adhesive capsulitis), or just a metallic taste in the mouth.

Recent research suggests that oral galvanism has the potential to affect the immune system; when all metals are removed from the mouth, several key indicators of immune function are significantly improved.[37] This is likely related to metal-induced chronic inflammation.

Over the last 15–20 years, my Sydney practice and many others have tried to eliminate the use of metals in the mouth. Materials available in dentistry today, when placed carefully, are just as strong and durable as the old metal-based restorations. When I hear dentists say, 'There is no proof that mercury in particular or metals in general have the potential to effect human health,' I can't help thinking it would be far more accurate or honest for them to have said, 'I haven't read anything to that effect.'

Our body is a marvel of biochemical and bioelectrical reactions; we need to respect the subtlety and balance of these reactions if we want to maintain our health and wellness.

Water fluoridation

The human body requires many chemical elements to optimally support life — around 60, in fact. Fluoride is not one of them. It begs the question: if it is not an essential nutrient the body requires, then shouldn't it be considered a medicine?

Fluoride is the only substance added to the water supply to treat the entire population for a health condition (tooth decay) without the permission of the individual. It is the only medicine prescribed without patient monitoring or regard to the age, weight, health, or nutritional status of the user. Fluoride is also the only medicine administered without control over the dose. These are important ethical issues.

The most commonly used fluoride additive to the water supply is not the medical-grade sodium fluoride found in toothpastes or mouth rinses that you would expect. Instead, it is fluorosilicic acid, an inexpensive liquid waste by-product of the fertiliser industry.

The level of fluoride added to the water supply ranges from 0.7 to 1.2 mg/L (milligrams per litre, equivalent to parts per million). A glass of tap water doesn't distinguish between an 80-year-old woman weighing 50 kilograms and a 30-year-old man weighing 100 kilograms. And what of the labourer who, in sweltering conditions, consumes in excess of ten litres of water per day?

The only valid argument to support water fluoridation is a reduction in tooth decay. However, according to the WHO, over the last 40–50 years the rate of tooth decay in populations without fluoride in their water supply has declined at the same rate as those that added fluoride to the water. As outlined in Figure 8-25 and Figure 8-26, the trends showing the reduction in decayed, missing, and filled teeth (DMFT) for those countries that have chosen to fluoridate the water is remarkably similar to those countries that have not fluoridated.

Let's examine one of the best foods known — a baby's first meal, breast milk — and use it as an example of fluoride exposure. A nursing mother's body eliminates all but a miniscule amount of fluoride to pass onto the baby. This is a good indication of how much fluoride is required in the human body. By comparison, babies who are formula-fed using fluoridated tap water receive up to 250 times the amount of fluoride, at a dose of one part per million (ppm) in the water supply. Surely nature hasn't got this so wrong.

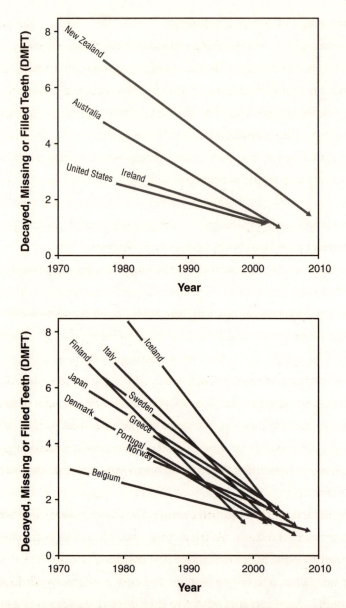

Above: Figure 8-25. DMFT for 12-year-olds in countries that fluoridate most of their water.
Below: Figure 8-26. DMFT for 12-year-olds in countries that do not fluoridate their water.

The book *The Case Against Fluoride*, authored by three scientists, Paul Connett, James Beck, and H.S. Micklem, reveals that research into water fluoridation is flawed.[38] In a recent meta-analysis, researchers from the Harvard School of Public Health and China Medical University in Shenyang examined 27 different studies and found that fluoride may adversely affect cognitive development in children.[39] Based on the findings, the authors say this risk should not be ignored and that more research on fluoride's impact on the developing brain is warranted. In 2014, one of the authors, Philippe Grandjean, classified fluoride as a developmental neurotoxicant.

The problem is, there are specific issues when it comes to children and the ingestion of substances:

- an infant's blood–brain barrier is not properly formed, and is therefore particularly vulnerable to toxic exposure
- relative to body size, infants consume proportionally more fluids than adults
- infants absorb and uptake a higher proportion of ingested fluoride than adults.

The vast majority of countries across the globe don't add fluoride to their water supplies. In fact, 97 per cent of the world's population has chosen not to fluoridate its water supply, and some countries, such as Israel, a country renowned for being advanced in technology and science, recently stopped the practice because of concerns over its safety and effectiveness.

In the first half of the 20th century, the use of fluoride had nothing to do with oral health. At that time, it was an accepted form of treatment to suppress an overactive thyroid, because fluoride belongs to the same chemical family as iodine and thus competes with iodine in the thyroid. An under- or overactive thyroid is an increasingly common health problem, with many possible causes, but the potential influence of fluoride on thyroid function and cancer should not be ignored.

Studies suggest that thyroid disease affects 10 per cent of the Australian population but warn that many cases are undiagnosed.[40] In Australia between 1982 and 2018, the incidence of thyroid cancer increased from one in 100,000 to five in 100,000 in men, and from four in 100,000 to almost 16 in 100,000 in women.[41] In the US, the incidence of thyroid cancer has risen by 168 per cent since 1975.[42]

Meanwhile, iodine deficiency is the largest deficiency in the world.

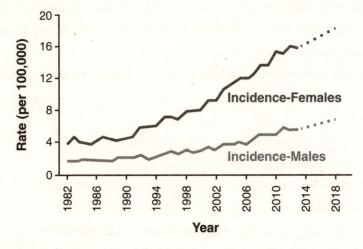

Figure 8-27. Incidence and mortality of thyroid cancer, by sex, 1982–2014 (projected to 2018)

Like so many other potential environmental stresses, I believe the precautionary principle should be applied here; apart from the potential health risks, it's ethically questionable to impose a medication on an entire population. Given our exposure to chemicals throughout the environment and in our food supply, we do not need to add to the burden, particularly with something as basic as water.

The public health approach to water fluoridation is another excellent example of the linear way in which western medicine approaches a health problem. The solution to tooth decay is supposedly to make the tooth harder. The real issue is that tooth decay happens because of what we eat — not how hard our teeth are. The effect of what we eat goes much further than tooth decay, so why not address the bigger picture in a constructive way?

A good example of how policymakers can make positive changes can be seen in Scotland, a country that does not fluoridate its water, where in 2005 a more holistic approach saw the introduction of a public health measure called the Childsmile program.[43] Along with the offer of dental check-ups and treatment, the program set out to educate children and parents on oral hygiene and to give advice about healthy snacks and drinks. It seems to have had a significant impact: the proportion of children aged from four to six without obvious tooth decay has risen from 42 per cent in 1996 to 67 per cent in 2012; for 10-to-12-year-olds, it has risen from 53 per cent in 2005 to 73 per cent in 2013. And even better, changes in diet and hygiene have had far-reaching positive effects, not only on tooth decay rates, but also on obesity and other health conditions.

Oral cancer

Another important dental stress is oral cancer, which is now ranked as the 11th-most-common cancer in the world. In Australia, the rate is especially high because of sun exposure on the lower lip, but the disease can also be caused by smoking, alcohol consumption, and the human papilloma virus (HPV). Oral cancer is notoriously difficult to detect because the patient is often unaware, as they generally don't feel any discomfort. In a comprehensive oral examination, your dentist inspects lips, tongue, cheeks, palate, floor of the mouth, and back of the throat. Oral-cancer screening is another reason why it's important to have regular visits to the dentist. We do more than check for holes in your teeth!

The key to minimising what can be complex and debilitating intervention is early detection. Otherwise, treatment often involves surgery and radiation. This radiation can cause reduced saliva flow, leading to a permanently dry mouth — and the list of problems caused by a dry mouth is long and uncomfortable: patients are more susceptible to tooth decay and gum disease; they may have problems with chewing and swallowing food; taste and the enjoyment of food is compromised; and patients may have difficulty speaking. Have I convinced you yet that it's important to regularly visit the dentist?

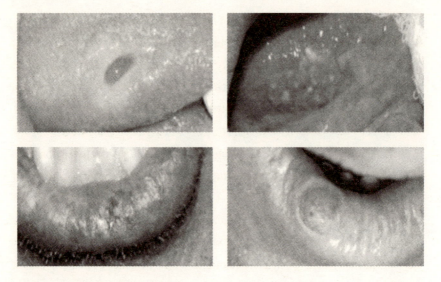

Figure 8-28. What dentists see when doing an oral cancer screening: the common ulcer (non-cancerous), non-homogenous leukoplakia (biopsy subsequently revealed squamous-cell carcinoma), actinocheilitis (common in Australia and pre-cancerous), and squamous-cell carcinoma (malignant cancer).

A PATIENT'S STORY — ANDRE

Andre, 32, was concerned about a tooth on the upper right side of his mouth that he felt was loose. When I checked his teeth, it was immediately apparent to me that every tooth in this corner of his mouth was loose. An X-ray revealed complete bone loss around the teeth here. Andre had a rare malignant myofibroblastic tumour, requiring every tooth, and part of his jaw (maxilla) on the upper right side of his mouth, to be removed.

After an incredible 14-hour operation with a highly skilled team including a maxillofacial surgeon, plastic surgeon, ENT (ear, nose, and throat) surgeon, and oncologist, his face was reconstructed. After five years and extensive reconstruction, together with a removable partial denture, he is enjoying good health.

Detecting oral cancer is rarely as straightforward as that, but it highlights how dramatic the treatment can be.

Conclusion

Eating, talking, and smiling are just some of the vital functions performed by the mouth. What you don't see, or necessarily feel, are the connections between your mouth and the rest of your body. You may not feel an infection in your tooth or jawbone, or realise that your gums may be contributing to heart disease or other degenerative diseases. The metal restorations in your mouth may be contributing to symptoms you have never connected. How well you actually chew your food is something you rarely think about, but it has implications for your digestion. The shape and size of your mouth and how crowded your teeth are may also affect how well you breathe, the quality of your sleep, and even your posture. Chronic tension headaches or neck aches may be connected with clenching and grinding of your teeth.

At the risk of sounding biased, I hope I have alerted you to the importance of your mouth, and the potential impact of dental stress on your health and wellbeing! Take oral health seriously. Your body already does.

CHAPTER 9

Postural Stress

Do you tightly grip the steering wheel when driving? Do you hunch over a keyboard at work, stare in your lap as you look at your phone, or slump on the couch at home while watching TV? What position do you sleep in at night?

As a rule, we simply don't pay enough attention to our posture. For most of us, we only focus on posture when we are in chronic pain, experiencing back ache, neck ache, headaches, and so on. But postural stress has a dramatic impact on our health and wellbeing every single day — slumping while sitting, for example, restricts our ability to breathe, makes digestion more difficult by squashing the intestines, and places more wear and tear on the body. Moreover, this stress affects our ability to maintain homeostasis — the healthy balance our body constantly strives for.

Postural stress can be brought on by:

- **Head posture.** How you hold your head affects breathing and spinal alignment, which not only affect body chemistry, which I will discuss more in Chapter 11: Breathing, but can also strain the muscles of the neck and spine.
- **Spinal alignment.** This has the potential to cause imbalances in the nerves, muscles, and joints, and the functioning of the internal organs.
- **Craniosacral rhythm.** This relates to the subtle bodily rhythms of cerebrospinal fluid moving through the cranium and spine, which

can also be affected by the beating of the heart and the taking of a breath. When muscles that attach to the skull are strained through imbalances in the jaws, the spine, or even the pelvis, this rhythm can be disrupted.

- **Sleeping position.** Stomach, side, or back? Sleep is something we spend so much time doing yet give so little thought to. Sleeping position can affect head, neck, jaw, and structural muscles, as well as the ability to breathe well. It is also implicated in digestive problems. Poor sleeping posture can frustrate the healing of muscles and joints, and is related to many chronic musculoskeletal pain problems, such as chronic tension headaches, neck aches, and lower back pain.

- **Work posture.** Sitting at a screen with your head forward; balancing a phone under your chin while writing or typing on a computer; looking down at a laptop or phone; spending hours with poor chair and desk position — all place stress on your body.

- **Walk.** Foot mechanics and discrepancies in leg length can affect pelvic stability, spinal stability, and alignment throughout the body, and potentially frustrate the healing of chronic or acute musculoskeletal problems.

- **Over-training.** This occurs when a person performs more training than their body can recover from, to the point where performance declines and injuries persist.

- **Being sedentary.** Yes, sitting for long periods of time at work or at home can cause you harm and is an increasingly significant problem for young and old.

- **Toilet position.** And yes, this can compromise your ability to have a full and comfortable bowel movement, which is essential for good health.

Fibrous tissue — which includes muscles, tendons, ligaments, fascia, joint capsules, or periosteum (the attachment of these structures to bone) — all have the potential to maintain an inflammation for many years after an accident or trauma has occurred. So if you are suffering from chronic musculoskeletal pain (this is at least 20 per cent of the population), the following could be causing postural stress:

- **Accidents or physical traumas.** Car accidents, sporting injuries, falls, or knocks to the body, which may have occurred many years ago, are often overlooked or forgotten but can be significant.
- **General anaesthetic.** Even this can be traumatic to the soft tissue, particularly the attachment of muscles at the base of the skull if the head is not well supported when being moved under anaesthetic. The normal opening for the mouth is 45–55 millimetres; when intubating under general anaesthetic, it can be as much as 70 mm, which can strain the muscles and tendons around the jaw.

Posture and mood

One of the more surprising facts about posture is that its effects can go far beyond the physiological. This was highlighted in an experiment undertaken at the University of Auckland in New Zealand. Seventy-four volunteers were placed in two groups and put through a job interview process where their heart rate and blood pressure were monitored. There was one key difference between the groups: half of the volunteers had their backs strapped with physiotherapy tape to create a slumped posture; the other half were strapped in order to make them sit up straight. Participants were told a story to disguise the intention of the study so that they wouldn't consciously adjust their posture one way or the other.

The results are fascinating. Those who had their backs taped into an upright posture reported higher self-esteem, better mood, and lower fear compared with those who were taped into a slumped position. The researchers concluded: 'This is the first study to show that holding an upright seated posture during a psychological stressor can have protective effects on mood, compared to a slumped posture. The upright participants reported feeling more enthusiastic, excited and strong, while the slumped participants reported feeling more fearful, hostile, nervous, quiet, still, passive, dull, sleepy, and sluggish.'[1] This is just one of many experiments showing a link between posture and mood, and is an excellent example of the mind–body connection. If you walk or sit with hunched shoulders and an arched back, research suggests you are more likely to report feeling unhappy.

The effect of long-term sitting

Unfortunately, our modern daily life sees many of us, including our children, spending far too much time at jobs, tasks, or 'leisure' that promote poor posture — sitting is a perfect example of just how far-reaching the health repercussions of bad posture can be. According to James Levine, obesity researcher at one of America's top hospitals, the Mayo Clinic, the biggest difference between people of average weight and those who are overweight isn't related to diet or exercise, but to the amount of time they are seated.[2] According to Levine, this is because of an enzyme called lipoprotein lipase, found in the cells that line the tiny blood vessels of muscles and in fatty tissue, where it plays a critical role in the breakdown of fat.

When you stand, the postural muscles that support your weight — mostly in your legs — release this enzyme, which helps burn fat. But when you sit still and don't shift every 30–90 seconds, as the body is inclined to do naturally, the fat remains in the arteries and can be stored as body fat. Studies have shown that a typical day of sitting lowers lipoprotein-lipase activity in animals by 90–95 per cent,[3] and we can safely assume that the effect is similar in humans.

'When we are sitting, there are no muscle contractions,' said David Dunstan, from the Baker IDI Heart and Diabetes Institute, on ABC TV's *Catalyst* program.[4] He went on to explain why this is so important: 'Muscle contraction helps the body's efficiency to clear blood-sugar levels and blood-fat levels. It's known that elevated glucose levels can lead to inflammation, which if repeated on a number of days or weeks can lead to heart disease and a host of other conditions, such as cancer.' A gentle walk for two minutes every 20 minutes can lower blood-glucose levels by around 30 per cent. 'It's the physical movement that's important,' according to Dunstan. 'What we need to start to incorporate is more movement throughout the day. I think the problem is that we have people just sitting throughout the day.'

There are studies that have tracked a large number of people over several years and found an association between longer sitting times and impaired brain function. While not going so far as to say that sitting increases the risk of dementia, they conclude that limiting sedentary behaviour and engaging in moderate exercise promotes healthy cognitive aging.[5]

The problem with postural stress

'Body stressors such as sitting too much, not moving enough, and poor posture may not be very big on their own,' reveals physiotherapist Anna-Louise Bouvier, creator of the Happy Body at Work program.[6] 'But collectively, they can lead to headaches, neck tension, backaches, fatigue, weight gain, digestive problems, and even constipation.' Bouvier believes it's important to recognise the signals our body gives us to alert us to the fact it's overloaded. 'Once you recognise these signals, you can use strategies to release some of the load before it becomes a problem.'

Signs of postural stress vary: they could be headaches and back pain or an upset stomach, or even a compromised immune system reflected in mouth ulcers and cold sores — all of which may also affect your mood. 'Many people find they just feel tired and as though they are getting by on a half-flat battery,' explains Bouvier. Small changes such as sitting less and moving more will reduce fluctuations in blood-glucose levels, giving you more energy.

In fact some studies show that moving lightly periodically throughout the day may be more effective at controlling blood sugar levels that just one session of structured exercise.[7] The problem is that poor posture and sitting for long periods have become normalised in today's world.

American spinal and orthopaedic surgeon Ken Hansraj measured the impact of the typical posture when writing a text message on a phone.[8] The weight of the average adult's head is between four and five kilograms, but when it is tilted forward its effective weight increases, placing greater pressure on the neck. A 30-degree tilt of the head is the equivalent of holding 18 kilograms of weight. Hansraj believes this posture could lead to 'early wear, tear, degeneration and possibly surgeries'.

As you travel on a bus or train or even just walk down a street, the majority of people nowadays have their heads down looking at the phones or other digital devices, so the implications of this imbalance are potentially widespread. This exaggerated yet common head position may also be exacerbating some chronic musculoskeletal pain conditions.

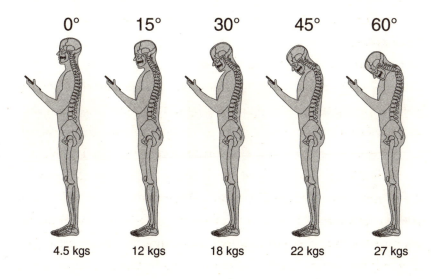

Figure 9-1. The impact of the head's tilt on its effective weight.

The issue of spinal alignment, balanced musculature, and improved blood flow is the focus of manual therapists — chiropractors, physiotherapists, osteopaths, and massage therapists — all of whom use a wide variety of techniques to eliminate pain and postural imbalances, and to restore function. Just as the body constantly strives to maintain homeostasis by regulating body chemistry, heartbeat, blood pressure, and breathing rate, it also tries to maintain a balance that is pain-free and comfortable. Often this involves compensations.

If the body is strained from over-compensating for bad posture, a nerve may be impinged upon. This can give rise to symptoms that may at first not seem connected, such as blurred vision, dizziness, or even excessive mucous production.

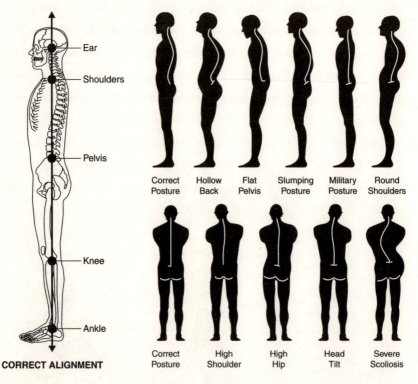

Left: Figure 9-2. Correct alignment of the ear, shoulders, pelvis, knee, and ankle, placing minimal strain on the neck, spine, pelvis, and joints.
Right: Figure 9-3. Variations on body posture.

Mouth breathing and head-forward posture

One of the most important functions of breathing is to regulate the amount of carbon dioxide in your lungs. These levels are critical in establishing and maintaining the biochemical acid–alkali balance of your entire body, ensuring you get the right amount of energy from oxygen that your body needs. There are definite postural considerations to breathing, but, again, breathing is something we often give little thought to — as I will demonstrate in detail in Chapter 11: Breathing.

Air is the most important thing we consume. It's so important that the body will always compensate to ensure we are able to breathe as best we can with the body structure we have. Even if our posture isn't optimal, it keeps us alive.

Are you a shallow breather or do you fill your lungs deeply using your diaphragm? As anyone who has trained in resuscitation knows, tilting the head back will open the airway. If you breathe primarily through your mouth, your body tries to open and improve the airway by doing just that. But we can't walk around with our head tilted up; we need to keep our eyes forward and parallel to the horizon in order to maintain our balance; and so the head moves forward on the spine. A head tilted forward off the centre of the spine, as I noted, also increases its relative weight.

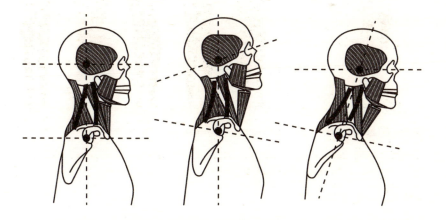

Figure 9-4. Left: nasal breathing, good head posture. Middle: mouth breathing with head tilted back to open the airway. Right: trying to keep the eyes parallel to the horizon for balance, but, wanting to maintain a more-open airway, the head is positioned forward of the spine.

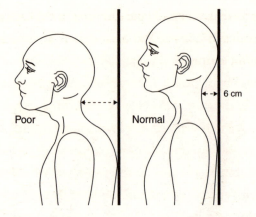

Figure 9-5. Left: poor posture of the head, which places a strain on the muscles of the neck and shoulder. Right: ideal balanced head posture.

Do you use your diaphragm?

The diaphragm is a thin muscle at the base of the rib cage separating the thoracic and abdominal cavities that draws air deeply in and out of the lungs. When you engage your diaphragm, air is drawn deeper into the lungs, utilising the entire available capacity and greater surface area of the lungs for optimal oxygen and carbon-dioxide exchange.

If you don't engage your diaphragm when breathing, it also places additional strain on the neck and shoulder muscles, specifically the scalene, sternocleidomastoid, and trapezius muscles as they try to lift the rib cage. All of these muscles are commonly associated with chronic tension headaches or neck aches or even pain into the arms, hands, and fingers. It's often overlooked that the pain may actually originate from these neck and shoulder muscles.[9]

Sleeping position

Many people find it natural to sleep on their stomach — I used to count myself among them. However, this position puts strain on muscles of the head, neck, jaw, and spine, and can also restrict the airway. What about sleeping on your back? The news still isn't good — if you sleep on your back, the lower jaw and tongue can drop to the back of your throat and, again, restrict the airway. You need to look after your posture, but you also need to breathe.

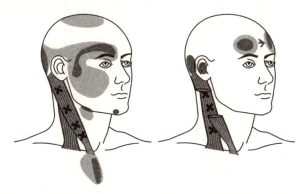

Figure 9-6. Sternocleidomastoid muscles with their trigger points and the pain-referral patterns.

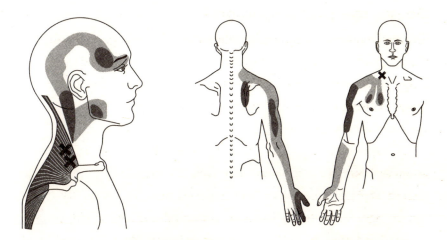

Left: Figure 9-7. Trapezius muscles with their trigger points and the pain-referral patterns.
Right: Figure 9-8. Scalene muscles with their trigger points and the pain-referral patterns.

A PATIENT'S STORY — JANE

Stomach sleeping is a problem for many reasons, as one of my patients, Jane (aged 42), discovered. For many years, Jane suffered from chronic tension headaches and neck pain, particularly in the morning. Regular chiropractic adjustments relieved the discomfort, but, after a few weeks, the pain would return and another adjustment was needed. When she visited my practice, I alerted her to the problem of stomach sleeping — and its potential impact on head and neck pain — and I advised her how to change her position. Jane committed to retrain herself to sleep on her side. After only a few days, her pain dissipated, and after a few weeks it disappeared completely. Stomach sleeping had been placing constant strain on her neck and shoulder muscles, which were the source of her headaches. Again, it's not always as straightforward as Jane's case, but participating in a cure, taking control, and changing something you are doing to yourself means that, like Jane, you can become part of the healing process, and get the complete and lasting benefit of other treatments such as chiropractic, physiotherapy, or osteopathic sessions.

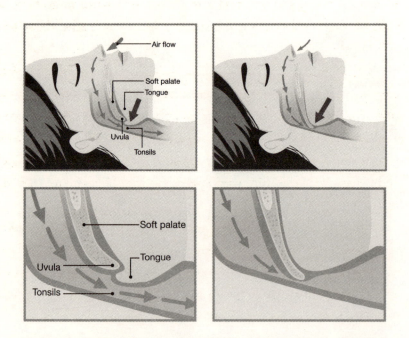

Figure 9-9. Left: restricted airway (hypopnoea), resulting in snoring. Right: obstructed airway, resulting in obstructive sleep apnoea (OSA).

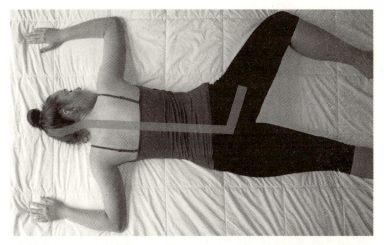

Figure 9-10. Shows stomach sleeping and how it twists and strains the muscles of the jaw, neck, shoulders, and lower back.

As a stomach sleeper for the first 30 years of my life, I know this habit isn't easy to break. Depending on your age, it could take up to six weeks to change, but it is well worth the effort. Once you have broken the habit, you will find it too much of a strain to go back on your stomach — a position and strain you may once have thought of as 'normal'.

My suggestion is to use a pillow to snuggle into while you sleep on your side, creating a similar comforting feeling to sleeping on your stomach. Bend your uppermost leg and place it atop the pillow. Choose a pillow with the same thickness as your leg. If the pillow is too thick, your uppermost leg will be raised too much, twisting your lower back and pelvis. If it's too thin, your uppermost leg will rotate towards the mattress.

Side sleeping will help keep your head, jaw, neck, airway, spine, and pelvis well aligned. It also helps maintain your airways and reduces stress on muscles, so that you'll wake feeling more refreshed. It doesn't always solve chronic pain, but it's an essential first step in healing soft-tissue lesions.

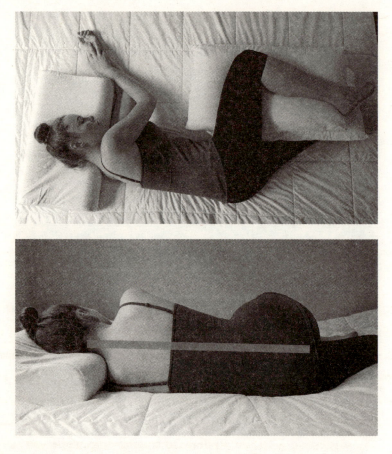

Above: Figure 9-11. Use a pillow to snuggle into while you sleep to create a similar comforting feeling to sleeping on your stomach.
Below: Figure 9-12. Side sleeping with a pillow by your side to give you comfort and support helps keep your head, jaw, neck, airway, spine, and pelvis well aligned.

PAIN DEFINED

The International Association for the Study of Pain (IASP) defined pain as 'an unpleasant emotional experience caused by the activation of pain receptors'. So there are two parts to this definition:

* Our emotional state influences the experience of pain. When you are rundown and emotionally stressed, you are more

likely to facilitate and feel pain. When you are calmer, you inhibit and experience less pain.

- Pain receptors (nociceptors) need to be activated in order for pain to occur.

Pain receptors are mainly located in soft tissues, and are stimulated by:
- temperature — both hot and cold
- mechanical stimulation — compression, tension, and twisting (targeted by manual therapists)
- chemicals — produced in response to chronic inflammation or an allergic reaction (targeted by many medications and also manual therapists).

Important points:
- pain indicates tissue damage is occurring or has occurred
- soft tissue has 'memory', which means the injury or inflammation can be maintained many years after the original trauma or injury
- acute pain is pain that lasts for less than three months; the location of the pain is often closely linked to the site of the original injury
- chronic pain lasts more than three months, and the location of the pain *may not* be the same as the original source of that pain.

Chronic musculoskeletal pain — what's the underlying cause?

Chronic musculoskeletal pain is a frustratingly common problem and a major postural stress, yet it is poorly understood. Our musculoskeletal system includes our muscles, bones, cartilage, joints, ligaments, tendons, and other connective tissue that supports our body. Over three million

Australians suffer from chronic musculoskeletal pain, costing over AU$34 billion a year.[10]

The treatment for acute musculoskeletal pain is usually through rest, the application of ice or medication to reduce inflammation, or the attention of a manual therapist, who focuses on restoring balance to the spine, muscles, nerves, and joints, improving the restorative benefits of blood flow, and increasing lymphatic drainage to remove inflammatory chemicals. In most cases, this successfully reduces and resolves the acute pain, although, depending on the nature of the problem, the treatment can take weeks or months.

Chronic pain has become a huge and costly problem, with many sufferers and their families resigning themselves to years of ongoing pain and treatment. These patients may be frequently taking painkillers or anti-inflammatory medications to control the symptoms, while being regularly treated with ongoing manipulation, adjustments, or massages. Even though they may then feel relief for days or weeks, the pain ultimately returns. In this scenario, I think we should ask the question: why does the pain recur?

Understanding chronic musculoskeletal pain

The hypothesis I have worked with for over 35 years is that soft-tissue lesions cause chronic musculoskeletal pain. I would define these soft-tissue lesions as tear or damage to a muscle, tendon, ligament, fascia, joint capsule, or periosteum. Soft-tissue lesions are caused by trauma. This can be macroscopic trauma, such as whiplash, a fall, or a blow to the body — or even a general anaesthetic — or microscopic trauma, which includes teeth clenching or grinding, shin splints, and other repetitive postural strains and stresses.

Soft-tissue lesions cause the body to release inflammatory chemicals such as bradykinins, prostaglandins, and substance P, which are signals to pain receptors to fire — this is then felt as pain. Substance P is a particularly interesting compound as, apart from being involved in chronic pain, it also regulates moods, anxiety, nausea, and respiratory rate; it is particularly involved as a response to stressful situations.

I believe many postural stresses prevent soft-tissue lesions from healing, which ultimately causes recurring chronic pain such as headaches, neck aches, jaw pain, or back problems, as well as several repetitive strain injuries. These pain conditions are frustrating and often debilitating.

Repetitive strain injury (RSI)

Repetitive strain injury is a general term for a chronic musculoskeletal condition where pain is felt in the hands, wrists, forearms, elbows, neck, or shoulders. As the name implies, repetitive movements related to overuse or poor use of muscles and tendons in the upper body significantly increase the risk of developing such a condition. Common examples include carpel-tunnel syndrome, trigger finger or thumb, bursitis, tendonitis, and thoracic-outlet syndrome.

The symptoms associated with RSI can range from mild to severe. At first, you might only notice it when doing a particular activity, such as working at a desk or keyboard. It's easy to ignore or simply resort to medication.

Like all chronic musculoskeletal pain conditions, there are a multitude of factors to consider that undermine your resilience. Emotional stress, a cold or draughty work environment, a poorly designed workspace, poor form in a sporting activity, or vibrating equipment as in factory or construction jobs. Anything that may undermine your physical resilience, such as poor sleep or diet, surely increases your susceptibility.

Similarly, the treatment needs to be multifactorial, including: addressing the triggers by correcting or eliminating the postural stresses; engaging in manual therapy that is focused on restoring balance; performing stretching and strengthening exercises to improve range of motion; treatment with low-energy laser or ultrasound to increase lymphatic drainage and reduce inflammatory mediators of pain; focus on a nutrient-dense diet that facilitates healing; and engaging in some meditation, mindfulness, or cognitive behavioural therapy to encourage the inhibition rather than the facilitation of the pain response.

We need to understand the pain process, from those factors which trigger it, through those that modulate it, to those that frustrate its resolution. We need to think holistically.

Grinding — postural stress activating pain receptors in soft-tissue lesions

For several years, I conducted research at the University of New South Wales with one of Australia's leading podiatrists, Mark Ninio. Together, we showed that when you clench or grind your teeth, in addition to the contraction of the jaw muscles, important postural muscles at the back of the neck, shoulders, lower back, and even the abdomen also contract.[11]

The biggest effect occurred in the neck and shoulder muscles, the sternocleidomastoid and trapezius, commonly associated with chronic headaches and neck ache. If there are soft-tissue lesions in these muscles, the additional and frequent contraction when you clench your jaw frustrates the healing. Our review of the literature found research that links clenching or grinding of teeth to tightening of the calf muscles.[12] This additional contraction of muscles may act like a mechanical stimulus to activate the pain receptors, helping perpetuate chronic pain conditions.

Surprisingly, many people who grind their teeth, have a less than perfect bite, or even have clicking jaw joints do not experience any chronic pain. Perhaps it's a measure of how resilient the jaw and masticatory system is, but it may also be a question of degree. For example, you might pull on an elastic band for a week before it suddenly breaks. Does it break because of the last time you pulled on it or because you have been doing it for a week? Eventually, you exceeded its elastic limit. The same can occur with muscles. You strain a muscle until it produces enough inflammatory chemicals, exceeding a physiological limit — and you experience pain.

Foot mechanics

While clenching of the jaw can induce postural stress throughout the body, it's also important when thinking of postural stress to consider foot mechanics and imbalance in leg length. As with teeth grinding, many people with imbalances in leg lengths or foot mechanics still function well without any apparent chronic knee, hip, or back pain while developing long-term problems.

Foot instability, either in the ankle joint (subtalar) when your heel hits the ground, or the front half of the foot when you start to lift your heel, can lead to compensations throughout the entire body. I witnessed this when researching the effect of orthotics on both the jaw and feet.[13] Just as the jaw is often overlooked in chronic musculoskeletal upper-body pain, foot stability is also often overlooked when dealing with chronic musculoskeletal back, hip, or leg pain.

Imbalances in foot mechanics can cause instability in the pelvis and spine, which can perpetuate soft-tissue lesions and chronic musculoskeletal pain. In these chronic situations, it may be important to stabilise foot mechanics to support the pelvis, spine, neck, and head — and facilitate healing of soft-tissue lesions. A qualified podiatrist who understands the relationship between foot mechanics and chronic pain should be consulted for the best treatment.

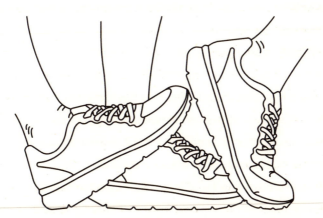

Figure 9-13. From left to right: rear foot heel strike; neutral position; fore foot lift off.

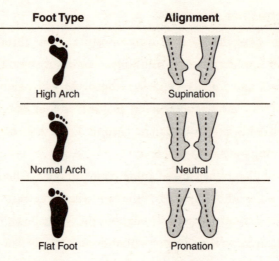

Figure 9-14. Different types of feet and alignment in supination (outward roll during normal motion), neutral position, and pronation (inward roll).

Leg-length discrepancies

Imbalance in the lengths of your two legs can also contribute to chronic pain and can be either:

- **Functional.** Caused by tightened, imbalanced muscles around the pelvis and lower back or by unilateral pronation (when the arch of the foot drops) giving the appearance of leg-length difference.
- **Anatomical.** An actual difference in the length of the major bones of the leg, the femur and tibia.

Most experts believe a difference of less than ten millimetres is not significant. But in my experience and in conversations with podiatrists and manual therapists focused on chronic musculoskeletal pain, when there is a persistent soft-tissue lesion a difference of between even one and two millimetres can be significant, at least while supporting the healing process.

Catherine, 37, was another of my patients who, with a more holistic approach to her dental care, saw an improvement in her overall health and wellbeing. She was suffering from terrible headaches when she started to notice her teeth touched only on the right side of her mouth when she ate. She also realised the teeth along the left side of her mouth didn't connect at all when chewing.

A dentist fitted a removable occlusal splint to stabilise her bite, and the headaches cleared. Unfortunately, after three months, they returned. The dentist adjusted the splint, and her headaches again subsided — before returning several months later. At this point, an oral and maxillofacial surgeon recommended she undergo extensive surgery to re-align both upper and lower jaws. This is when Catherine came to see me for a second opinion.

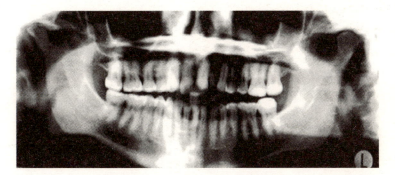

Figure 9-15. X-ray reveals different shape of the jaw joints from left to right. The left side (marked L) is rounded and well formed. The right side is flat and smaller. Note that the teeth only touch on the right side. The length of the jaw bone is also shorter on the right side than the left.

I set out to find the reason for the change in her bite. Why was she only able to bite on one side, something she had only become aware of in the last year or so? Why was a 37-year-old showing signs of degenerative arthritis in the right jaw joint? Why was there a lack of stability causing the chronic pain to recur?

Something was being overlooked. I suspected it was caused by a combination of factors, including: her job, which involved looking down a microscope for hours; excessive teeth grinding at night; and, because of my research with podiatrist Mark Ninio, possibly a leg-length discrepancy.

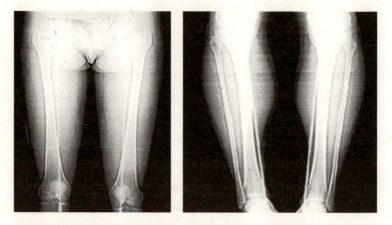

Figure 9-16. CAT scan is a very accurate way of measuring anatomical leg length of femur (left) and tibia (right). It is the most accurate way of measuring anatomical (actual) leg length as opposed to functional (perceived) differences, which are caused by tightened or imbalance muscles or unilateral pronation.

When a CAT scan measured the anatomical length of her legs, it showed the right leg was ten millimetres shorter than the left. This apparently had contributed to some serious osteo-arthritic changes to her right jaw joint only, which was certainly unusual for someone so young, but it did explain why her teeth only touched on the right side of her mouth. When you look at the X-ray in Figure 9-15, a head of the jaw bone (mandibular condyle) appears in each top corner. The left condyle is normal, rounded, and well formed; the osteo-arthritic right condyle is flattened.

Mark Ninio corrected both her anatomical leg-length discrepancy and the mechanics of her feet with a combination of custom fitted orthotics and right-sided heel lift. Additionally, I balanced her teeth by adding bonding resin to those on the left side of her mouth. Catherine's headaches stopped, and for the past five years she has been pain-free and stable. She avoided surgery, possible life-long headaches, and regular adjustments.

A solution to complex chronic pain is not always as easy, but it highlights the benefits of a holistic approach, looking beyond the location of the pain, or restricting treatment to the one focus.

Sitting on the toilet

I admit, it's unusual to think of sitting on the toilet as a postural stress — but as you know from reading Chapter 6: Nutritional Stress, a good bowel movement is important for our health and wellbeing. Considering how frequently we find ourselves in this position, ideally once or twice per day, it's worth adding to the list of postural stressors.

For most of history, humans squatted during a bowel movement, and the colon has evolved to work best in that position. The alignment of the anorectal angle associated with squatting allows smooth bowel elimination. The squatting position prevents excessive straining, which has the potential to damage the anal canal, rectum, and, possibly, the colon and other organs.

The first sitting toilet was invented for Queen Elizabeth I in 1596, but didn't really become widespread until the mid-1800s. While flushing toilets certainly are convenient and a great public health achievement, sitting (as opposed to squatting) on the toilet contributes to a range of not uncommon problems, including:

- constipation (defined as fewer than three bowel movements per week)
- haemorrhoids (swollen and inflamed veins in the anus and lower rectum)
- urinary tract difficulties and infections
- bloating and straining
- colon disease.

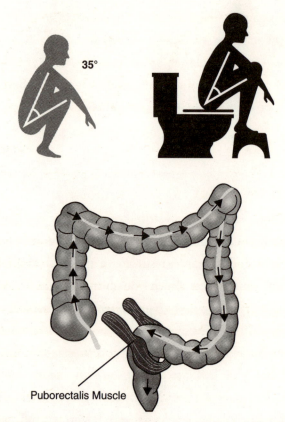

35°

Puborectalis Muscle

Figure 9-17. Diagrams show squatting position and ideal alignment of colon. The use of a low stool (no pun intended) facilitates using a modern toilet.

A more complete elimination helps maintain good colon health. Many studies point to faecal build up in the colon as a cause of diseases including colon cancer. When there is build up in the colon, the body can't absorb all the nutrients from the food, which in turn, affects energy levels.

One study compared three toilet-sitting positions and found that squatting was the most satisfactory, as a sitting posture requires greater strain.[14] Another study concluded that the more the hip is flexed (as occurs when squatting), the straighter the rectum and anal canal, and the less strain created.[15]

Try squatting when you go to the toilet. You'll be surprised at the difference this simple change can make.

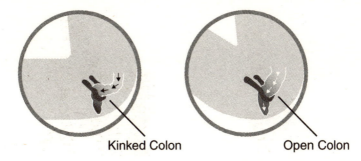

Kinked Colon   Open Colon

Figure 9-18. Left: kinked colon in sitting position. Right: open colon is squatting position.

Conclusion

There are many things to consider when we think about how we use or don't use our body, and the resulting impact on our health. Small changes to the positions in which you sleep, breathe, work, walk, or even go to the toilet can make a big difference. Repeated day after day, year after year, movements can have a dramatic impact on the stress they place on body and mind. Keep posture front of mind and be the best you can be.

PART 3

Taking Control
of Your Health

CHAPTER 10

Sleep

There is one crucial question I ask most of my patients: 'How well do you sleep?' More often than not, the answer is: 'Really well.' But when I go on to ask the even more pertinent question, 'Do you wake up feeling refreshed?', I'm often surprised by the answer: 'No.'

This reinforces the point that just putting your head on the pillow and shutting your eyes, even if it is for eight hours, does not necessarily constitute sleeping well. I am also surprised by how often people come to regard the way they sleep as normal — even if they wake up tired and continue to be tired throughout the day.

A good night's sleep is a daily opportunity to significantly improve and maintain your health.

I believe sleep is the most important pillar of wellbeing, and this is why I'm discussing it first and foremost in Part 3 of this book.

Every measure of health is affected by the quality of our sleep, with poor sleep implicated in almost every disease. When sleep is consistently interrupted, it predisposes our bodies to cardiovascular disease, obesity, thyroid problems, chronic pain, headaches and neck aches, depression and anxiety, and so on. In contrast, a good night's sleep provides the physical, mental, and emotional energy to face the stresses of modern life. Sleep refreshes and energises, giving us the mental and physical vitality to make optimal nutritional and exercise choices, and encouraging a more positive outlook on life. A consistently good night's sleep builds resilience in the mind, body, and immune system. If you don't sleep well, you are at a significant disadvantage. Sleeping is without a doubt the most important part of our day — something we should all be paying attention to. So, exactly how can we ensure a good night's sleep?

Let's begin by looking at our ancestors. The hunter-gatherer diet has become popular, so how about the hunter-gatherer sleep pattern? Does this hold clues for the optimal approach to sleep? When Emory University anthropologist Carol Worthman was asked about the ways in which different cultures approached sleep, she realised how little anthropologists had written on the topic, and made it her research specialty. She discovered that 'some cultures stretched it out, some chopped it up, and others, like our own, squeezed it into one big lump'.[1]

In pre-modern times, sleep was communal, bedtimes weren't regular, and the sleeping area could be relatively noisy. Sleep during the night was often interrupted, so napping was common during the day. In postmodern industrial societies, sleep is generally solitary or with one other person, there are scheduled sleeping and waking times, sleep takes place on a padded bed, with layers of bedding, and the room is ideally dark and silent.

Worthman wonders if modern habits place a high burden on sleep–wake regulation and contribute to problems sleeping. I most certainly agree, not only in that our modern world places added pressures on our ability to get a good night's sleep, but also because consistently getting a good night's sleep has never been more important, thanks to consistent daily performance expectations.

Our relationship with light is one major example that has dramatically affected our sleeping patterns, particularly in the last 20 years. Over millennia, our sleep patterns have been guided by daylight and darkness, but now our homes are brightly lit at the flick of a switch. There is also what is called 'blue light', on TV screens, phones, and computers, which compromises our ability to sleep well. It's under these environmental stresses — along with emotional, nutritional, dental, and postural stresses — that a good night's sleep has become such a challenge.

No matter the cultural background, one thing is certain: sleep is critical to health.

What happens during sleep?

Each day, the 37 trillion cells in your body cycle through two states in an effort to maintain homeostasis: building up (anabolic) and breaking down (catabolic). Sleep is an anabolic state and an opportunity for the body to rest and rebuild.

It has always been thought that the brain does not have a lymphatic system, which deals with waste throughout the rest of the body, but recent research has identified the glymphatic system, which does just that in the central nervous system.[2] Other studies show that in the deeper levels of sleep, the glymphatic system is more active, especially when sleeping on your side.[3] It's then that a common waste product in the brain, the protein amyloid beta, which is implicated in Alzheimer's disease, is cleared most efficiently.

During a good night's sleep, the body also releases growth hormone and melatonin, which not only aids growth (particularly important for children and teens), but also boosts repair of muscle mass, cells, and tissues. Melatonin is also a powerful antioxidant and has important immune functions. Its production and secretion is generated by the circadian rhythm, which is regulated by the 24-hour light–dark cycle. Melatonin has been described as the 'master hormone' and 'a candidate for universal panacea':[4] it reverses ageing, fights diseases such as cancer and heart disease, maintains your sexual vitality, and much more.[5]

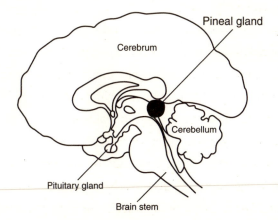

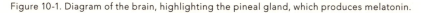

Figure 10-1. Diagram of the brain, highlighting the pineal gland, which produces melatonin.

Researchers now realise the vital role sleep also plays in the balance of two other important hormones — leptin and ghrelin. These signal hunger (ghrelin) and when you've had enough to eat (leptin). If you don't get enough sleep, levels of ghrelin go up and levels of leptin go down. It means your body and mind don't receive the signals that you've had enough to eat, while also reducing your ability to efficiently metabolise fat. Problems of overeating, building up fat, and difficulty losing weight relate to the imbalance in the levels of these hormones.

Lack of sleep also increases the likelihood of poor decision-making, particularly when choosing the type of food to eat and when to eat it. Of course, lack of sleep equals lack of energy, and in Chapter 9: Postural Stress I outlined how sitting around results in lowered levels of the enzyme lipoprotein lipase, which also contributes to weight gain.

Furthermore, sleep affects how your body reacts to the hormone insulin, which controls blood-glucose levels and fat storage. Sleep deficiency causes a higher-than-normal blood-sugar level, insulin resistance, and leptin resistance, increasing the risk of diabetes and an inability to control weight.

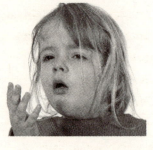

Figure 10-2. Some of the many effects of disturbed sleep.

I already discussed how poor sleep leads to increased cortisol levels in Chapter 5: Emotional Stress. This affects the immune system, making it more difficult to fight common infections.[6] The stress of not sleeping well also compromises the body's ability to digest and absorb nutrients in food, irrespective of how good your diet may be, or the supplements you may take. And if all of that isn't enough to convince you of the importance of a good night's sleep, poor sleep also affects the sex hormones, such as progesterone, oestrogen,[7] and testosterone,[8] reducing sex drive.

Common causes of insufficient sleep

- **Personal choice.** Many people simply don't realise that the body needs adequate sleep. True, people who sleep for three to four hours a night generally know they haven't had enough sleep, but those who sleep for six hours a night often don't think they are missing out. Rather than go to bed at a reasonable hour, they prefer to stay up late, which is often a time when they believe they are 'at their best'. They socialise, check emails or social media, watch television, or read a book. Research shows, however, that people who consistently sleep for only six hours a night have cognitive impairment similar to those who sleep for three to four hours a night.[9]
- **Work.** People who work shifts regularly disrupt their sleep–wake cycle. Frequent travellers, such as airline crews, also have erratic sleeping patterns. Even when not physically working shifts, it's sometimes hard to switch off, and all too often we become virtual shift workers.
- **Poor sleep hygiene.** Inadequate preparations for sleep — with habits such as drinking coffee, smoking cigarettes, or interacting with technology close to bedtime — stimulate the nervous system and make sleep more challenging.
- **The sleeping environment.** Sleep can be disrupted by environmental reasons such as a too-hot or too-cold bedroom,

traffic, a noisy neighbour, or (very commonly) a bed partner who snores.

- **Illness.** When you are sick with a cold or ear, nose, or throat infection, it can cause snoring, gagging, and frequent waking, which fragments sleep.

- **Sleep disorders.** Common problems such as snoring, periodic limb-movement disorder (or 'restless legs'), and sleep apnoea can disturb sleep throughout the night.

- **Insomnia.** This is a common sleep disorder and is defined as difficulty falling asleep (sleep onset) or staying asleep (sleep maintenance). Acute insomnia is brief, often happens because of life's circumstances, and tends to resolve without any need for treatment. Chronic insomnia is defined as when sleep is disrupted at least three times a week for at least three months. A 2005 US study showed that 51 per cent of women and 50 per cent of men experience a symptom of insomnia at least a few times per week, but only 10 per cent receive any treatment.[10]

- **Hormonal changes.** As discussed, poor sleep affects important hormones. Conversely, fluctuations in hormone levels during menstrual cycles, pregnancy, and menopause can also play havoc with women's sleep patterns. For both men and women, testosterone levels have been implicated in sleep-disordered breathing conditions, with low levels affecting sleep quality, particularly for men.[11]

- **Medications.** Some drugs used to treat disorders such as epilepsy or attention-deficit hyperactivity disorder (ADHD) can cause insomnia. The common use of antidepressants is also of concern, with studies showing that not all of these medications improve sleep — indeed, some worsen sleep disturbances in patients, which can only exacerbate depression and anxiety.[12] Whether sleep is improved or further disrupted is of high clinical significance, because persistent sleep problems elevate the risk of relapse, recurrence, or suicide.

- **Worry and anxiety.** Another common problem is to focus on events of the past, present, or future.

- **Babies, infants, and toddlers.** Most parents experience sleep
  deprivation, as young children wake frequently in the night for
  feeding, for comfort, or even with their own often-undiagnosed
  night-time breathing problems. One of the greatest challenges of
  parenthood is teaching your child to sleep, but the rewards are
  worth it for the whole family.

So what is a good night's sleep?

Before the invention of artificial light, sleeping patterns were guided by
the rising and setting of the sun. For 90 per cent of the population, the
ideal amount of sleep is between seven and nine hours a day.

A night's sleep is made up of cycles. Each sleep cycle is made up of
five stages. The first four stages account for 75 per cent of the cycle and
are categorised as non-rapid eye movement (NREM). When you begin
to fall asleep, you enter NREM sleep. The remaining 25 per cent of the
cycle is spent in stage 5 — rapid eye movement (REM). REM occurs
about 90 minutes after falling asleep and recurs approximately every 90
minutes, with the cycles becoming longer each time.

Stage 1
- Between being awake and falling asleep
- Light sleep

Stage 2
- Onset of sleep
- Becoming disengaged from surroundings
- Breathing and heart rate is regular
- Body temperature drops (sleeping in a cool room is helpful)
- Note that the first stages are very light, and, when people are
  disturbed from them, they will often report that they haven't even
  been asleep.

233

Stages 3 and 4

- Deepest and most restorative sleep
- Blood pressure drops
- Breathing slows
- Muscles are relaxed
- Blood supply to muscles increases
- Tissue repair occurs
- Energy is restored
- Hormones are released, including growth hormone

Stage 5 — rapid eye movement (REM)

- Provides energy to brain and body
- Supports daytime performance
- The brain is active and dreams occur
- Eyes dart back and forth
- Body becomes immobile and relaxed, as muscles are turned off
- Ideally, you should complete five cycles each night. The deepest levels of sleep should occur between 11.00 p.m. and 4.00 a.m.

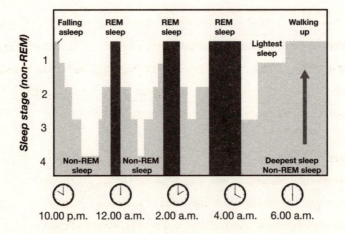

Figure 10-3. The four stages of NREM sleep followed by REM sleep. Each cycle is approximately 90 minutes.

It's about quantity and quality

If you've ever slept for eight hours but woken feeling tired, you will understand it's not just the *quantity* but also the *quality* of your sleep that counts. One of the main contributors to sleep quality is the way you breathe, which again is one of those things people give very little thought to.

People are often surprised when, as a dentist, I am so focused on their sleeping habits. They're also surprised at my dental practice's involvement in treating sleep and breathing disorders. But just as teeth led to my interest in the whole person, the crowded teeth that the vast majority of us have led to problems with breathing, which is the most critical factor affecting sleep quality.

These problems are often compounded by exposure to environmental toxins, dust mites, moulds, and certain foods, which can further restrict the airway through allergies and asthma. As sleep-disordered breathing can be the result of a variety of factors, it's good to find out if any are affecting your sleeping patterns, by consulting a health practitioner aware of the issues involved, working in consultation with a sleep physician.

Sleep-disordered breathing

The International Classification of Sleep Disorders lists more than 80 distinct sleep disorders, divided into eight categories, including insomnia, sleep-related movement disorders, and sleep-disordered breathing.[13]

Problems with breathing while sleeping include:

- **Snoring.** This is caused either by vibration of the soft palate or when the tongue falls to the back of the throat, restricting the airway. Snoring is often dismissed as a nuisance but is now recognised by most health practitioners as an early indicator of potentially serious health problems. Snoring affects 19–37 per cent of the population, and more than 50 per cent of middle-aged men; these figures refer to the snorer and not the partner who has to listen to the noise and have their own sleep disturbed as well. The prevalence of snoring increases with age and obesity. Men tend to snore more than women, but young men and women who are not overweight can also snore, as can children.

- **Obstructive sleep apnoea (OSA).** This can occur when the tongue drops towards the back of the throat and blocks the airway. Your breathing may be restricted (hypopnoea) or completely blocked (apnoea). An episode of hypopnoea or apnoea may last anywhere from ten seconds to three minutes. This may be particularly distressing to the sufferer's partner.

- **Central sleep apnoea (CSA).** Another condition where breathing is restricted or stopped. CSA occurs if there's a fault in the brain's control centre for breathing, and episodes may last ten seconds or longer. There's overlap between OSA and CSA.

- **Upper-airway resistance syndrome (UARS).** This term is used to describe patients who are excessively sleepy during the day but without a clear cause. UARS is characterised by repeated arousals or waking because of airflow resistance in the upper airway. This may be a function of the biochemistry of the person's breathing pattern, with the level of carbon dioxide in the lungs (end-tidal CO_2) affecting smooth muscle when it goes out of balance. UARS may also relate to the lack of production of nitric oxide, an important regulator, when people breathe predominantly through their mouth. Snoring is sometimes present but is not necessary for identification of UARS. Given the prevalence of narrow jaws, crowded teeth, and mouth breathing, it's not surprising that this condition is common. It's often overlooked during diagnosis once the more serious OSA is eliminated, and so there may be an even larger number of undiagnosed patients suffering from UARS.

Most snorers will know they snore — thanks to complaints from their suffering partner, housemates, or friends — but how do you know if this has tipped into something more serious, such as OSA or UARS? A sleep physician will conduct a sleep study, referred to as polysomnography, which is a comprehensive recording of several physiological changes that can occur during sleep. It measures many body functions, including brain activity (EEG), heart rhythm (ECG), eye movements (EOG), muscle activity (EMG), respiratory airflow (AHI), and oxygen saturation (pulse oximetry).

The Apnoea-Hypopnoea Index (AHI) is used to diagnose OSA and counts the number of times in the space of an hour that you stop breathing, or when breathing is restricted, for more than ten seconds — described as an 'episode'. An AHI of five episodes per hour and below is considered normal. If the AHI records more than five episodes in an hour, the sleeper's condition is categorised as OSA, and then categorised again as to how severe:

- 5–15 AHI episodes per hour = mild OSA
- 15–30 AHI episodes per hour = moderate OSA
- 30+ AHI episodes per hour = severe OSA.

Another measure in sleep studies is the respiratory-disturbance index (RDI). This measures the total number of apnoeas, hypopneas, and respiratory-effort related arousals (which don't quite qualify as hypopneas or apnoeas, but occur when there is a sudden transition between a deeper stage of sleep to a shallower stage).

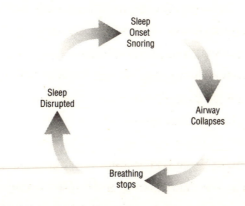

Figure 10-4. Cycle of obstructive sleep apnoea.

If CSA or UARS is suspected, the sleep physician may do a split-night sleep study. In the first half of the night, you are monitored as before; in the second half of the night, you are additionally fitted with a CPAP (continuous positive airway pressure) mask, which both helps and monitors your breathing. Diagnosis may require consultation with neurologists, cardiologists, or other specialists.

A PATIENT'S STORY — BRENDA

Diseases and illnesses have many causes — but not always obvious ones — as Brenda, 65, discovered. Brenda suffered from chronic fatigue and depression, and had been on antidepressants for several years. One of her many health practitioners believed Brenda's chronic fatigue could be the result of mercury leaching from fillings in her teeth, so she came to see me.

As part of my routine comprehensive dental consultation, I asked her how well she slept. Brenda replied 'reassuringly': 'Oh, Dr Ron, sleeping is not a problem. I could fall asleep anywhere, anytime.' In fact, she described herself as being able to 'sleep like a log, anywhere, anytime, even with chronic fatigue and depression'. I told her I felt that, rather than mercury fillings being the problem, it was far more likely her sleep quality was the reason for her fatigue. I also explained that this could be a major contributor to her depression. I suggested she visit our sleep physician and have him conduct a comprehensive sleep study.

The results revealed Brenda had an incredible 58 AHI episodes in an hour. With only 60 minutes in an hour, it was clear that Brenda spent a good deal of her sleeping time either not breathing well or not breathing at all. It's no wonder she felt tired and depressed. Like many, Brenda assumed her sleeping patterns were 'normal' — that this was 'just the way it was and had always been'. Health practitioners also often overlook the issue of sleep quality, either ignoring it or reaching too quickly for the prescription pad.

Brenda's severe OSA was treated and her fatigue improved considerably, as did her depression. Within 12 months, Brenda's energy had improved dramatically and she was happily off all medication.

Sleep disorders in children

Children can also suffer from sleep-disordered breathing and obstructive sleep apnoea. If your child is a noisy breather, this is often an indication of early-stage sleep-disordered breathing. The condition is surprisingly common, and has implications for a child's mental and physical development, IQ, and performance at school.

As with adults, sleep quality is far too often overlooked when treating children, particularly those with behavioural problems — an ever-increasing issue in our modern world. Paradoxically, sleepy or tired children who are not good sleepers can often 'speed up' rather than slow down. Symptoms of sleep-disordered breathing in children include:

- moodiness and irritability
- temper tantrums
- a tendency to emotionally 'explode' at the slightest provocation
- over-activity and hyperactive behaviour
- daytime naps
- grogginess when they wake
- reluctance to get out of bed.

In Australia, a 2001 study showed that 11.2 per cent of children are diagnosed with ADHD, with the incidence much higher in boys (15.4 per cent) than girls (6.8 per cent).[14] A 2015 study put the figure at 7.2 per cent.[15] In the UK, the figure is 3.6 per cent,[16] while in the USA it varies from 5 to 11 per cent depending on which state's data is used.[17]

Perhaps the variations are an indicator of how subjective the diagnosis of ADHD is, but I digress.

According to paediatric respiratory physician Jim Papadopolous, 48 per cent of those children with ADHD also have sleep disorders and often go undiagnosed.[18] The point is, if your child has been diagnosed with ADHD, before opting for pharmaceutical treatment, ask your doctor for a referral to a paediatric sleep specialist to test their sleep patterns.

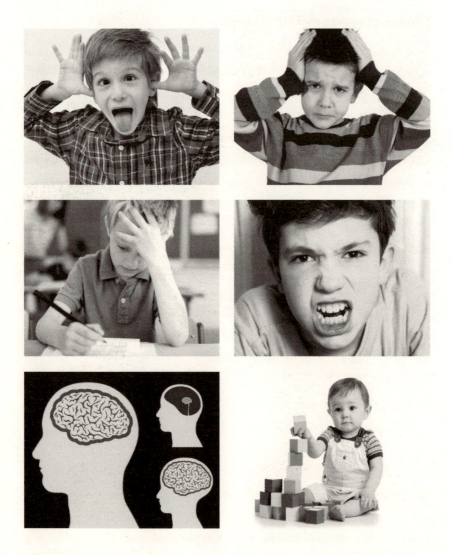

Figure 10-5. Poor sleep or sleep-disordered breathing manifests in children in many ways.

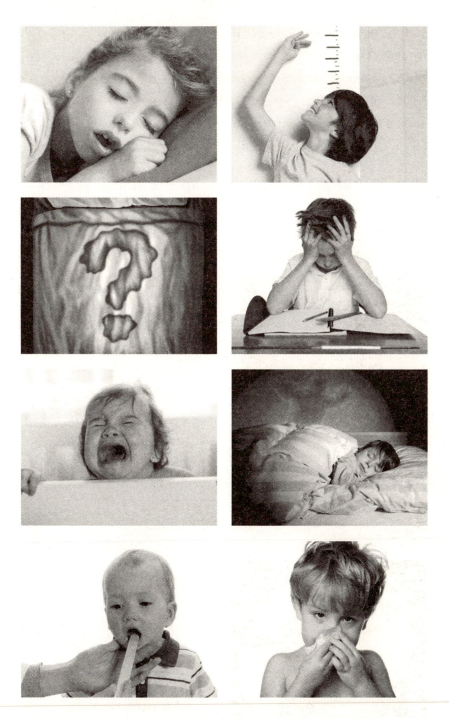

Figure 10-6. Symptoms of obstructive sleep apnoea (OSA) in children.

The incidence of childhood cancers, diabetes, obesity, and depression has more than doubled in the last 20 years, and while I have outlined many stresses that could be contributing to this problem, the importance of sleep to a child's physical and mental health, as well as their immune system, should always be considered.

How do I know if I have a sleep problem?

The Epworth Sleepiness Scale is an internationally recognised questionnaire that helps people to work out if they're getting enough sleep. It was developed at the Epworth Hospital in Melbourne, Australia.

The rating for each scenario is on a scale from zero to three, where:

- 0 = no chance of dozing
- 1 = slight chance of dozing
- 2 = moderate chance of dozing
- 3 = high chance of dozing.

Take a moment to do this quick quiz. How likely is it you would doze or fall asleep in the following situations?

Situation	Chance of Dozing
Sitting and reading	
Watching TV	
Sitting inactive in a public place (e.g. theatre or a meeting)	
As a passenger in a car for an hour without a break	
Lying down to rest in the afternoon when circumstances permit	
Sitting and talking to someone	
Sitting quietly after a lunch without alcohol	
In a car, while stopped for a few minutes in traffic	

How did you score?

- **9 and over.** You could have an underlying sleep problem such as obstructive sleep apnoea. It is recommended that you seek the advice of a sleep specialist.
- **7 to 8.** Interestingly, this is considered by the Epworth Sleepiness Scale to be 'average', but I believe it reflects that the average person often has a problem with sleep quality or quantity.
- **2 to 6.** Even more interestingly, this is officially considered an acceptable level of sleep. It is considered 'normal', but have we set the bar too low? I believe it still indicates a problem with sleep quality or quantity, even though it may not constitute a diagnosable condition.
- **0 to 1.** This should be the goal and, to me, indicates adequate sleep.

A word of caution: it's important to realise that the Epworth Sleepiness Scale is only a very basic screening questionnaire and *does not* detect all sleep-disordered breathing conditions or even obstructive sleep apnoea. You could score well on the scale, report feeling tired, and still have a serious problem; it's just that your form of tiredness may not cause you to doze during the day.

The stereotypical image of someone suffering from OSA is an overweight, middle-aged man, but I have seen many cases of young women and men in my dental practice who look fit yet suffer from some form of sleep-disordered breathing condition. Insomnia affects many people, and a significant number of those with obstructive sleep apnoea go undiagnosed.

It surprises me when taking a medical history that many patients with longstanding physical or mental-health concerns have never been questioned about or tested for the quality of their sleep. There are a number of reasons why you might not fit the typical picture of an OSA sufferer. For instance, you are a TOFI — 'thin-outside-fat-inside'. This describes a person who appears thin and yet has a substantial and often significant build-up of fatty tissue around their internal organs, particularly the liver and the heart. 'TOFI' was coined by Professor Jimmy Bell from Imperial College London, who developed a simple, non-invasive scanning technique to identify the condition.[19]

But let's focus on good sleep hygiene.

Sleep hygiene — three key questions

I see a regular six-monthly check-up at my dental practice as a great opportunity to check on more than just oral hygiene, brushing, and flossing; it's also an opportunity to check on your sleep hygiene, too. There are three basic questions I ask about sleep at these biannual check-ups:

1 . Is it easy for you to fall asleep? If the answer is 'no', I explore issues around sleep hygiene, routine, and possibly insomnia.
2. Do you wake during sleep? If the answer is 'yes', I consider sleep hygiene, including eating and drinking habits, exposure to bright lights or blue screens (laptops, mobile phones, and tablets), and breathing patterns such as mouth breathing.
3. Do you wake up feeling refreshed? If the answer is 'no', I look at first the quantity — are you getting enough sleep? I then look at the quality of sleep, focusing on breathing patterns during sleep. Depending on the severity of the tiredness, I may refer patients to a sleep physician for a comprehensive sleep study.

Good sleep hygiene — make this the habit of a lifetime

Now that you understand how vital good sleep is to our health, and how poor sleep plays a central role in disease, energy levels, obesity, and so much more — it is time to put together a plan for achieving a good night's rest.

PRIORITISE

If you don't prioritise sleep and take it seriously, it's unlikely you'll take the necessary steps to change your habits. This is something I discovered over ten years ago, after changing my own sleep habits: you just don't realise how much better you can feel from a good night's sleep until you make the change and experience the difference yourself. I encourage you to find out how much better you can feel. If you haven't slept well for a long time, you may have accepted your sleep cycle as normal. It will take a while for you to make up for the sleep deficit that accumulates after extended periods of poor sleep — you may have a lot of sleep to catch up on — but the rewards are well worth it.

The fact that your own health practitioner hasn't mentioned the importance of sleep to you may mean they haven't prioritised it in their own personal or professional lives yet either. They should. A good night's sleep is life-changing and can also be lifesaving.

The issue of how much sleep, and when to sleep, varies depending on your age and from person to person. The National Sleep Foundation recommends:[20]

- newborns, infants, and toddlers (0–2 years) need 14–17 hours
- preschool to school age (3–10 years) need 11–12 hours
- teens (11–18 years) need 9–10 hours
- adults (18–65 years) need 7–9 hours
- seniors (over 65 years) need 7–8 hours.

BREATHING

The most critical part of sleep is breathing well during sleep. Even if you sleep for a full eight hours, if you don't breathe well, you won't feel rested.

Poor breathing patterns or disordered breathing during sleep can cause unexpected problems with health, such as bedwetting for children or night-time urination (needing to get up in the middle of the night for the toilet) in adults. This is why my regularly checking-in with my patients about their sleep is so important.

If you, as an adult, wake in the middle of the night to visit the toilet, it could be from mouth breathing or irregular breathing throwing the body's chemistry out of balance. Mouth breathing affects the smooth muscle in blood vessels and has been connected with high blood pressure that's resistant to medication. In fact, there are smooth muscles throughout the body, and the effect of relaxing them can be profound. Breathing in a calmer way, as nasal breathing promotes, also helps switch on our parasympathetic nervous system. I'll cover this more in Chapter 11: Breathing.

ROUTINE

When our first daughter was born, the paediatrician suggested we get her into a good sleep routine. It would be good for her health, and we'd be happier and healthier parents. Looking back, it was a great piece of advice — perhaps the best piece of preventive health advice we could have ever received — and it applies not only to newborns but to every one of us, at any age. A good routine when preparing for sleep is the cornerstone of a good night's sleep. It involves making good choices with food, drink, artificial light, stimulation, noise, temperature, mood, and breathing.

As an example of organising yourself for sleep, if you accept the goal of eight hours of sleep a night and you want to wake up at 6.00 a.m., you need to be sleeping by 10.00 p.m. Set a 'mental alarm clock' for an hour before you want to be asleep, say 9.00 p.m. From that time, start to wind down, dim the lights, and prepare for sleep. Going to bed at the same time and waking at the same time also helps establish a better routine for a consistently good night's sleep.

FOOD AND DRINK

Ideally, you should finish eating dinner two hours before going to bed and avoid eating heavy or spicy foods. I know this is challenging for people who don't arrive home from work until seven o'clock at night or even later, so if this is you, you'll need to do some planning. Prepare meals beforehand, such as a slow roast or stew, or eat a bigger meal at lunch. Avoid or limit alcohol. Caffeine is a stimulant and counter-productive to a restful sleep, so it's best not to have caffeine from coffee, tea, cola, or chocolate after one o'clock in the afternoon. Remember that many decaffeinated products still contain caffeine.

If you fill up on fluids before going to bed, you'll be more likely to wake during the night. Hydration is critical to our health, but drink most of your water throughout the day. It is fine to have a cup of herbal tea or hot water with a slice of lemon after the evening meal. Remember that many teas are diuretics and will also make you go to the toilet.

LIGHT AND ELECTROMAGNETIC RADIATION

During the day, melatonin levels vary and are controlled by our body clock and exposure to light. Ideally, your blood melatonin level starts to rise around two hours before you go to sleep as the natural light begins to fade, but exposure to bright lights, or blue lights from electronic devices such as TVs, mobile phones, laptops, and tablets, lowers melatonin levels, affecting your ability to get to sleep and enjoy the many benefits of this important hormone.

If you decide to set your own mental 'I'm-preparing-for-sleep' alarm clock an hour before your bedtime, this is the time to dim the lights and stop using electronic devices. Your bedroom should be dark and you shouldn't have a digital clock sitting by your bed with a green light. Try going for an alarm clock that has an amber or orange light, with these warmer lights making for a better more restful sleep. Don't use your phone as an alarm clock, or as a sleep monitor for that matter. In fact, keep your mobile phone out of bedroom. There shouldn't be TVs or other electronic equipment in the room either, or at least within two metres of the bed. Ensure your bed isn't placed against a wall that backs onto a power board, fridge, or item that produces high levels of electromagnetic radiation (EMR). This EMR can affect the quality of your sleep.

On the other hand, getting out in the sun during the day, particularly the middle of the day for 20–30 minutes, can help regulate circadian rhythms and melatonin, vitamin D, and nitric-oxide production at night.

NOISE

Consider the impact of living in a noisy home. This poses a challenge in our urban environment with noisy neighbours, street noise, or even housemates. I've mentioned my own life-changing experience with the annoying call of the koel.

Soundproofing of walls, floors, ceilings or windows may seem like a big expense, but, if you had to put a price on a good night's sleep and all its benefits, you may find this a worthwhile investment. Simple earplugs may also help.

Of course, the most common and annoying sleep-disturbing noise includes the noise made by your partner. The problem of a partner's snoring is often dismissed or trivialised, but because it disturbs your own sleep it can have a profound impact on your health, too. I confess: my snoring affected my wife's sleep patterns, and I eventually took steps to fix it for the benefit of us both. I then realised what a good night's sleep actually was, and my wife had a better night's sleep as well.

SLEEPING POSITION

As I mentioned in Chapter 9: Postural Stress, the ideal sleeping position is on your side with a pillow by your side to keep the head, neck, spine, and pelvis well aligned, while helping to maintain an open airway.

TEMPERATURE

Feeling too hot or too cold affects the quality of your sleep, and it's particularly challenging if your bed partner likes a different temperature to you. Choose bedding that's appropriate for each of you. Before bed, try taking a hot shower or a relaxing bath with Epsom salts — a great way to detox and unwind while preparing your body and mind for sleep. It helps to establish the conditions for sleep as you come from the hot shower into a cool room, with reductions in your core body temperature signalling to your body it's time to rest, slowing down heart rate, breathing, and digestion.

ENVIRONMENTAL TOXINS

As building biologist Nicole Bijlsma points out, mould can be a serious issue, with one of the first symptoms being fatigue that isn't alleviated by rest.[21] Moulds typically affect the lungs and the immune system. Dampness is the key, so perform a thorough search for signs of mould behind furniture, under beds, in wardrobes, and under carpets. If gyprock walls or ceiling have every been exposed at some stage to damp, they can also harbour mould. If in doubt, it's worthwhile engaging a home biologist to do a more thorough assessment.

Dust mites are the most common cause of childhood asthma and allergies worldwide. For dust mites to thrive, they require moisture, warmth, and food, all provided by us when we get into bed. According to Bijlsma, each person sheds enough skin to feed one million dust mites per day, while a queen-size bed can be home to two billion dust mites, and a two-year-old pillow can contain 10 per cent of its weight in dust-mite faeces and carcasses. Point made. The regular use of a high-efficiency particulate air-filter (HEPA) vacuum cleaner and the placing of bedding in sunshine are great ways to control this common problem. Once you eliminate these moulds or dust mites, you will breathe and sleep better.

BEDDING

Considering you should spend a third of your life in bed, your bedding should be a priority and is a very worthwhile investment in your health. The bed and pillows should be good quality, provide good support, and be low allergenic. The bed should be regularly turned and vacuumed (using a HEPA vacuum cleaner), and the bedding should be regularly cleaned and sunned.

BE POSITIVE

If you are fortunate enough to share a bed with a loved one, finish the day by describing three positive events, no matter how small or insignificant. It could be beautiful weather, a wonderful conversation, a great breakfast, or a funny comment or moment at work. If you sleep alone, write three positive things in a journal. I'll describe the benefits of positive psychology, expressing gratitude, focusing on appreciation rather than expectation, journaling, and the power of thoughts on physical, mental, and emotional wellbeing in Chapter 14: Thought. Focusing on being positive just before going to sleep has value. Don't try to solve the problems of the world just before going to sleep, and don't check email or Facebook — these are far too stimulating.

SEX

Sex has a positive effect on sleep. It lowers the stress hormone cortisol and increases the 'hugging' hormone, oxytocin. Sex is a wonderful release of energy and even counts as exercise! It increases oestrogen levels, which can enhance a woman's REM cycle for a deeper, better night's sleep.[22] Men's ability to sleep better after sex is legendary.

Interventions

Having implemented a good sleep routine, you may still be tired. There are several interventions for sleep-disordered breathing:

SLEEP STUDY

An initial screening by your dentist or medical practitioner may lead them to review your sleep hygiene or work closely with a specialist sleep physician. A sleep physician will thoroughly examine your relevant medical history in the context of your sleep, and conduct a comprehensive sleep study, either at home or in a dedicated sleep clinic. As I've mentioned, this study measures your body's response to sleep, including respiratory airflow, heart rate, the blood's oxygen saturation, number of sleep arousals, and time spent in different stages of sleep. It's an important test that can literally save your life.

NUTRITION

Excessive weight and obesity are associated with decreased sleep quality and duration. Stimulants such as caffeine, the consumption of alcohol, and food allergies or sensitivities can all have an impact on your sleep quality. Nourish yourself.

EXERCISE

Exercise improves every measure of health, and I'll cover this more in Chapter 13: Movement.

It has been suggested that not exercising in the two hours before bed is a good idea, but I think common sense plays a role here. If you're unable to exercise in the morning, and you've tried going to bed earlier so that you can build exercise into your morning routine, evening workouts may be the only solution. Obviously, you should listen to your body; get into bed once you've properly cooled down.

One interesting study showed that rather than exercise influencing sleep, the quality of your sleep influences the next day's exercise.[23] In other words, a better night's sleep encourages better exercise participation. This is certainly my own experience.

You may still need help in getting a good night's sleep

CONTINUOUS POSITIVE AIRWAY PRESSURE (CPAP)

If diagnosed with moderate or severe OSA, a ventilator providing continuous positive airway pressure is considered the treatment of choice. Basically, when sleeping the patient wears a mask that fits over the mouth and/or nose; this pumps in air, keeping airways continuously open with positive airway pressure. The health benefits are significant and often lifesaving, but compliance (wearing it) is often a challenge. In studies to determine whether the CPAP is actually being used, adherence is defined as greater than four hours of nightly use.[24] However, 46–83 per cent of patients with OSA have been reported to be non-adherent to treatment — that is, many people find wearing the CPAP difficult or uncomfortable and simply don't use it. The better-quality machines are quiet and less bulky, but their mask is still awkward to some. On a positive note, improvements are always being made to the masks and delivery systems, and the potential benefits are often obvious to the user, and profound, so it's worth persisting with if you can.

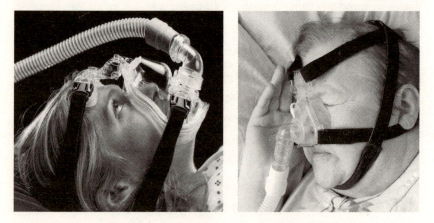

Figure 10-7. Continuous positive airway pressure (CPAP).

MANDIBULAR-ADVANCEMENT SPLINT (MAS)

These anti-snoring devices look a little like a mouth guard — they are custom-made by a dentist and fit over your upper and lower teeth. MAS is the treatment of choice for snoring or mild OSA, but can also be part of moderate or severe OSA treatments. By supporting the lower jaw (mandible) in a slightly forward position, it prevents the lower jaw and tongue from falling back and restricting or blocking the airway. The fitting dentist would perform regular check-ups on its use and effects:

• Jaw joints and occlusion can change quite dramatically when using the device.

- The way in which the upper and lower jaws are positioned in the construction of the appliance is also important, to ensure positon of the plate provides you with the best possible airway.
- If you suffer from headaches, neck aches, and jaw-joint problems, a poorly designed MAS may aggravate these conditions.

People often find an MAS easier to wear than the bulkier CPAP mask and accompanying tube connected to a machine. A recent study showed MAS had health outcomes similar to CPAP.[25] This was probably because more people tended to actually use the splints, unlike CPAP masks and machines — compliance was higher.

A study in 2011 revealed that after one year, 77 per cent of patients consistently used an oral appliance for the whole night, whereas only 46 per cent of those on a CPAP machine maintained at least four hours of therapy over more than 70 per cent of nights.[26] Given that 50 per cent of people diagnosed with OSA won't even agree to a CPAP trial, MAS is an important option or addition for people with moderate or severe sleep apnoea.

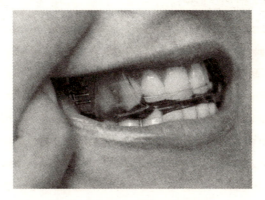

Figure 10-8. A mandibular-advancement splint (MAS) in place.

THERAPY

Insomnia is a common problem: 13 per cent of adults are estimated to suffer from chronic insomnia, and an additional 25–35 per cent have occasional insomnia.[27] While many of the things I have covered in

Part 2 and will cover in Part 3 are important in establishing good sleep hygiene, the problem of insomnia can be addressed with a combination of cognitive behavioural therapy (CBT). This is a form of psychotherapy that helps to change negative or unhealthy thoughts and habits, re-training the way we feel and behave. The aim of this non-pharmaceutical approach is to associate going to bed with a restful night's sleep, and relates to many of my sleep-hygiene recommendations. It is also referred to as 'stimulus-control therapy'.

Another relatively new treatment, intensive sleep retraining (ISR) is also showing encouraging results — treating sufferers of insomnia as effectively as CBT but in a fraction of the time.[28] In this technique, patients are deprived of sleep for a night and then, over a 24-hour period, encouraged to fall asleep every 30 minutes. By 'teaching' the patients to fall asleep over and over again, ISR helps them quickly re-learn how to sleep. It provides rapid benefits and maintenance of those benefits after a six-month follow-up.

A life-changing decision for my wife and for me

For many years, like far too many men, I casually dismissed my wife's complaints about my snoring. This changed at the age of 50, when she announced she'd had enough and suggested I move into another bedroom. That got my attention. Suddenly, 'her problem' became my problem, which I soon came to learn had really been a potentially more serious problem for me all along. It was time to do something about it.

I decided to make a custom-made mandibular-advancement splint (MAS), which thankfully stopped me from snoring — and to my relief, I maintained my place in the bedroom. But the most interesting thing for me was that even though I had never even considered that I slept badly, within a few days of not snoring I was amazed at how much more energised I felt. An added and significant bonus was that my wife also slept more soundly, waking more refreshed and happier than usual. A win-win situation.

We also changed our sleeping times — having always gone to bed around midnight, or even later, we began to go to bed earlier, at 9.00 p.m., and wake up earlier, at 5.30 a.m. This left me with enough time to visit the gym, something I had always promised myself I would do, but never really had the energy for first thing in the morning.

We both felt more refreshed, energised, and fitter — we had both learned what a new 'normal' really was. It also allowed me to share the importance of sleep quality with my patients.

Conclusion

Remember: there is no magic bullet. Take a step back and review all of the factors that may be having an impact on your sleep. Take a new approach. Doing the same thing that you've always done and expecting things to change is setting you up for failure.

A good night's sleep gives you physical, mental, and emotional energy. It builds resilience, helping you deal with the stresses of our modern world and get the most out of your life. Sleeping well is a function of both quantity (getting enough sleep and making up for the years of lost sleep) and quality (breathing well while you are asleep). Make it the most important part of your day.

CHAPTER 11

Breathing

According to yoga tradition, 'life is in the breath'. We all know that as long as we breathe, we are alive, but one of the 'secrets' to a longer, healthier life is to breathe *well*. Breathing well, in a controlled and relaxed way, is central to what makes meditation or mindfulness practices so beneficial — and it can also have far-reaching benefits to many aspects of our everyday lives.

After the heartbeat, breathing is the second-most-frequent bodily function, with the average person taking 12–20 breaths per minute, which equates to 17–30,000 breaths per day. Optimal breathing delivers the right amount of oxygen to each cell and ensures our body maintains an ideal pH balance with minimal effort. The act of breathing is a complex one, involving physiological and psychosocial factors. It can also be affected by emotional, nutritional, environmental, dental, and postural factors.

Dysfunctional breathing has been defined as the presentation of breathing patterns that do not perform its primary or secondary function, and may produce a long list of symptoms[1] — something we should all, including healthcare professionals, be more focused on. These may include: coughing, breathlessness, dry mouth, fatigue, 'foggy head', dizziness, gastric problems, frequent urination, high blood pressure, headaches, a feeling of not being able to breathe or 'being short of breath', hearing sensitivity, sighing, visual problems, poor concentration, throat-clearing, tingling, yawning, palpitations, joint stiffness, chest pain, postural imbalance, aches and pains, anxiety, and panic attacks.

Breathing — a question of balance

Most of us take breathing for granted — until there is a problem. One popular technique that examines how well we breathe is the Buteyko breathing method, developed in Russia in the 1940s to combat over-breathing, hyperventilation, and mouth breathing.[2] Its practitioners argue that optimal breathing has a significant impact on body chemistry and health. It can help with:

- asthma
- snoring and sleep apnoea
- chronic tiredness
- bedwetting in children
- night-time toilet trips in adults
- digestive disorders (heartburn, constipation, bloating)
- anxiety and panic attacks
- high blood pressure.

The Buteyko method employs a series of exercises that focus on carbon-dioxide levels in the lungs that in turn balance body chemistry — including acid and alkali levels. Both levels require carbon dioxide for their maintenance, and if CO_2 levels are out of balance, there are problems. But as we are learning when it comes to health, focusing on just the one factor — in this case CO_2 levels in the lungs, or end-tidal CO_2 — oversimplifies what constitutes and causes dysfunctional breathing and how to restore it. There is much more to this picture.

When it comes to breathing well, there are several basic factors that are universal. You should do the following:

- Inhale and exhale through the nose rather than the mouth, resting your tongue on the roof of your mouth (the palate) just behind the upper teeth.
- Employ nasal breathing, because it stimulates the production of nitric oxide, an important regulator of body functions, as well as

filtering the air you breathe.

- Engage the diaphragm (80 per cent of the effort), which allows you
to draw air deeper into the lungs and utilise the entire lung capacity,
with a minimum amount of effort from neck and shoulder muscles
(20 per cent of the effort).

- Breathe slowly — between eight and 12 breaths per minute is ideal.
Slowing down your breathing in a controlled way also affects your
autonomic nervous system.

Carbon dioxide holds the key to pH balance

pH is a measure of acidity and alkalinity and is represented on a scale
from one (highly acidic) to 14 (highly alkaline). The neutral point is
seven, which is the approximate pH of water — it is also close to the
optimal pH level of our blood, which sits between 7.35 and 7.45. While
this range isn't big, it is critical to biochemical balance and homeostasis,
your lifelong friend. When the pH levels of blood fall out of this range,
there can be significant impacts: from oxygen in red blood cells not
being released properly, to waste products not being removed from cells.
Below 6.8 or above 7.8, cell death occurs.

The breathing control centre in the brain carefully monitors pH
levels. The moment the level goes above or below the optimum range,
a sensor in the brainstem — the medulla — restores balance through
a process known as buffering in the respiratory system. If blood is too
acidic, bicarbonate, which is an alkali, is released. If it's too alkaline,
carbonic acid is released. Both substances require carbon dioxide for
their manufacture. While most people think the key to breathing is
oxygen, carbon dioxide is the key to maintaining pH balance, which
in turn is vital in transporting and releasing oxygen throughout the
body.

Oxygen transport and delivery — a delicate balance

How is oxygen transported around the body and delivered to each of its 37 trillion cells? A simple way of understanding the importance of carbon dioxide and buffering is to view the bloodstream as a transport system, like a railway. Its job is to deliver nutrients (such as oxygen) and remove waste from cells (such as carbon dioxide). There are about 250 million molecules of haemoglobin in each red blood cell. Each haemoglobin molecule has four iron (haem) atoms that allows an oxygen molecule to attach to it.

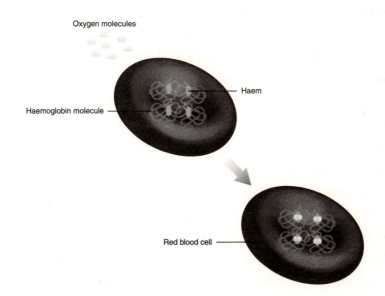

Oxygen molecules

Haem

Haemoglobin molecule

Red blood cell

Figure 11-1. Diagram shows oxygen molecules attaching to the four iron atoms that are part of the haemoglobin molecule, the key component of a red blood cell.

These transport carriages will only load the oxygen when the pH of the blood in the pulmonary alveoli of the lungs is 7.45. Once the oxygen molecule is attached to the haemoglobin, it is then transported around the body to where it's needed by cells. The oxygen molecules will only be released from the haemoglobin if the pH is 7.35. So the loading and unloading of oxygen is determined by very specific pH, and that pH is kept balanced by carbon-dioxide levels.

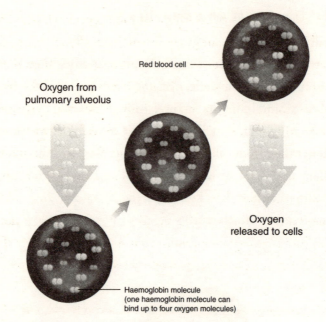

Figure 11-2. Four oxygen molecules attach to each haemoglobin molecule at pH 7.45; the haemoglobin is transported via the blood stream throughout the body; the oxygen is released at the cellular level at pH 7.35.

You can now see how maintaining carbon-dioxide levels in the lungs is important, particularly when you consider there is only 0.03 per cent CO_2 in the air we breathe. There is more than enough oxygen in the air we breathe (21 per cent) compared to how much we use (5 per cent). The only way you can be sure you have adequate CO_2 is to make and maintain it yourself — through exercise, digestion, balanced breathing, and other metabolic processes. Unlike oxygen, CO_2 has to be stored in the body, mainly in the lungs.

	Inhaled air at sea level	Body needs	Exhaled air
Oxygen (O_2)	21	5	16
Carbon dioxide (CO_2)	0.03	6.5	3.7

Figure 11-3. Percentage oxygen and carbon-dioxide levels.

At the ideal rate of 8–12 breaths per minute, optimal levels of oxygen and carbon dioxide in the lungs are maintained. If you over-breathe or hyperventilate, you push out too much carbon dioxide from the lungs, which affects its ability to effectively buffer the pH of the blood. If taken to an extreme, you can end up fainting when you hyperventilate. This is the brain and body's way of forcing you to slow your breathing down so that the carbon-dioxide level can build up in your lungs again and restore balance. Breathing in and out of a paper bag for a minute or two does the same thing.

Over-breathing, at say 15–25 breaths per minute, may not cause you to pass out but may compromise your health, particularly if that is the 'normal' way you have breathed over weeks, months, or even, as can commonly occur, years.

How does the brain respond to this constantly changing level of carbon dioxide and pH? One effect is a narrowing of the smooth muscle in the respiratory system in order to limit the amount of CO_2 loss. This could be felt as a tight chest, a difficulty in catching your breath, or breathlessness. In some cases, it is diagnosed as asthma.

There's also smooth muscle in other parts of the body, including the digestive (stomach, intestines), circulatory (arteries, veins, capillaries), and the urinary (bladder, urethra) systems. Some night-time toilet trips or bedwetting can be traced to over-breathing, with breathing imbalances causing low end-tidal CO_2, resulting in constriction of the smooth muscle in the bladder.

Another way in which the brain regulates CO_2 levels is through a 'breath hold', or apnoea. This is a quick and efficient way to build the end-tidal level of CO_2 in the lungs. Many people unconsciously hold their breath during the day, forget to breathe, or while concentrating. This is called daytime apnoea. At night, if there is heavy, faster breathing, the end-tidal level of CO_2 drops sharply in the lungs, and a signal is sent to stop breathing until the CO_2 level is restored. Having this protective mechanism go out of balance is one suggested mechanism for central sleep apnoea.

Noses are for breathing

Noses have evolved for the purpose of getting air to the lungs at the right volume. Most importantly, the nose filters, humidifies, and warms the air before entering the lungs, allowing them to function more efficiently. Lungs are extremely delicate and sensitive organs, so 'processing' the air is important. Just as food has an impact on the immune system, so do toxins or microbes in the air affect the lungs, potentially triggering allergies and asthma.

When you inhale air through your nose, it controls the quality and quantity of air that enters your lungs. It's a multi-level filtration system:

1. fine hairs in the nasal passages filter and trap airborne particles and dust
2. enzymes in the mucus lining of the nasal passages kill viruses and bacteria
3. the turbinates (ridges inside the nostril) and the sinuses control temperature and humidity
4. the adenoids (glands located in the roof of the mouth behind the soft palate, where the nose connects to the throat) produce white blood cells that help fight infections
5. the tonsils also fight infection and are the final fine filters, ensuring the purest possible air enters the lungs.

Conversely, if you predominantly breathe through the mouth, you bypass the first four steps of nasal filtration. This makes you more susceptible to colds, flus, allergies, asthma, and other upper-respiratory infections. Enlarged and frequently infected tonsils are often connected to chronic mouth breathing. Removal of tonsils was once a common occurrence, but not so any more. It's better to find out why the nasal and sinus passages are blocked in the first place.

Well-balanced breathing through the nose can have positive effects on sleep, the digestive and immune systems, skin, and even mental health. In some cases, removing tonsils and adenoids improves a child's ability to breathe, but it may be worth considering other options first:

identifying food allergies or sensitivities; locating environmental toxins, dust mites, or moulds; exploring why teeth are narrow and crowded; and looking at poor swallowing patterns — all of which predispose children to mouth breathing and make them more susceptible to disease.

Possibly even more significant than all of that, nasal breathing also allows the sinuses to produce nitric oxide (NO), which shouldn't be confused with nitrous oxide (N_2O), also known as laughing gas. Nitric oxide is an important body regulator, and the sinuses produce 60 per cent of the body's supply — when you breathe through your nose. Among nitric oxide's many important functions:

- assisting memory and behaviour by transmitting information between nerve cells in the brain
- assisting the immune system in fighting bacteria and defending against tumours
- regulating blood pressure by dilating arteries
- reducing inflammation
- improving sleep quality
- increasing sense recognition, such as smell
- increasing endurance and strength
- assisting in the movement of food through the digestive tract
- assisting in sexual arousal by vaso-dilation, or engorgement, which helps maintain erections.

Breathing through your nose can also enhance emotional judgement: it activates the amygdala, the part of the brain involved in empathy, particularly the recognition of fear in others.[3]

Finally, breathing through your nose maintains your sense of smell, which is important for safety, for enjoying life, and for social acceptance — just in case you are unaware of your own bodily odours. Smell influences behaviour, memories, and many autonomic nervous system functions at a subconscious level. This is because receptors in the nose, called olfactory bulbs, are direct extensions of the hypothalamus, which is considered the 'brain's brain', in charge of the autonomic nervous system. The hypothalamus is also responsible for generating chemicals that influence memory and emotion, as well as being critical to fight-or-flight response.

Diaphragms are for breathing

Along with nasal breathing, a well-balanced breathing pattern also uses the diaphragm, located under the ribcage. As Figure 11-4 reveals, during inhalation the abdomen should expand; during exhalation, the abdomen should contract.

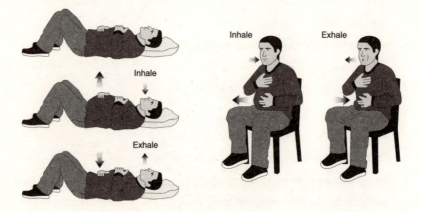

Figure 11-4. A useful exercise to practise diaphragmatic breathing in the lying and sitting positions.

If you breathe through your mouth, you primarily engage the muscles in the upper chest and neck. As outlined in Chapter 9: Postural Stress, this contributes to postural imbalance such as a head-forward posture, and may contribute to common chronic musculoskeletal pain such as tension headaches and neck aches or even RSI.

Breathing through your mouth also means you use only around one-third of your lung's total or available capacity. Breathe through your nose and engage your diaphragm to ensure you utilise the entire volume of your lungs. This also provides rhythmic pressure to the abdomen, assisting digestion.

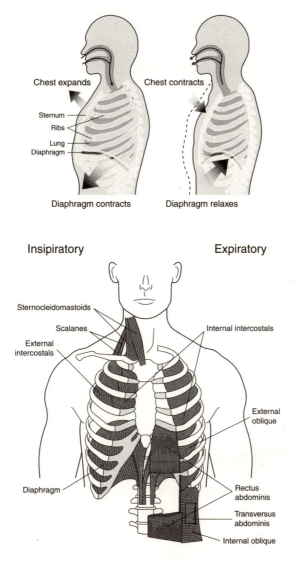

Chest expands

Sternum
Ribs
Lung
Diaphragm

Diaphragm contracts

Chest contracts

Diaphragm relaxes

Insipiratory

Expiratory

Sternocleidomastoids

Scalanes

External
intercostals

Internal intercostals

External
oblique

Diaphragm

Rectus
abdominis

Transversus
abdominis

Internal oblique

Above: Figure 11-5. The action of inhalation (left) and exhalation (right).
Below: Figure 11-6. Most of the effort in breathing should come from the diaphragm (80 per cent) and less from the neck and shoulder (20 per cent).

Optimal breathing — let's recap

Optimal breathing is imperative to overall health and wellbeing because it:

- strengthens the diaphragm, making it easier to breathe

- filters the air for particles and microbes
- allows the lungs to fill completely with greater capacity and less effort
- requires less energy than over-breathing
- moves air into the lower sections of the lungs, which increases the exchange of oxygen from the lungs to the bloodstream, utilising the full capacity
- maintains the correct balance of carbon-dioxide levels
- maintains the ideal level of pH in the bloodstream
- assists digestion
- improves mood, empathy, and memory
- stimulates the production of nitric oxide, an important body regulator
- improves posture and reduces strain on the muscles of the neck and shoulder
- provides the energy to function at your best.

At between eight and 12 breaths per minute, the movement of the diaphragm also helps to 'massage' and detoxify our inner organs, and pump the lymph more efficiently through our lymphatic system, an important part of our immune system.

Let's take a moment to consider this holistically once more. Imagine this scenario: you take short, shallow breaths and have tried to breathe through your nose; you've never really thought about your diaphragm as weak or under-utilised; food sensitivities and environmental toxins restrict your nasal breathing; your nose often feels blocked; unconsciously, you start breathing through your mouth to get more oxygen; the mouth breathing alters your posture into a head-forward position; this strains your neck muscles; the continual strain causes pain receptors to fire; cortisol is released throughout your body; inflammation is triggered; you can't sleep and the situation worsens; chronic inflammation leads to chronic pain. It's all connected. And there are many more possible sequences of events with similarly negative results, not all revolving around chronic pain.

That's why optimal breathing is a pillar of your health.

What causes breathing-pattern disorders?

Biomechanical	Biochemical	Psychological
Postural maladaptations	Lung disease	Anxiety
Upper-limb movement	Metabolic disorders	Stress
Chronic mouth	Allergies	Panic disorders
breathing	Diet	Personality traits (e.g.
Cultural practices (e.g.	Exaggerated response	perfectionist, high
'tummy in', 'chest out',	to decreased CO_2	achiever, obsessive)
tight-waisted clothing)	Drugs, including	Suppressed emotions
Congenital defects	recreational drugs,	Conditioning/learned
Overuse, missuse,	caffeine, aspirin, alcohol	response
or abuse of	Exercise	Anticipation
musculoskeletal system	Speech and laughter	History of abuse
Abnormal movement	Chronic low-grade fever	Sustained concentration
patterns	Heat	Sustained boredom
Braced posture	Humidity	Pain
Occupational hazards	Altitude	Depression
(e.g. for divers, singers,		Phobic avoidance
swimmers, etc.)		Fear of symptoms/
		misattribution of
		symptoms

Figure 11-7. Some of the causes of breathing pattern disorders.[4]

As you can see from Figure 11-7, the list of possible causes or influencers behind breathing-pattern disorders is extensive — but it doesn't stop here. There are other significant factors, areas I've looked at already in this book, that also affect our breathing:

- **Function.** By this I mean how you sit, stand, sleep, and talk. If there's postural imbalance, or nagging aches and pains, or weakness or tightness in the breathing muscles, you will compensate by over-breathing. If you talk too quickly, you engage your upper chest rather than your diaphragm. There's simply not enough time for the exhaled air to refill your reservoir.

- **Ingestion or exposure.** Eating too quickly and what you eat, drink, sniff, and inhale can all cause over-breathing. Are you exposed to solvents or chemicals? The body will remove those that it registers as inappropriate.

- **Emotional stress.** How do you manage the day-to-day frustrations of modern life? Do you react, become upset, over-breathe, and lower your resilience? Or do you take a moment, pause, switch on the parasympathetic nervous system, think it through, and create a solution?
- **Pathology.** Of course, illness and impairment affects breathing, e.g. respiratory or cardiovascular diseases, chronic pain, obstructed airways from asthma or allergies, or sleep apnoea.

One of the best ways to show just how important good breathing techniques are to our body is to look at some case studies. Here are a few remarkable stories.

A PATIENT'S STORY — AMANDA

At the age of 12, Amanda came to my clinic for advice on orthodontics. She had narrow upper and lower jaws and crowded teeth, and was also clearly breathing through her mouth as she sat during my discussion with her parents. Another of her symptoms was bedwetting — which in medical terms is referred to as enuresis. Following visits to the family GP, a paediatrician, a urologist, a neurologist, and a psychologist, she was prescribed various medications to suppress urine production. Drugs commonly prescribed for bedwetting include desmopressin (Stimate or Minirin), imipramine (Tofranil), and anticholinergic drugs (Ditropan or Levsinex) — all have limited success, but many have a range of side effects, such as irritability, insomnia, drowsiness, reduced appetite, dry mouth, facial flushing, headache, nausea, and vomiting. These are some of the drugs recommended by the National Kidney Foundation.[5]

I knew that enuresis and frequent night-time urination are often indications of sleep-disordered breathing. Capnometer breathing tests, which measure breathing rate and CO_2 in the lungs, revealed Amanda was taking between 22 and 25 breaths per minute, an incredible amount (remember the optimal number is eight to 12 breaths per minute). Her end-tidal CO_2, which should have been at 35–40 mmHg, was at 28 mmHg, which was affecting the ability of her smooth muscles to relax. Because her breathing was out of balance, it affected the CO_2 levels in her lungs as well as nitric-oxide production, her body chemistry, and, ultimately, her ability to control her bladder.

The solution was remarkably simple, and part of the Buteyko breathing program. I recommended she apply a thin, paper-like, low-allergenic tape (sometimes called Micropore) over her mouth as she slept. In this way, we used the eight hours of sleep time to train her body to breathe through her nose. It also gave the breathing control centre in the brain an opportunity to recalibrate and get used to nasal breathing. This helped regulate Amanda's breathing rate, body chemistry, and pH balance — and her enuresis stopped within a couple of nights. She no longer wet her bed. No medication, just basic physiology and a two-dollar roll of tape.

A PATIENT'S STORY — CARLOS

Carlos, a 29-year-old former fitness trainer, wanted his dental mercury amalgam fillings removed, believing this was the cause of the chronic fatigue he had been suffering from for several years. In addition to a few heavily worn and cracked mercury fillings, which certainly required careful replacement, it was also clear that Carlos was grinding his teeth during sleep. The wear on his teeth would have been excessive for someone 30 years his senior — it was significant.

Clenching or grinding teeth often reflects sleep-disordered breathing. When he completed the Epworth Sleepiness Scale, he had a score of 13 (remember, a score over nine suggests obstructive sleep apnoea). Being trim and seemingly fit, he didn't match the stereotypical picture of someone with OSA, so I suggested he try non-irritating paper tape over his mouth at night to encourage nasal breathing.

When he returned three weeks later, he said he felt terrific — 'never better'. When he rated himself on the Epworth Sleepiness Scale again, his score was three. It was a significant difference from just one simple intervention.

Taping your mouth — it's not that crazy

As a recent study showed, the simple use of tape can significantly reduce the number of significant breathing restrictions when sleeping (AHI) and has been successful in treating mild OSA (5–15 AHI per hour).[6]

I have personally been using Micropore tape for many years, and find it very helpful. When I suggest it to my patients, they typically fall into two categories. The first look at me in a rather bemused way to see whether I am seriously suggesting this for them — and think nothing more of it.

The second category give it a go, and return more often than not to say that they can't believe that something as simple as this can make such a difference. The more I learn about optimal breathing in general and the importance of nasal breathing in particular, the more I am reminded of how interconnected the body is.

Gentle paper tape — it is such a simple exercise and well worth a try. Use the eight hours of sleep to retrain your brain and body to breathe through your nose and the benefits can flow over to your day time breathing patterns.

First, you must ensure that you don't have major nasal obstructions, or food sensitivities and allergies causing inflammation, or swelling resulting in blockage or restriction of your airway. A visit to your doctor can help. Breathing patterns can be assessed by a respiratory physiologist, and breathing-retraining courses are available online with straightforward techniques.

If you'd like to try the paper tape but are concerned about it being a little difficult to get used to, follow these helpful tips before wearing it while you sleep:

- Put it on as you watch TV or read. Even if your nose feels blocked, apply the tape. Keep calm and, as breathing becomes regulated, in the majority of cases, you will be surprised to find that your nose will unblock.
- Fold the end of tape over itself to create a tab to make it easy to hold, and to assist in its removal.
- Before removing the tape, poke your tongue into the tape to moisten and loosen it. Ripping the tape off will traumatise the lips, particularly after a few nights of using the tape. (However, dry or cracked lips are one of the most obvious signs of chronic mouth breathing. By practising nasal breathing and making it your norm, lips should be moist and supple, not requiring the application of lip balm or moisturisers.)

Once you are wearing the paper tape as you sleep, you can expect calm, refreshing rest, with fewer interruptions and fewer urges to go to the bathroom.

Practising mind–body medicine

Stress is a major focus of my practice and this book. When we are stressed, the sympathetic nervous system is active, prepared for fight or flight. Ideally, we should spend our time dominated by the parasympathetic nervous system, resting and digesting.

As I pointed out at the very start of this chapter, many meditation or mindfulness practices focus on the importance of the breath. Controlling your breathing in this way is one of the simplest and most effective ways of switching on the parasympathetic nervous system, allowing your body to conserve energy, improve your immune system, improve your digestion, and improve your mood. No pill, no supplement, totally free — just controlling how you breathe. The following simple breathing technique, which can take as little as one to two minutes, is the most effective way of engaging this restorative part of your nervous system.

A simple breathing exercise to relax your nervous system

I call this the 4:4:4 breathing exercise:

1. With your lips lightly touching, your tongue resting against the roof of your mouth, your teeth only lightly touching or slightly apart, and a hand on your stomach, take a slow, deep breath from your diaphragm through your nose for four seconds. Your hand and stomach should go out as you inhale.
2. Slowly and gently exhale through your nose for four seconds. Your lips should remain lightly closed and your tongue stay against the roof of your mouth, while your hand and stomach should go in as you exhale.
3. Hold the exhaled breath for four seconds.
4. Repeat eight to ten breaths.

You can practise this simple yet powerful exercise a few times a day, including just before going to sleep.

It's as simple as that.

Conclusion

We are seldom conscious of the way we breathe, but it is one of the most basic bodily functions of human life — and as I have shown, there is a significant difference between just breathing and breathing well.

Breathing well means breathing from the diaphragm and through the nose to ensure body chemistry is well balanced and oxygen is delivered to cells and organs throughout the body. Inadequate breathing affects energy levels, blood pressure, bedwetting in children, and night-time urination in adults.

Life is in the breath. Integrate breathing awareness into your life. Breathing well during the day is important, but it is the night-time breathing that defines a good night's sleep and ignoring it has the potential to cause significant health problems. Breathing is an important part of being the best you can be. Breathe well, sleep well, and there's a very good chance you will be well.

CHAPTER 12

Nutrition

Everything you place in, on, or near your body has the potential to nourish, but it equally has the potential to harm. The most obvious source of nutrition is food and water: the fuel of life. Making healthy food choices, though, can be difficult. Public health messages about 'what you should eat', or talk of the latest 'superfood' or 'breakthrough', are all too often influenced by profit — and not by health.

So the question then has to be: when nutrition advice from public health bodies is questionable, how do you work out what you should be eating? The good news is, it isn't all that complicated — there are some basic principles based on lessons from the past and some common sense to work by. Read on!

Principle 1 — 'nutrient-dense food' should be your guiding principle

In the 1930s, Weston A. Price ran a dental practice in Cleveland, Ohio, but travelled the world to discover the cause of tooth decay. In the villages and developing cities of non-industrialised countries, he found the answer, as I've explained: a nutrient-dense diet, absent of white flour and sugar, not only maintained a full set of perfectly aligned, decay-free teeth, but also warded off degenerative diseases such as heart disease, cancer, and arthritis, which, even in the 1930s, were becoming common in many western industrialised countries; meanwhile, those consuming a more 'modern' diet were prey to all the problems of development, decay, and disease. This suggested that issues such as degenerative diseases and crowding of teeth were based more on diet and nutrition than on genetics, reinforcing the fact that most chronic disease is due to diet, lifestyle, and environmental factors.

As he travelled, Price also observed the wide variety of food eaten by different traditional cultures, including meat, organ meats, seafood, dairy, rye, oats, vegetables, broths, fermented foods, seasonal fruits, and more. The words 'Paleo', 'vegan', and 'vegetarian' were not then part of everyday vocabulary, and the 'diet' industry didn't even exist. Price was starting from ground zero, trying to sort out what the key was behind these varied traditional villages and their good health.

When he went on to analyse these traditional foods, he found they had ten times the amount of water-soluble vitamins (such as B-group vitamins) and minerals (such as calcium, magnesium, selenium, and zinc) than western foods that were typically consumed at the time. Even more importantly, they also had four times the amount of fat-soluble vitamins (A, D, E, and K), which are essential for the body to absorb the water-soluble vitamins and minerals. He specifically noted that the best source of fat-soluble vitamins came from animals raised on healthy pastures. When white flour and sugar entered the diet, so did tooth decay and many common degenerative diseases. Within one generation, the offspring raised on these western foods showed signs of narrow jawbones and crowded teeth.

This is why Price called his landmark 1939 book *Nutrition and Physical Degeneration*, because that's exactly what he had observed.[1] Remember, Price was making these discoveries in the 1930s, and since then dentistry has been warning of the effects of sugar. But are we seeing an improvement in narrow jaws, crowded teeth, and chronic degenerative disease — the problems Price was dealing with and warning us about eight decades ago? Today, while oral hygiene has become part of most people's daily routine, dramatically reducing the incidence of tooth decay, physical degeneration in the form of the epidemic of chronic degenerative diseases has become an even bigger problem.

And the reason for this rise in chronic disease? Undoubtedly, much of the reason comes down to the food we eat and how it is produced. With all the choice we have today, all the marketing and advertising, it can hard to know what we should eat and which foods we should avoid. But if we go back to Price's findings, we discover a wide and diverse list of nutrient-dense foods that were consumed around the world by those traditional — and healthy — cultures. There are some important lessons for us to be learned from the past.

Communities visited	Foods consumed by traditional cultures
Eskimos, North America	Fish, game meat, fish roe, marine animals, and seal-blubber oil
Indigenous Peruvians	Game meat, organ meats, glands, blood, marrow, and a variety of grains, tubers, vegetables, and fruits that were seasonally available
Melanesians, South Pacific	Seafood, tubers, and seasonal fruits
Gaelic Hebrides (Scotland)	Fish and various seafood, together with oats (porridge) and oatcakes
Isolated Swiss Alp Villages	Rich dairy products, dense rye bread, meat (occasionally), soups, and the few vegetables and fruits they could cultivate and preserve during the summer months

Figure 12-1. The variety of foods consumed in just some of the communities visited by Weston A. Price.

Nourishing Traditions is a cookbook that offers a contemporary perspective informed by Price's work,[2] and is supported by both the Weston A. Price Foundation[3] and the Price-Pottenger Nutrition Foundation.[4] Both organisations provide extensive resources and are well worth subscribing to on your path to a nutrient-dense future.

Over the last decade, there's been growing interest in the so-called Palaeolithic — or Paleo — diet. Proponents of this dietary approach argue that our modern stomachs are not suited to many of the foods that became available during the agricultural revolution. It took hundreds of thousands of years for the hunter-gatherer gut to evolve, but it's only been 10,000 years since the agricultural revolution. During that time, a relatively small variety of plants, grains, and animals have been domesticated, including wheat, rye, barley, millet, and rice, along with goats, sheep, cattle, pigs, and chickens. And records show our Palaeolithic ancestors had stronger teeth and bones than we do! So I think cookbooks that use the principles of Paleo diets are a good starting point for getting ideas about nutrient-dense foods.

Principle 2 — healthy fats are the key to combating disease

I can't emphasise this enough: fats are essential for the optimal working of our body. Every cell membrane throughout the body is fat; 60 per cent of the brain is fat; nerves have a myelin sheath made out of fat; fats are the building blocks of hormones; fat affects the absorption of minerals; fat affects bone density; 60 per cent of the heart's energy comes from fat; fat protects and insulates vital organs; fat is essential for healthy skin and hair; the lungs are prevented from collapsing by fat; fat aids digestion; fats are an alternative to glucose as a fuel source for the body; and fats are important for memory and cognition.

FATS DEFINED

Terminology is confusing when it comes to fats. Strictly speaking, fats are solid at room temperature, and oils are liquid at room temperature, and collectively they are referred to as lipids. I will include all lipids under the term 'fats', as that is what most people are familiar with when thinking about nutrition.

Fats are made up of so-called fatty acids, which in turn are made up of carbon-atom (C) chains (up to 24 atoms in length) bonded with hydrogen (H) atoms, with a carboxyl group (-COOH) at the end.

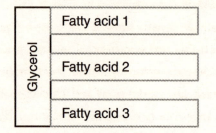

Figure 12-2. Fats are also known as triglycerides, the molecules formed when three fatty acids attach to a glycerol molecule.

The chemical structure of fatty acids falls into three different types: saturated, monounsaturated, and polyunsaturated. It's important to realise that we need them all and that one is not better or more important than the other. No food in nature contains only one type of fat; they are a combination of fats.

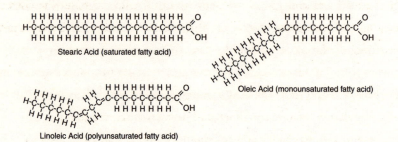

Figure 12-3. Examples of the three types of fatty acid.

In saturated fatty acids, each carbon atom in the chain has the maximum of four other atoms bonded to it, and is thus said to be 'saturated' (an unfortunately loaded word). These fatty acids vary in length and function, but have two main roles, one as structure and the other as energy.

We can manufacture our own saturated fat from carbohydrates in what is generally, in a healthy individual, an extremely minor pathway called lipogenesis. When we eat too many carbohydrates, this process becomes far more active, leading to obesity and metabolic disease. This process also expends energy that would otherwise be used for antioxidant defence and detoxification.

Monounsaturated fatty acids have one double, or 'unsaturated', carbon bond and one bend. They make up fats that are typically liquid at room temperature but solid when chilled. These oils, such as macadamia or olive oil, are relatively stable.

Polyunsaturated fatty acids have multiple double carbon bonds and therefore bends in the chain. They are highly reactive, particularly when heated. The term 'omega' refers to the last bend in the chain from the carboxyl group, e.g. omega-6 has a bend at the sixth link.

In Chapter 6: Nutritional Stress, I briefly looked at the importance of omega-3 and omega-6 fatty acids to our health. Getting the correct balance of these essential polyunsaturated fatty acids right is important because:

- omega-6 fatty acids help cell rigidity, assist with blood coagulation, help to store fats, and promote inflammation in response to external toxins or irritants (note: inflammation has an important purpose in the body; it's chronic inflammation that's the problem)
- omega-3 fatty acids are critical for the development of the nervous system, for flexible cell membranes, and for the reduction of inflammation.

There's a common belief that red meat causes inflammation and saturated fats are bad. But what sort of meat are we talking about? Processed meats and grain-fed, factory-farmed meats are lumped together with organic, free-range, pasture-fed-and-finished meats, as though they are all the same thing. They are not. What sort of fat are we talking about? All fat is not the same, just as all meat is not the same.

For instance, grass-fed beef usually contains less overall fat than grain-fed beef. And where grass-fed-and-finished beef contains an omega-3 to omega-6 ratio between 1:1 and 1:3, grain-fed beef may have 20 times more omega-6, making it the inflammatory red meat that many health authorities warn about. And the list of differences goes on, for other nutrients as well as fat.

In fact, *fat does not make you fat*. 'Healthy' fats not only make you feel full and less hungry, but also help control chronic inflammation and fluctuations in blood sugar — and therefore many chronic diseases. The same chronic diseases that are becoming major killers, killers we are having to contend with as a society. Meanwhile, despite years of public health warnings against saturated fats, there have been numerous meta-analyses, systematic reviews, and non-systematic reviews that have failed to find a clear link between saturated fats and heart disease or cardiovascular death.[5]

So which oils should we be using? The type of oil used in cooking and other food preparation is clearly important.[6] When cooking or preparing food, I ask myself these two questions:

1. Is it a naturally occurring fat? If not, avoid it.
2. Has the animal been naturally raised? If not, avoid it

Best for hot use (from highest to lowest temperature stability)	Best for cold use
Refined or unrefined Coconut oil	Extra virgin olive oil
Lard (pig fat), duck fat, tallow (beef or mutton)	Macadamia oil
Ghee	Avocado oil
Macadamia oil	Sesame oil
Avocado oil	Hazelnut oil
Sesame oil	Almond or walnut oil
Olive oil	Flaxseed oil
Almond or walnut oil	Butter
Butter	Unrefined Coconut oil

Figure 12-4. Fats best for 'hot use' in cooking (depending on the stability of the fat at raised temperature) and for 'cold use' as a dressing.

Principle 3 — be mindful about the source of your protein

Protein is an essential nutrient. We all need protein to rebuild and maintain body cells and biological processes.

PROTEINS DEFINED

Proteins are large, complex molecules that play many critical roles in the body. They are made up of amino acids, and, together, amino acids and proteins are the building blocks of life. When proteins are ingested, the body breaks them down into amino acids, which our genes then reassemble into the proteins we need to maintain life.

There are 22 amino acids, which are classified into three groups: essential, non-essential, and conditional.

- Essential amino acids cannot be made by the body, so they must come from food. They are histidine, isoleucine, leucine, lysine, methionine, phenylalanine, threonine, tryptophan, and valine.
- Non-essential amino acids can be produced by our bodies. They include alanine, asparagine, aspartate, and glutamate.
- Conditional, or semi-essential, amino acids become essential in times of illness and stress. They include arginine, cysteine, glutamine, tyrosine, glycine, ornithine, proline, and serine.

Your hair, skin, eyes, muscles, and organs are all made from protein. So are haemoglobin, antibodies, enzymes such as lipoprotein lipase, and hormones such as insulin.

Protein is also a major source of energy. If you consume more protein than you need for body-tissue maintenance and other necessary functions, your body will use it for energy. If it is not needed

due to sufficient intake of other energy sources such as carbohydrates or fats, the protein will be used to create fat and becomes
part of fat cells.

All meat, including seafood, and eggs are an excellent source of
all 22 amino acids. If you are a vegetarian, you can get the essential
amino acids you need by combining plant-based foods together, but it's
a challenge and takes vigilance to get it right. Your body is able to make
the other 13 amino acids on its own, provided there is a sufficient supply
of nitrogen and other molecules from a balanced diet.

So how much protein do we need? Much depends on your age, as
well as the amount and type of exercise you do, but, as a general guide,
0.8 grams of protein per kilogram of body weight should be sufficient.[7]
In the first three years of life, or if you are pregnant or lactating, or
if you exercise a lot, the figure might go as high as 1.25 grams per
kilogram of body weight.

As an example, I weigh 80 kilograms, which equates to a
recommended consumption of 64 grams of protein a day (0.8 × 80).

It's worth spending a week or two weighing and calculating your
protein intake and, while you're at it, measuring your carbohydrate
intake at the same time. It's an important exercise, and the results are
often surprising, with many people coming to the conclusion that,
ironically, we eat too much protein, and for that matter carbohydrate,
and not enough of the healthy fats.

There are many sources of protein. Below are examples with
approximate values showing actual served weight and protein content,
dependent on water content:

Source	% of protein by weight	Typical serve = protein intake
Beef, lamb, or pork	30	200g meat = 66g protein
Chicken or fish	20	200g meat = 40g protein

Eggs	10	70g egg = 7g protein
Cheese	15–40	100g feta = 15g protein 100g parmesan = 40g protein
Lentils	10	100g lentils = 10g protein
Tofu	10	100g tofu = 10g protein
Grains (wheat, oats, rye)	10–15	100g grains = 10–15g protein
Nuts	10–20	100g macadamia = 10g protein 100g almond = 20g protein
Quinoa	4	100g quinoa = 4g protein

Figure 12-5. Protein sources.

Just as not all fat is the same, not all protein is the same.

What is the protein's chemical load from antibiotics, growth hormones, fertilisers, pesticides, and herbicides? How was it grown — from a health, environmental, and ethical perspective? Reminding us of how interconnected we are with nature, it's reassuring to know the healthier and happier an animal is during its life, the more likely it is to produce protein and fat that is healthier for us.

Because of this and other reasons discussed in Chapter 7: Environmental Stress, I believe the consumption of industrialised meat represents too high a price, environmentally, is unsustainable in its current form, and is best avoided. Do not be drawn into the 'wonders' or 'high value' of beef that has been grain-fed for 100 days or more, which is commonly marketed as 'the best meat in the world'.

Extensively marbled meat, most often a reflection of how long an animal is grain-fed, ensures the predictability of meat flavour, overcoming seasonal variations but is essentially a marketing exercise to make it expensive and desirable — from a health perspective, the opposite is true: for both you and the animal. The grains that fatten animals are the same grains that have fattened humans over the last 40 years, as recommended by public health messages. While it's more commercially profitable to fatten cattle, and perhaps also humans, there is clearly a question of health and ethics for both.

I don't have a moral issue with eating meat provided the animal has enjoyed a life that is harmonious with nature — with due regard for the welfare of the animal and the planet. In addition to honouring the animal we kill and then consume, we should think about and use the *entire* animal. We have become preoccupied with muscle meat, which makes up almost the entire display in a butcher shop, the consequence of which is that we have missed out on many nutrients. In some traditional cultures, only organ meat was consumed, while the lean muscle meat was left for the dogs. Organ meats, or offal, are between ten and 100 times higher in nutrients than corresponding muscle meats, and are an excellent example of a nutrient-dense food. One we should be eating more of — and thus honouring the whole animal.

The liver, for instance, is a storage organ for many important nutrients (vitamins A, D, E, K, B12, folic acid; minerals such as copper and iron) and should truly be considered a 'superfood'. As always, provenance is important: the liver is involved in detoxification, so a food animal exposed to toxic chemicals will have a chemical-laden liver, and should be avoided.

	Apple	Carrots	Red meat	Beef liver
Calcium	3.0 mg	3.3 mg	11.0 mg	11.0 mg
Phosphorus	6.0 mg	31.0 mg	140.0 mg	476.0 mg
Magnesium	4.8 mg	6.2 mg	15.0 mg	18.0 mg
Potassium	139.0 mg	222.0 mg	370.0 mg	380.0 mg
Iron	0.1 mg	0.6 mg	3.3 mg	8.8 mg
Zinc	0.05 mg	0.3 mg	4.4 mg	4.0 mg
Copper	0.04 mg	0.08 mg	0.18 mg	12.0 mg
Vitamin A	None	None	40 IU	53,400 IU
Vitamin D	None	None	Trace	19 IU
Vitamin E	0.37 mg	0.11 mg	1.7 mg	0.63 mg
Vitamin C	7.0 mg	6.0 mg	None	27.0 mg

Thiamin	0.03 mg	0.05 mg	0.05 mg	0.26 mg
Riboflavin	0.02 mg	0.05 mg	0.20 mg	4.19 mg
Niacin	0.10 mg	0.60 mg	4.0 mg	16.5 mg
Pantothenic acid	0.11 mg	0.19 mg	0.42 mg	8.8 mg
Vitamin B6	0.03 mg	0.10 mg	0.07 mg	0.73 mg
Folate	8.0 mcg	24.0 mcg	4.0 mcg	145.0 mcg
Biotin	None	0.42 mcg	2.08 mcg	96.0 mcg
Vitamin B12	None	None	1.84 mcg	111.3 mcg

Figure 12-6. The many nutrients provided by liver compared with other foods (100 gram servings).[8]

The choices we make about the things we consume are perhaps our greatest contribution to environmental health and animal welfare, let alone our own health. Beyond what I have already discussed, there are numerous specific health benefits of pasture-fed-and-finished beef, including:

- it contains ten times more beta-carotene, which is important for stimulating the immune system and maintaining healthy vision, skin, and bones
- it has three times more vitamin E, helping prevent cancer and cardiovascular disease
- it has up to 15 times more omega-3 fatty acids, which help reduce blood pressure, maintain brain function, prevent cardiovascular diseases, prevent arthritis, prevent and slow the growth of many cancers, and prevent and treat depression
- it contains twice the conjugated linoleic acid, which lowers the risk of diabetes, heart disease, and many cancers
- it should contain less chemicals, antibiotics, and hormones.

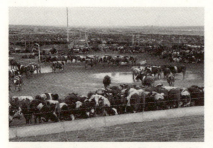

Feedlot beef.

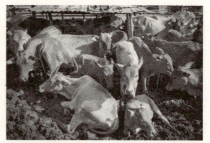

Manure — seen as a toxin, not a resource.

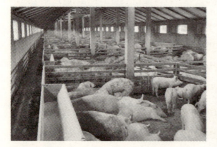

Industrial pork.

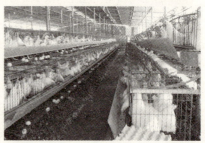

Industrial chicken.

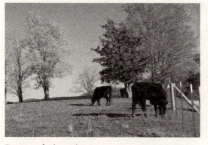

Pasture-fed cattle.

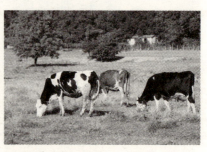

Pasture-fed dairy cows.

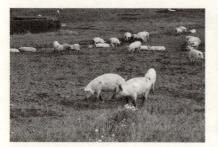

Free-range pigs.

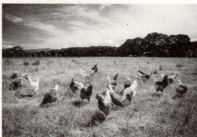

Free-range chickens.

Figure 12-7. These images speak for themselves. You have a choice.

WHAT ABOUT SEAFOOD?

There are many reasons why ancient communities decided to live near the sea, including the availability and abundance of seafood, which, as we are often reminded, is an excellent source of protein and healthy fats. However, while there are many health benefits to eating seafood, there are also risks from toxins. In advice to pregnant women, one of America's top hospitals, the Mayo Clinic, warns: 'Seafood can be a great source of protein, and the omega-3 fatty acids in many fish can promote your baby's brain and eye development. However, some fish and shellfish contain potentially dangerous levels of mercury. Too much mercury could harm your baby's developing nervous system.'[9] Not to mention all the other chemicals, human effluence, plastics, and even radioactive waste that find their way into the rivers and oceans and become an integral part of the food chain.

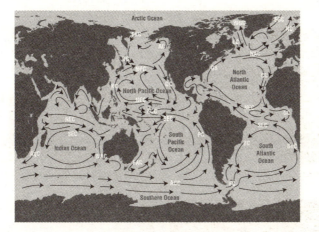

Figure 12-8. We are, via these global ocean currents, all connected, so we are all affected. Pollution on one side of an ocean will invariably affect waterways on the other side.

The sustainability of seafood is also a huge and growing problem, with one study estimating an alarming 90 per cent reduction in sea stocks.[10] In Chapter 7: Environmental Stress, I briefly looked at the issues surrounding fish farming and how feed is sourced, the type of feed, antibiotic use, and the ethics of keeping migratory fish in a confined enclosure. Some people refer to farmed fish as the caged-chicken or feedlot-cattle of the sea. I agree and personally avoid eating farmed fish as well.

ISN'T ALL SALMON GOOD FOR YOU?

The flesh of wild salmon is pink because of the carotenoids they consume; it is darker or lighter depending on the amount of krill and shrimp they eat during migration. Farmed salmon are pink because they are fed artificial dyes. It also takes at least 1.7 kilograms of fishmeal (which, as I mentioned, is gathered using vast nets to trawl the ocean, capturing unintended 'bykill' along the way) to produce around one kilogram of farmed Atlantic salmon. In Australia, salmon producers have reduced the amount of wild fish used in fishmeal, replacing it with poultry, grains, and vegetable proteins.

Farmed fish are kept in small sea pens. High stocking rates in these pens create problems such as:

- high levels of fish effluent in the water
- algal blooms in the surrounding sea
- outbreaks of disease, which can spread beyond the pens and into wild fish stocks
- chemicals and antibiotics finding their way into wild fish — and humans.[11]

So what do you do if you want the nutritional benefit of fish without the ethical and sustainability problems and the chemical load? I suggest eating small sardines, which are an excellent, low-toxicity, nutritious, sustainable choice, particularly when marinated in olive oil. Sardine populations are abundant in most parts of the world, and low down the food chain, making them a sound ecological choice. Sardines have fewer contaminants than larger fish further up the food chain such as tuna, swordfish, farmed salmon, and most other fatty fish.[12] Herring and mackerel are also a rich source of omega-3 fats — richer than many fish-oil supplements. Anchovies are another great choice.

WHAT ABOUT DAIRY?

Many people are allergic to a protein in dairy called casein. Their immune system mistakenly thinks the protein is harmful and creates antibodies that may result in an allergic or autoimmune response. It's not surprising then that many people report feeling healthier without dairy. Walter Willet, head of nutrition at the Harvard School of Public Health, and one of the most cited authors in nutritional-research journals, makes the following points:

- Milk doesn't reduce fractures, and eating dairy products has never been shown to reduce fracture risk. According to the Nurses' Health Study, dairy may actually increase risk of fractures by 50 per cent.[13]
- Countries with the lowest rates of dairy and calcium consumption (such as Africa and Asia) have the lowest rates of osteoporosis.
- Calcium isn't as bone-protective as once thought. Studies of calcium supplementation show no benefit in reducing fracture risk. Vitamin D appears to be more important than calcium in preventing fractures.
- Excess calcium may raise cancer risk. Research shows that a higher intake of calcium and dairy may increase the risk of prostate cancer by 30–50 per cent.[14] Dairy consumption increases the body's level of insulin-like growth factor (IGF-1), which promotes cancer.
- Many people are unable to properly digest milk and other dairy products — whether they are clearly lactose intolerant or lactose sensitive, or they simply notice they just feel better avoiding dairy products.

Clearly Walter Willet, one of the world's most respected independent-of-industry researchers doesn't agree with the advice that daily consumption of dairy is important for our health.

There's no doubt that human infants thrive on breast milk — as do calves and lambs and piglets, but they all eventually stop needing that milk, and go on to live with healthy bones and no 'dairy'. It's also worth mentioning that bones are not just calcium. In fact, they are made up of calcium, zinc, potassium, selenium, magnesium, boron, manganese, phosphorous, silica, iron, chromium, and over 60 trace elements. Having too much calcium has the potential to cause those other minerals to go out of balance, which may go some way to explaining what Willet and others have observed.

Having said that, while I don't drink milk, I do occasionally consume some dairy. If you are consuming dairy, then cultured dairy such as kefir and yoghurt and some softer cheeses may be fine. These products incorporate and utilise their microbes' ability to assist in the digestion of proteins and sugars, which may be otherwise difficult for the body to tolerate.

Principle 4 — vegetables should be the foundation of your nutrition

Vegetables are truly the foundation of a nourishing, nutrient-dense diet — those grown above ground, such as leafy vegetables, are preferable because those grown underground tend to be higher in carbohydrates. Vegetables contain a range of vitamins, minerals, antioxidants, natural fibre, and other important nutrients, and fall into five different colour categories: red, purple/blue, orange, green, and white/brown. Each has its own set of unique disease-fighting compounds, called phytochemicals.

Phytochemicals, or phytonutrients, are biologically active compounds that give fruit and vegetables their bright colour and are associated with healing properties. There are more than 1,000 known phytonutrients and many have important antioxidant and anticancer properties. When you eat vegetables, you counteract the effects of environmental chemicals and toxins, electromagnetic radiation, and stress. Given what we are exposed to in our modern world, think of building resilience as being synonymous with a diet high in a wide variety of vegetables with a wide variety of colours, and therefore phytonutrients.

Phytochemical	Food source	Protective action
allyl sulphides	garlic, onions, shallots, chives	lower risk of stomach and colon cancer
sulphoraphanes, indoles, isothiocyanates	broccoli, cabbage, Brussels sprouts, cauliflower, kohlrabi, watercress, turnips, Chinese cabbage	lower risk of breast, stomach, and lung cancers
carotenes	carrots, dried apricots and peaches, cantaloupe, green leafy vegetables, sweet potatoes, yams	lower risk of lung and many other cancers
lycopenes, p-Coumaric acid, chlorogenic acid	tomatoes	lower risk of prostate and stomach cancer
monoterpenes	cherries, essential oils, orange-peel oil, citrus-peel oil, caraway, dill, spearmint, lemongrass	lower risk of breast, skin, liver, lung, stomach, and pancreatic cancers
polyphenols	green tea, berries, cherries	lower risk of skin, lung, and stomach cancers, and heart disease
phytoestrogens	soybeans, fermented tofu, miso and tempeh, herbs such as thyme, licorice, and verbena	can interfere with tumour-cell growth, which may help prevent cancer

Figure 12-9. Eating by colours provides a wide range of benefits.

WHAT ABOUT FRUIT?

While I never put a limit on the number of above-ground vegetables I eat, I do restrict my fruit intake. As you now know, many modern fruits have been bred to be sweeter, resulting in a higher sugar content. When eating fruit, I choose mainly berries, apples, and bananas — and when they're in season, figs, stone fruits, and mango. When it comes to fruit juices, many boast they have 'no added sugar', but they can still contain as much natural sugar as a 600 mL soft drink — they are best avoided. Think of it this way: you couldn't possibly eat the five to six apples that go into a glass of apple juice, and you would also be missing out on the fibre.

WHAT ABOUT GRAINS?

In previous chapters, I have spent a good amount of time exploring grains; they have come under a great deal of scrutiny and criticism in recent years. An ever-increasing number of people are gluten intolerant (suffering coeliac disease) or gluten sensitive. The gluten that seems to be the main problem is found in the modern varieties of wheat, barley, rye, and some oats.

If you are gluten intolerant with coeliac disease, total elimination is critical to your health. You can't be a little bit intolerant — it's like describing yourself as 'a little bit pregnant'; it's all or none. If you believe you have non-coeliac gluten sensitivity, it is worth visiting an integrative medical practitioner, nutritionist, or naturopath who can assist and investigate with appropriate testing and an elimination diet.

For those who have a sensitivity, depending on how much gluten you find you can tolerate without compromising your health, try sourdough, which uses traditional grains such as emmer and einkorn. Other alternatives are ancient grains such as spelt or kamut.

Sourdough contains a combination of lactobacillus culture in combination with yeast, making it more easily digested and more nutritious. These microbes neutralise the potentially damaging phytic acid, or phytates, also present in grains, which can interfere with the absorption of vitamins and minerals. They also convert sugars to lactic acid, which slows down the rate at which glucose from the carbohydrate in the bread is released into the bloodstream. This may make the gluten protein in bread more digestible and less likely to cause problems, but limiting intake may still be preferable.

If you can, avoid breads made with the modern, high-yield, high-gluten semi-dwarf variety of wheat, and ensure the bread has been allowed to rise overnight. Other grains such as corn, rice, soy, millet, and sorghum belong to a completely different subfamily of grass plants, and their gluten proteins are very different, too, making them somewhat more tolerable for consumption.

Many people around the world eat rice, which is the least reactive of the grains and obviously has a significant role to play in literally feeding the world. Completely dismissing all grains as a food source is a first-world option, which many people around the globe don't have the luxury to be 'confused' about.

LEGUMES

Legumes comprise some 13,000 species, such as peas, beans, lentils, and soybeans — they are characterised by their ability to take nitrogen from the air and convert it into protein within the plant's seeds. They play an important role in bringing nitrogen into the soil and have played a critical role in maintaining soil quality and fertility in agriculture over the millennia. Yet as the consumption of grains has gone up in the western world, consumption of legumes has decreased.

The relatively high protein content (for a vegetable) in peas, beans, and lentils make them an important food source in many parts of the world. Legumes are high in fibre and contain a vast range of vitamins and minerals that help maintain good health. The minerals magnesium, phosphorus, iron, and molybdenum, as well as B-group vitamins such as folate and thiamine are all present in legumes. The high level of the B-group vitamin folic acid, along with B6 and B12, helps the body convert homocysteine, an important inflammatory marker of heart disease, into an innocuous form in the bloodstream. Legumes also contain omega-3 and omega-6 fatty acids, with kidney and pinto beans particularly high in omega-3.

Like grains, legumes contain antinutrients to protect the grain; these include phytic acids (which affect our ability to absorb nutrients) as well as complex carbohydrates (which can pose a painful challenge in the form of wind in the human gut). This antinutrient problem requires preparation, which usually involves soaking the legumes in slightly warm water with a tablespoon of apple-cider vinegar for several hours or overnight, draining them, and then slow cooking, combining with herbs and spices.[15]

GO NUTS — AND SEEDS!

Nuts are a whole, unprocessed food containing protein, fats, vitamins, and fibre with many proven health benefits. They are the perfect snack food, and I love them. In order to neutralise the phytic acid that occurs in nuts, soak them overnight in water with a touch of salt, then thoroughly strain and dry roast in an oven heated to 100–120°C for three to six hours, depending on the type of nut and heat of your oven. This process is called 'activating'. You need to know your own oven and experiment to get the best results, but the nuts should be dry, crunchy, and delicious. Store the activated nuts in a glass jar in the fridge.

Nut	Nutrition
Walnuts	High in omega-3 fatty acid (fights inflammation) and manganese (which may reduce PMS symptoms)
Brazil nuts	High in selenium (assists in creating antioxidants) and zinc (for healthy skin and ageing)
Almonds	Have the nutritional benefits of other nuts plus the highest amount of healthy vegetable protein (six grams per serving), the highest amount of calcium, and a generous dose of vitamin E, which boosts memory and potentially reduces cognitive decline
Pecans	High in phytosterol, which assists prostate health and can reduce prostate and urinary symptoms in older men
Pistachios	Contain L-arginine, which can make the lining of arteries more flexible and potentially reduce heart-attack and stroke risk
Peanuts	Contain folic acid and vitamin E for improved brain health. If eating in butter form, ensure it has no added sugar. This spread is rich in vitamin E, niacin, folate, protein, and manganese.

Pine nuts	Contain manganese, an important co-factor for some of the body's most powerful antioxidants. Manganese ensures healthy bone structure, bone metabolism, and creates essential enzymes for building bones. It also acts as a co-enzyme for metabolic activity.

Figure 12-10. Which nuts should you be eating? Which offer the best nutrition?.

In Chapter 6: Nutritional Stress, I asked the question, 'What does your poo say about you?' I have found an excellent addition to my diet that helps with regular bowel movements, which as I've said is our body's way of sending us an important 'message' each and every day. This addition is thanks to holistic nutritionist Sarah Britton. It is relatively high in protein, flourless, filled with nutrient-dense ingredients, and optimistically (but accurately) called 'The Life-changing Loaf of Bread'.[16] While not strictly 'bread' as you may know it, it delivers on its promise; we have been making loaves of it for over two years at home. If you accept that your bowel movements are a good reflection of gut health, then I would recommend you give this a go — there is a very good chance your body will thank you.

This loaf uses whole grains, nuts, and seeds. It is relatively high in protein and clearly high in fibre. It is gluten-free and vegan-friendly.

The life-changing loaf of bread

(Copyright © Sarah Britton 2013, mynewroots.org)

INGREDIENTS

Makes one loaf

1 cup (135 g) sunflower seeds

½ cup (90 g) flaxseed (linseed)

½ cup (65 g) activated hazelnuts

   (all soaked and dry roasted beforehand)

1½ cups (145 g) rolled oats

2 tbsp. chia seeds

4 tbsp. psyllium seed husks (or 3 tbsp. psyllium husk powder)

1 tsp. fine-grain sea salt (add ½ tsp. if using coarse salt)

1 tbsp. maple syrup

3 tbsp. melted coconut oil or ghee

1½ cups (350 mL) water

INSTRUCTIONS

1. In a flexible, silicone bread pan, combine all dry ingredients, stirring well.
2. Whisk maple syrup, oil, and water together in a measuring cup.
3. Add this to the dry ingredients and mix very well until everything is completely soaked and dough becomes very thick (if the dough is too thick to stir, add one or two teaspoons of water until the dough is manageable).
4. Smooth out the top with the back of a spoon.
5. Let sit out on the counter for at least two hours, or all day or overnight. To ensure the dough is ready, it should retain its shape even when you pull the sides of the bread pan away from it.
6. Preheat oven to 175°C.
7. Place bread pan in the oven on the middle rack, and bake for 20 minutes.
8. Remove bread from bread pan, place it upside down directly on the oven rack and bake for another 30–40 minutes. Bread is done when it sounds hollow when tapped.
9. Let cool completely before slicing (difficult, but important).
10. Store bread in a tightly sealed container for up to five days. Freezes well too — slice before freezing for quick and easy toast!

NOTES

*   You rule the bread, not the other way around. Dump all the ingredients into the bread pan, stir, and let it sit for a couple of

hours. Or overnight. Or all day. Or however long or short you find convenient.

- It responds well to being cooked for an extra 15–20 minutes, and this makes it easier to cut thinly.
- Out of maple syrup? Use honey! The only thing to emphasise is to replace the ingredients in the same proportion and with a similar ingredient for the best results. The rest is your call.
- If you don't have hazelnuts, you could use almonds. I've also sometimes used cashews or brazil nuts. The bread holds together better if you break up or grind the nuts.
- According to the University of Chicago's Coeliac Disease Centre, a large body of scientific evidence accumulated over more than 15 years has proven that oats are completely safe for more than 99 per cent of coeliac sufferers. Oats are not related to gluten-containing grains such as wheat, barley, and rye.
- If you don't like oats, you could use rolled spelt, but it does contain gluten.
- Each loaf yields approximately 180 grams of carbohydrate. If you can cut 15 slices, this makes 12 grams of carbohydrate per slice (relevant to the next Principle).

Principle 5 — how many carbs?

To have a 'healthy' diet, we are taught that it is important we maintain or sustain a consistent blood-sugar level. This in turn creates the metabolic system of a 'sugar burner', where your body runs on glucose for fuel. You could be excused for thinking that glucose was the only fuel our bodies used. It is not. The alternative is to be a 'fat burner', where your body's primary source of fuel is fat. Yet when dietary fat is consumed in conjunction with a sugar-burner diet, it is far more likely to be stored as excess.

Nutrition expert Nora Gedgaudas uses the analogy of a fire

to explore the role of macronutrients in our diet and metabolism.[17] Carbohydrates can be seen as metabolic 'kindling' — whole grains as 'twigs'; white rice, bread, and pasta as 'paper' — and alcoholic beverages as 'kerosene'. And although all these elements can keep a fire alight, you would need to sit by the fire and continually load it up. In contrast, you could place a nice big 'fat' log on the fire and you wouldn't need to think about it too regularly and your fuel wouldn't take up much space.

So how much carbohydrate should you be consuming?

When making a decision, it is good to know who you are listening to, and what interests these experts and agencies are supporting. As I explored in Chapter 6: Nutritional Stress, the United States Department of Agriculture (USDA) developed the Food Pyramid, the foundation of which was between six and 11 serves of grains per day (as is still endorsed by the National Health and Medical Research Council).

According to the Dietitians Association of Australia, the recommended daily intake of carbohydrate is 310 grams per day. And so it's worth going to the USDA Interactive DRI Calculator for Healthcare Professionals and asking, 'Is this an exercise in marketing or is this sound health advice?'

After I entered my age, weight, height, and activity level, and ticked all the boxes for macronutrients, it gave me my 'Recommended Intake per day' for carbohydrate: it came in at a staggering 329–475 grams per day. Recommendations such as this have created entire nations of sugar burners, where we constantly need to graze (not unlike cows) to maintain our moods, emotions, energy levels, weight, lifestyle, and so on.

The advice that the USDA suggests health practitioners should be giving their patients sounds very similar to the advice one might have got from the 1992 Food Pyramid and 2011 MyPlate, which I have already discussed; basically high-carb, low-fat, and avoid cholesterol. Clearly, things have not really changed, at an official level at least.

Macronutrient	Recommended intake per day
Carbohydrate	329–475 g
Total fibre	30 g
Protein	67 g
Fat	65–114 g
Saturated fatty acids	As low as possible while consuming a nutritionally adequate diet
Trans fatty acids	As low as possible while consuming a nutritionally adequate diet
alpha-linolenic acid	1.6 g
Linoleic acid	14 g
Dietary cholesterol	As low as possible while consuming a nutritionally adequate diet
Total water	3.7 litres (about 16 cups)

Figure 12-11. The recommended daily macronutrient intake for me according to the USDA.

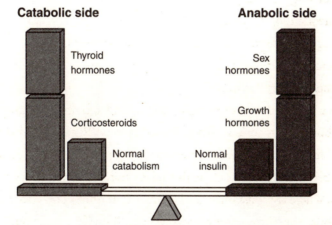

Figure 12-12. The balancing act between anabolic hormones on the right and catabolic hormones on the left. When we eat the right amount of carbohydrates per day, we keep these hormones in balance.

In the landmark book *Life Without Bread*, Austrian physician Wolfgang Lutz, who with over 50 years of independent clinical experience in this area and, importantly, no ties to industry, recommends that for most people the ideal amount of carbohydrate is 72 grams a day.[18] This, he says, not 310 grams, is the ideal level for important regulatory hormones such as insulin, the thyroid hormones, and other anabolic and catabolic hormones. From my own experience, 70–80 grams per day is very doable and sustainable. It's a good target to aim for.

To work out the carbohydrate content of food, I suggest measuring and calculating your servings using various carbohydrate-counter apps or booklets. As with proteins, the weight of the serve is different to the actual carbohydrate content of what you are eating.

Food	Actual CHO content (grams/100g serve)	Dietary fibre (grams/100g serve)
Broccoli	7	2.6
Cauliflower	5	3.5
Eggplant	3	2.5
Peas	6	3
Pumpkin	7	0.5
Potatoes	19	2.2
Sweet potatoes	20	3
Carrots	10	2.8
Onions	9	1.7
Beetroot	10	2.8
Spinach	3.6	2.2
Lettuce	2.9	1.3
Tomatoes	3.9	1.2
Oranges	12	2.4
Apples	14	2.4
Bananas	23	2.6
Strawberries	8	2
Mango	15	1.6

Figure 12-13. Total carbohydrate (CHO) and dietary fibre per serve of food. This highlights the difference between above-ground and below-ground vegetables, as well as the carbohydrate content of fruits.

To put Figure 12-13 into perspective: a medium-sized potato is 200 grams, which would contain about 40 grams of carbohydrate; an average orange weighs 250 grams and contains 30 grams of carbohydrate; and 200 grams of broccoli contains 14 grams of carbohydrate.

You should only need to measure and weigh food over a one-to-two-week period to learn the approximate carbohydrate amount you are actually consuming.

When lowering the carbohydrate or protein content of your meals, it's important *not* to also go low-fat. Many people believe they are being extra 'diligent' and doubling their health benefit by appeasing both health messages, eating low-carb and also low-fat. It won't work; you'll be hungry.

Like so many things in health, people often enthusiastically embrace a new concept and overdo it. It's a bad scenario when someone has eliminated processed foods and sugar, but continues to embrace the recommended carbohydrate intake and also decides to enthusiastically embrace 'healthy fats'. The health outcomes will be poor and so will the waistline.

Instead, become a fat burner. A low-carb diet is often referred to as a ketogenic diet, as the liver breaks fat into ketones, which can be used instead of glucose for energy. As a general rule, healthy fats are your friends, from so many health perspectives — but when you are eating low-carb, they ensure you will also, and importantly, not be hungry.

Principle 6 — cultivate healthy gut bacteria

There are 37 trillion cells in the human body, but we share our bodies with ten times that number of microbes, the vast majority of which are beneficial bacteria, and most of which occur in the gut.

We have become very focused on our own human genetic code, made up of 23 pairs of chromosomes and over 20,000 genes, but, when we put that into a broader perspective and take into account the genetic information we carry in our bodies, we see that our microbial partners'

DNA runs into millions of genes. In fact, 99 per cent of the genetic code in our body is microbial, so it really is in our best interests to ensure the bulk of the cells and genetic code in our body is working for us and not against us.

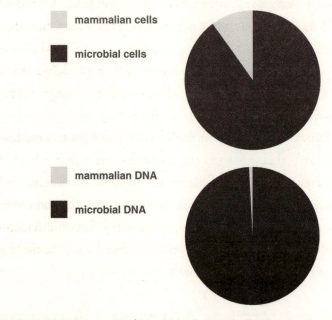

mammalian cells

microbial cells

mammalian DNA

microbial DNA

Above: Figure 12-14. Percentage of microbial cells in our body (90 per cent).
Below: Figure 12-15. Genetic code in our microbial DNA (99 per cent).

The number and type of bacteria that live in the digestive tract are now recognised as critical to our physical and mental wellbeing. There is a strong case to say that when you eat and drink something, it is best to first consider and prioritise the bacteria in your body. Are you feeding your friends or your foes? They will either keep you healthy or make you sick, physically and mentally.

The gut itself is also referred to as the 'second brain' because it contains over 100 million neurons, more than either the spinal cord or peripheral nervous system.[19] The nervous system that controls the gut (the enteric nervous system) uses more than 30 neurotransmitters, just like the brain, and 95 per cent of the body's serotonin (an important neurotransmitter that stabilises mood and is implicated in depression and other mental health issues) is found in the gut. In addition, 80 per cent of the body's immune system is also located in the gut. One of the key factors in promoting a healthy gut biome is dietary fibre, found in vegetables, nuts and seeds, legumes, and some fruits.

Fermented foods, a traditional way of preserving food (and another important lesson from the past), are also beneficial for a healthy gut biome. Most vegetables can be fermented to provide good nutrition year-round. This is beautifully presented in a book called *The Art of Fermentation* by Sandor Katz, which outlines a huge range of fermentation possibilities.[20]

When fermenting food, begin with lacto-fermentation, a method of food preservation that enhances the nutrient content of the food. The action of the bacteria makes minerals in cultured foods more readily available to the body. The bacteria also produce vitamins and enzymes that are beneficial for our digestion. One of my favourite fermented foods is sauerkraut, and there are many variations. It's easy to make and a great accompaniment to many meals.

Sauerkraut

INGREDIENTS

1 medium head of organic cabbage
1–3 tbsp. sea salt
Tiny pinch of caraway seed

INSTRUCTIONS

1. Chop or shred cabbage. Sprinkle with salt.
2. Knead the cabbage with clean hands, or pound with a potato masher or large pestle, until there is enough liquid released to cover the cabbage (approximately ten minutes).
3. Stuff the cabbage into a glass jar, firmly pressing the cabbage to

ensure it is covered by the liquid. Keeping the cabbage covered is very important in the fermentation process. If necessary, add a little bit of water to completely cover the cabbage (or knead/pound for longer). Don't fill the jar to the top.

4. Cover the jar with an airtight lid.

5. Sit at room temperature (15–21°C is preferred) until desired flavour and texture is achieved (at least three to four days, but up to one to two weeks). If using a tight lid, unscrew and allow the culture to 'burp' daily to release excess pressure. Ensure the cabbage remains covered with liquid. You may want to place the jar on a plate should any liquid escape as the fermentation process continues.

6. Once the sauerkraut is finished, put the jar into the fridge. It will keep for months. The sauerkraut's flavour will continue to develop as it ages.

I grew up with my mother's chicken soup as a panacea for all ailments, and, every time I hear people listing the many wonders of bone broth, I am reminded of my mother's wisdom — and, for that matter, my grandmother's, too. Bone broth has been a part of many traditional diets and is a rich source of nutrients — minerals, collagen, glutamine, and many other amino acids — particularly when sourced from animals raised on healthy pastures. It's a great way to support the immune system, rebuild a healthy gut, help with joint pain, maintain healthy skin, and boost detoxification. Broth is soothing and delicious.

Broth is also an ideal way to honour the whole animal, by making use of its bones. It can be consumed as a drink or added to slow-roasted meat, soups, stews, and braised vegetables for extra flavour. Apart from its many health benefits, bone broth is easy to prepare and inexpensive. There are many ways to make broth, but ensure you use organic, grass-fed bones — they're better for you, and you'll taste the difference.

Bone broth

INGREDIENTS

2 kg beef marrow, knuckle bones, or leftover bones from a roast

1 kg meat rib or neck bones (I like to use chicken bones
   or chicken feet)

10 L cold water

¼ cup apple-cider vinegar

Add garlic or Celtic sea salt near the end of cooking for
   added flavour

INSTRUCTIONS

1. Place all ingredients in the pot and bring to boil.
2. After it comes to the boil, skim off the top, and simmer for
    between eight and 12 hours. The longer it cooks, the richer the
    flavour.
3. Once all cooked, remove the bones with tongs and strain the
    broth into a large bowl.
4. The broth can keep in the fridge for a week or in the freezer for
    six months.

Principle 7 — water is still the best drink of all

Sanitation and clean water are two of the greatest breakthroughs ever made in public health. As humans, we are made up of 65 per cent water and have been drinking it along with the rest of the animal kingdom for millions of years. Water is vital.

Filtering water is a philosophical and health issue based on reducing your overall chemical load. In modern cities, people don't die from drinking tap water, but I choose to lower my chemical load by filtering it with a reverse-osmosis filter. I do this to remove what can seem to be an overwhelming list of chemicals that can be found in the tap water we drink: aluminium, barium, cadmium, chlorine, copper, cryptosporidium, *E. coli* bacteria, giardia parasites, heavy metal, hydrocarbons, iron, lead, manganese, mercury, microbial cysts, nitrate, oestrogen, polychlorinated biphenyl (PCBs), potassium, radium, selenium, and sodium. And, of course, here in Australia, fluoride.

In the morning on waking, I add one tablespoon of organic, raw apple-cider vinegar to a 250 mL glass of warm water, which I drink while preparing breakfast. Apple-cider vinegar is an excellent remedy for digestive distress, helps in detoxification and digestion, and reduces intestinal bloating. The acetic and butyric acids promote gastrointestinal health by balancing pH levels and encouraging friendly bacterial growth in the gut.

At other times in the day, I add just a few grains of Celtic sea salt or Himalayan rock salt to a large glass of reverse-osmosis-filtered water to provide healthy trace elements. If I can taste any salt, I've added far too much. It's my version of home-made, pure 'mineral water'. I avoid plastic bottled water and prefer to have a stainless-steel refillable bottle or a glass bottle at my desk or at work.

For effective digestion, it's best to avoid drinking water for 20 minutes before a meal, during a meal, and for 20 minutes after a meal. Stomach acid has a lower pH and is very acidic for a reason: it needs to be acidic for effective digestion. Diluting acid by drinking water while you eat reduces your ability to effectively digest your food, particularly proteins. The habit of wait staff in restaurants constantly topping up your still or sparkling water may look like good service, but it's not good for your digestion.

The growing popularity of alkaline water is a good example of a linear way of approaching health. The solution to high acidity isn't to drink alkaline water. A glass of water with a squeeze of lemon juice or a glass of apple-cider vinegar 20 minutes before a meal makes the water mildly acidic and promotes good digestion: the mild acidity of the water sends important messages to the gut that food is on its way.

Alkaline water sends the wrong message.

Sports drinks, carbonated drinks (diet or otherwise), and fruit juices are also best avoided completely. Freshly prepared, organic vegetable juices, on the other hand, can be a good source of antioxidants and phytochemicals, and form part of many health regimens and detox programs.

CAFFEINE

Many people can't imagine starting the day without drinking a cup of coffee. Coffee is a complex brew, containing chemicals that have both protective and adverse effects on various systems throughout the body, such as the skeletal, reproductive, nervous, and cardiovascular systems.[21] It contains some antioxidant, certainly improves energy levels, and may help with diabetes, various cancers, Parkinson's disease, and Alzheimer's disease.[22]

But you need to remember it is a stimulant — it affects insulin levels, blood-sugar levels, and the stress hormones adrenaline and cortisol. If you must drink coffee, moderation is the key, which to me would mean one to two cups of real coffee per day. Avoid drinking coffee after lunch because it affects the ability to get a good night's sleep.

Keep in mind that caffeine is also found in many teas — and decaffeinated products may still contain caffeine. Avoid energy drinks, which contain high caffeine and sugar levels, preservatives, and very low pH (high acidity) levels, as well as high-fructose corn syrup (HFCS) or artificial sweeteners such as aspartame.

Food or drink	Caffeine content (mg)	Serve
Instant coffee	60–80	250 mL
Cafe coffee (e.g. latte or cappuccino)	113–282	250 mL
Espresso/short black	25–214	1 shot
Energy drink	80	250 mL
Cola	36–48	375 mL

Iced coffee	30–200	500 mL
Starbucks Breakfast Blend brewed coffee	300–564	600 mL ('Venti')
Black tea	25–110	250 mL
Green tea	30–50	250 mL
Milk chocolate	20	100 g

Figure 12-16. Caffeine content of various beverages and milk chocolate.

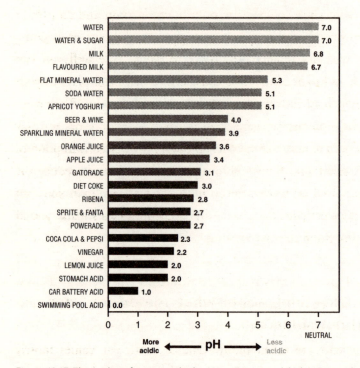

Figure 12-17. The acidity of common drinks. Note: 7 is neutral; below 7 is acidic. pH is not a linear scale, meaning the difference between 6 and 7 is very significant. Clearly, I'm not suggesting car battery acid and swimming pool acid is a common drink — these have been included as a reference.

ALCOHOL

There are many reasons we choose to drink alcohol: relaxation, as part of a social gathering, at celebrations or funerals, as a way to deal with stress, or to help us get to sleep. I enjoy drinking a glass of wine, but I don't think drinking is good for my health, for the reasons I described in Chapter 6: Nutritional Stress.

My approach to nutrition is a percentage game. I aim to make healthy choices at least 80 per cent of the time. When I'm in great form, I make them 90 per cent of the time. Should I ever reach 100 per cent, I would probably irritate my family, friends, and patients, and perhaps even become a social outcast. But when diagnosed with a disease, as I have been, I certainly aim for the higher percentages, to build resilience into my immune system.

As I've said, you should drink only in moderation and aim for at least four to five alcohol-free days per week. The benefits of avoiding alcohol are well documented. In order to gauge how well you can actually feel, and to become more conscious of the role it plays in your life, give up alcohol for several weeks. It will surprise you. Try not to become sanctimonious or evangelical during this period, or you may lose friends. Be content just to observe. Stopping your consumption of alcohol will almost-certainly improve your sleep, certainly reduce the load on your liver, and provide you with more energy than you ever imagined. It's worth seeing what a difference it makes so that you at least have something to compare it to.

Principle 8 — think about what you put on your skin, and get some sun

Not all nutrients are taken orally. One in particular comes mostly through our skin after it receives the rays of the sun.

Our relationship with the sun has changed since I was young, when the aim at the beginning of each summer was to get the first 'burn' out of the way. In those days, and I'm going back to the 1960s, once the skin peeled you were 'set' for an endless summer of sun, surf, and a great tan. Thankfully, this is not the approach taken today, although I feel we have moved too much in the opposite direction. The message to stay out of the sun has led to widespread vitamin D deficiency — a worldwide pandemic with far-reaching health consequences.[23]

For millions of years, we evolved under the warmth of the sun. In the last 30–40 years, sunshine has been demonised, becoming something to avoid because of fears of melanoma. Ironically, while staying out of the sun is good advice to deal with the incidence of skin cancer, vitamin D deficiency is now associated with ill health and many common diseases that are remarkably prevalent in our modern world: low bone density and broken bones due to osteoporosis, muscle weakness, diabetes, multiple sclerosis, cardiovascular disease, colon cancer, dementia, depression, and an overall increased risk of dying prematurely.[24] Sunlight is the best and most available source of vitamin D, with experts suggesting 20 minutes of exposure in the middle of the day to be ideal — and it's free.

In a discussion about vitamin D in 2013, it occurred to me that I had never been tested. I was alarmed when I realised that I was in fact deficient, very deficient. I had a reading of 40 nmol/L compared with a normal range of 51–140 nmol/L; around 90 nmol/L is ideal for most, but if you have a history of cancer your level should be on the higher end of the range. Because of my work and indoor gym-based exercise routine, I had probably been at that low level for over 30 years!

Along with vitamin D, sun exposure is also an important source of nitric oxide, which as I've also discussed is a simple yet vital compound central to the regulation of many biochemical and biological processes in the body, including improving blood flow and thus oxygen to the brain, heart, and other organs, while also decreasing blood clotting and a build-up of plaque in the blood vessels.

The next time you have a blood test, ask your doctor to check out your vitamin D levels. Until then, make sure you get some sun.

THE SUNSCREEN EXPERIMENT

Protecting ourselves from skin cancer by not getting too much sun exposure is, of course, important, but most sunscreens contain chemicals that are chosen to be absorbed into the skin, and, while they do protect from the sun's UV rays, they can also cause harm. As anyone using a nicotine or hormone patch would know, skin is an excellent pathway to the internal body.

Ingredient	Effect
oxybenzone	can cause an eczema-like allergic reaction disrupts hormones 97 per cent of Americans have this chemical circulating in their bodies; it can accumulate more quickly than our bodies can get rid of it
octinoxate	disrupts hormones affects the oestrogen of other humans and wildlife, too, should they come into contact with the chemical once it gets into water produces free radicals, which are toxic to cells, damage DNA, and may lead to cancer
retinyl palmitate (vitamin A palmitate)	when exposed to the sun's UV rays, breaks down and produces free radicals may speed the development of malignant cells and skin tumours when applied to skin before sun exposure
homosalate	disrupts hormones accumulates more quickly than our bodies can get rid of it
octocrylene	when exposed to the sun's UV rays, breaks down and produces free radicals accumulates within your body in measurable amounts can be toxic to the environment
paraben preservatives	can induce allergic reactions disrupts hormones can cause problems with development and reproduction

Figure 12-18. Six common ingredients in commercially available sunscreens.

In the last 10–15 years, sunscreen has incorporated nanoparticles, products engineered on a molecular scale. This is a whole new area where the science is far outstripping our ability to determine the exact health and environmental impacts. Experts are unsure about the risks to health, so I return to a simple idea: let's go back to the precautionary principle again — if something has the potential to cause harm, avoid it. Until it is proven to be safe, avoid it.

When we are talking about total chemical load, the precautionary principle is again important. Each day in our modern world, our bodies are exposed to thousands of chemicals. Why add to the load by applying toxic chemical and nanoparticles through sunscreen? I want my skin to be exposed to the sun to get the many health benefits, while ensuring I don't overdo that exposure and burn my skin, but I also want to avoid applying chemicals. I don't want to be part of the sunscreen experiment.

SENSIBLE SUN ADVICE

The best ways to get the benefits of sunshine and vitamin D and at the same time protect yourself:

- get 20 or more minutes of sunshine daily, preferably when your shadow is shorter than you are
- cover up with light clothing and a hat before you get burnt
- wear natural, organic sunscreen or zinc-oxide-based sunscreen if you're going to stay out for a long period of time
- eat a nutrient-dense diet to build resilience, health, and wellbeing and also to protect your skin
- if you get burnt, use a mixture of aloe, coconut oil, and vitamin E on your skin.

PERSONAL-CARE PRODUCTS

Personal-care and homecare products are also a major source of antinutrients to our bodies. Be aware of the ingredients in products and make choices that 'nourish' you with a lower toxic load. An excellent resource is *The Chemical Maze* by Bill Statham, available as a book or smartphone app.[25] There are many others. Essentially, avoidance is the best app-roach (if you'll excuse the 'dad joke').

Another excellent resource comes from building biologist Nicole Bijlsma, whose website and book *Healthy Home, Healthy Family* deals with how your home and the products you choose affect your health.[26] Again, I have interviewed Nicole on my podcast, and I would highly recommend her expertise to alert you to the potential problems that we can face on a daily basis in our own homes. She also offers some very simple steps to minimise the effects on your health:

1. **Take your shoes off before you enter the home.** This will significantly reduce the dust load.

2. **Use a vacuum cleaner fitted with a HEPA filter and motorised head.** Vacuum cleaners that are *not* fitted with a HEPA filter will exacerbate exposure to allergens like mould, dust mites, and dander by causing them to become airborne. Investing in a good vacuum cleaner is important in establishing a healthy home for children and is critical if anybody in the household suffers from asthma or allergies.

3. **Air your home by opening windows.** Do this as often as you can (unless you live near a major road, heavy industry, an open-cut mine, or fields during crop-dusting season). A healthy home smells like fresh air!

4. **Reduce the number of chemicals to clean your home.** Damp microfibre cloths are great for dusting and to reduce the microbial load in the home.

5. **Use the sun.** Put chopping boards, soft toys, pillows and mattresses, pet bedding, and other fabric furnishings out to air on a regular basis.

6. **Store food and beverages in glass, stainless steel, and lead-free ceramics.** Avoid plastics, pewter, highly coloured ceramics, ceramics with a corroded glaze, and leaded crystal.

7. **Avoid air fresheners, pesticides, and artificial fragrances.** Many are lung irritants and may also contain hormone-disrupting chemicals.

8. **Make space for your electrical appliances.** Ensure they are at least one metre away from your bed, favourite couch, and any other area where you spend time, to reduce your exposure to electromagnetic fields.

9. **Use a water filter.** Chlorine and fluoride in drinking water are associated with health risks, not to mention the long list of potential ingredients that find their way in to tap water.

10. **Remove visible mould.** Use a damp microfibre cloth that has been soaked in a solution of 80 per cent white vinegar to 20 per cent water.

To prevent the mould coming back, find and address the source of moisture.

Your choice of personal-care products, detergents, and other cleaning products around the house, just like your choice of foods, has the greatest potential to limit the effect of chemicals on you. Take the time to lessen the load. We have enough to contend with that we have no control over, so why not make the best choices about those things we do have control over?

Principle 9 — fasting

I'm not sure there was ever a time in human history when three meals a day, together with morning and afternoon tea, were part of a person's daily routine or expectation. It is something, however, that became an absolute necessity once the unprecedented demonisation of fat became part of the accepted public health message — and we all became hungrier.

Let's face it, lose the fat in your diet and follow the recommended Food Pyramid of the last 30 years, and you were bound to be hungry. This dovetailed nicely with the tsunami of processed and fast food that has characterised the same period.

Fasting has been a ritual in so many religious and cultural practices, a period of 'cleansing' for both the spiritual and physical being. More recently, the issue of intermittent fasting has gained popularity with the 5:2 concept of normal eating for five days and restriction to 500–600 calories for two days.[27] When you think about it from a historical and evolutionary perspective, it makes so much sense.

There are many benefits, including positive effects on the following areas:

- **Insulin levels.** Blood levels of insulin drop significantly, which facilitates fat burning. Remember: the lower your insulin, the healthier you will be.

- **Human growth hormone.** The blood levels of growth hormone may increase as much as fivefold. Higher levels of this hormone facilitate fat burning and muscle gain, and have numerous other benefits.
- **Cellular repair.** The body induces important cellular-repair processes, such as removing waste material from cells.
- **Gene expression.** There are beneficial changes in several genes and molecules related to longevity and protection against disease.

It doesn't get much cheaper or more accessible than fasting. Again, there are clearly lessons to be learned from the past, where cultures have used fasting as a purification and an opportunity to reflect mentally and physically. Over the millennia, our ability to fast would have helped ensure our survival. Perhaps it still holds true today.

Principle 10 — detoxing

In Chapter 7: Environmental Stress, I outlined some of the problems we face from environmental chemicals, and also raised concerns about the ubiquitous nature of electromagnetic radiation in our modern world. Building resilience is the key, and, fortunately, our bodies have built-in mechanisms to help us detox. It's easy to feel overwhelmed by the barrage of information about the toxins we are exposed to, but, with careful choices, you can eliminate most of your exposure. Here are some key points:

- What you consume and put on your skin or in your home can significantly reduce your toxic load. Some estimates suggest you can reduce the toxic load by as much as 80–90 per cent simply by making wise choices.
- Your kidneys are an excellent filtration system, so drink lots of purified water.
- Consuming herbal teas (such as organic green, dandelion, and milk

thistle) aids your body's ability to eliminate toxins.

- Sweating is one of the best ways of detoxifying the body. Exercise comes with extra benefits, but dry saunas are also good for building up a sweat.

- Vegetable juicing concentrates the phytonutrients. These vitamins and minerals regulate detoxifying enzymes in the liver, increase antioxidants, and reduce inflammation.

- Regular bowel movements are essential to removing toxins — remember to squat.

- The liver is a major detox organ, so look after it by reducing your chemical load, limiting your alcohol intake, and eliminating seed oils, sugar, preservatives, and all processed foods.

- Keep an open and positive mind. Elevated cortisol and adrenaline levels compromise your internal organs, including your liver, and your ability to absorb nutrients and eliminate toxins.

- Remember to breathe through your nose!

- Dry skin brushing is a traditional health practice in which a dry brush made from natural material is rubbed over a dry body, brushing towards the heart (the same direction your lymph flows). I've done it for over 25 years, and the benefits are more than skin deep. It is invigorating, removes dead skin, improves blood flow, and assists lymphatic drainage with benefits to the immune system. As an added bonus, it feels great!

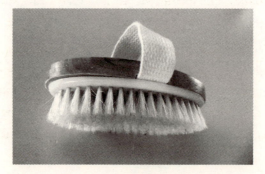

Figure 12-19. Natural fibre brush. Fits in the palm of your hand — brush towards your heart.

DETOX BATH

A detox bath is also an excellent, simple, and inexpensive way of detoxing and relaxing. Add two cups of Epsom salt (magnesium sulphate) to a hot bath, and stay in the bath for 20 minutes. This has benefits that go beyond flushing toxins:

- helping muscles and nerves to function properly
- regulating activity of over 325 enzymes in the body
- helping prevent artery hardening and blood clots
- making insulin more effective
- reducing inflammation to relieve pain and muscle cramps
- improving absorption of nutrients
- helping prevent or ease migraine headaches.

Apart from that, a detox bath feels fabulous and will help you get a better night's sleep.

Some other issues to consider

REMEMBER YOUR TRACE ELEMENTS

Trace elements, also referred to as minerals, include iron, zinc, copper, selenium, iodine, boron, molybdenum, and chromium. The major minerals are sodium, potassium, calcium, phosphorus, magnesium, manganese, sulphur, cobalt, and chlorine. Minerals provide structure in forming bones and teeth; help to maintain heart rhythm, muscle function, nerve conductivity, and acid–alkali balance; and aid the regulation of cellular metabolism and hormones.

Of all the 118 elements in the periodic table, the human body requires about 60 to function optimally. Remember: fluoride is not one of them; in fact, fluoride is not required for any biological function of the human body. Below is a table of just some of those essential elements.

Minerals	Men	Women	Sources
Calcium	700 mg	700 mg	milk, cheese and other dairy foods, green leafy vegetables, bok choy, broccoli, cabbage, and okra (but not spinach), soybeans, tofu, nuts, fish with edible bones such as sardines and pilchards
Iodine	0.14 mg	0.14 mg	sea fish and shellfish, eggs, milk, vegetables, sea vegetables
Iron	8.7 mg	14.8 mg	liver, meat, beans, nuts, dried fruit such as dried apricots, whole grains such as brown rice, most dark-green leafy vegetables such as watercress and curly kale
Beta-carotene	7 mg	7 mg	yellow and green leafy vegetables such as spinach, carrots, and red peppers, yellow fruit such as mango, melon, and apricots
Boron	< 6 mg	< 6 mg	green vegetables, fruit, nuts
Chromium	0.025 mg	0.025 mg	meat and whole oats, lentils, spices
Cobalt	0.0015 mg	0.0015 mg	fish, nuts, green leafy vegetables such as broccoli and spinach, cereals such as oats
Copper	1.2 mg	1.2 mg	nuts, shellfish, offal
Magnesium	300 mg	270 mg	nuts, spinach, fish, meat, dairy foods
Manganese	< 0.5 mg	< 0.5 mg	tea, nuts, green vegetables such as peas and runner beans
Phosphorus	550 mg	550 mg	red meat, dairy foods, fish, poultry, rice, oats
Potassium	3,500 mg	3,500 mg	fruit such as bananas, vegetables, pulses, nuts and seeds, milk, fish, shellfish, beef, chicken, turkey
Selenium	0.075 mg	0.06 mg	brazil nuts, bread, fish, meat, eggs
Zinc	9 mg	7 mg	meat, shellfish, milk, dairy foods such as cheese

Figure 12-20. Recommended daily requirements of minerals for men and women.[28]

ORGANIC VS NON-ORGANIC — IS IT WORTH IT?

Some people are put off by the higher price tag of organic food, but I think there are good reasons to choose it, particularly with some meats, vegetables, and fruits. As I've explained, organic food has greater nutrient density because of the higher-quality soil in which the food is grown. Yet it's not just a question of what's *in* the food (trace elements), but also what is *not in* the food: herbicides, pesticides — and antibiotics. Our greatest exposure to antibiotics is potentially through the food we eat, and antibiotic-resistant harmful bacteria are a major and growing problem.

Food production is a multi-billion-dollar industry that employs 'thought leaders' to conduct 'independent' research, which then tells the public that buying organic food isn't worth the extra money. I hope by now you'll see that it is. In addition, I justify the additional cost of buying organic food by moderating how much I eat, particularly meat and eggs.

The Dirty Dozen	The Clean Fifteen
Apples	Asparagus
Blueberries	Avocado
Capsicum (bell pepper)	Cabbage
Celery	Eggplant
Cucumbers	Grapefruit
Grapes	Kiwi
Lettuce	Mangoes
Nectarines	Mushrooms
Peaches	Onions
Potatoes	Pineapples
Spinach	Rockmelon (cantaloupe)
Strawberries	Sweet corn
	Sweet peas
	Sweet potatoes
	Watermelon

Figure 12-21. Sourced from the Environmental Working Group.

Some food carries more chemicals than others. Washington-based environmental research organisation the Environmental Working Group (EWG) has created a list of foods they dub the 'Dirty Dozen'[29] and 'Clean Fifteen'.[30] This is a great guide to reducing the chemicals we ingest, and forms the basis of our advice for patients at my Sydney dental practice. By avoiding the 'Dirty Dozen', we can reduce exposure to pesticides by up to 80 per cent.

Ultimately, the benefits of organic foods need to be judged across several criteria, including the impact on your health, the long-term savings in medical costs, and, of course, the long-term health of you and the planet.

Nurturing the soil in which our food is grown is critical for long-term sustainability. Some argue the choice of organic versus non-organic food is a first-world problem. Given that many in the world struggle to find enough food just to survive, this is certainly a point, but I am lucky enough to live in the first world and I do have a choice. So do you.

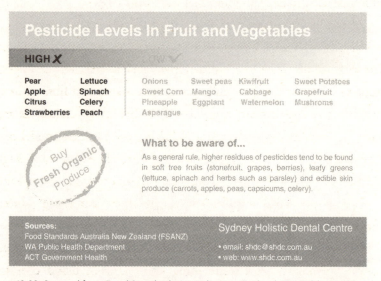

Pesticide Levels In Fruit and Vegetables

HIGH X   LOW ✓

Pear	Lettuce	Onions	Sweet peas	Kiwifruit	Sweet Potatoes
Apple	Spinach	Sweet Corn	Mango	Cabbage	Grapefruit
Citrus	Celery	Pineapple	Eggplant	Watermelon	Mushroms
Strawberries	Peach	Asparagus			

Buy Fresh Organic Produce

What to be aware of...

As a general rule, higher residues of pesticides tend to be found in soft tree fruits (stonefruit, grapes, berries), leafy greens (lettuce, spinach and herbs such as parsley) and edible skin produce (carrots, apples, peas, capsicums, celery).

Sources:
Food Standards Australia New Zealand (FSANZ)
WA Public Health Department
ACT Government Health

Sydney Holistic Dental Centre
• email: shdc@shdc.com.au
• web: www.shdc.com.au

Figure 12-22. Sourced from Food Standards Australia New Zealand, WA Public Health Department, and ACT Government Health.

FARMERS SHOULD BE HONOURED BY US ALL

This bears repeating. Food is essential for survival. Apart from the air we breathe, nothing is as important for human existence and wellbeing as a sustainable, nutrient-dense diet and clean water supply. The problem today is that food and even water has become a commodity. I believe farmers should be the most revered and honoured members of our community because not only do they grow the very food we need to survive (and hopefully thrive), but they are also the custodians of the land. Well-managed land creates the best medicine of all — nutrient-dense food, for us now, and for future generations.

SUPPLEMENTS — TO TAKE OR NOT TO TAKE?

We have become accustomed to taking a pill to cure or manage a health problem, so supplements are, in many ways, an extension of that paradigm, and we're happy to pay. The wellness supplements market, which includes dietary supplements, functional and fortified foods and beverages, as well as gluten-free and lactose-free foods, will be worth US$249.4 billion by 2020.[31] Supplements are clearly another multi-billion-dollar industry, but are they worth the cost?

After billions of years of 'research and development', nature seems to have the vitamins, minerals, co-factors, phytochemicals, and more that we probably haven't even discovered, let alone isolated yet, in perfect proportion. These complex collections of nutrients and fibre cannot be found in any supplement, regardless of its quality or claims. In many ways, the supplement industry is following the business model of the pharmaceutical industry. Find an active ingredient, isolate it, package it, and market it — suddenly you have a new 'superfood' or super supplement.

But as the word 'supplement' suggests, it is a thing added to something else in order to complete or enhance it. That 'something else' ideally should be what I focused on in the 10 Principles. To truly benefit from supplements, we require some knowledge of blood chemistry, medical history, and other clinical and sub-clinical signs and symptoms, together with awareness of the soils in which food is grown and some of the stresses we face in our modern world. Consulting an integrative doctor, nutritionist, or naturopath who is trained in nutritional and environmental medicine and is aware of all of these factors is the best way forward.

In Australia, our ancient and depleted soils are deficient in selenium, magnesium, and zinc. Iodine is essential for healthy thyroid function and metabolism, yet two billion people worldwide are deficient in it, making it the most common deficiency of all. And as I've noted, vitamin D deficiency is also at epidemic proportions. Meanwhile, we almost all live in a less than ideal world of chemicals, electromagnetic radiation, and other stress, all adding to the burden on our bodies.

Note: 50% (2,500 IU) of vitamin A is supplied as β-carotene, while the rest (2,500 IU) is supplied as retinol.

Supplement Facts

Serving Size 1 Tablet

Each Tablet Contains	% Daily Value
Vitamin A 5000 IU (50% as s β-carotene)	100%
Vitamin C 60 mg	100%
Vitamin D 400 IU	100%
Vitamin E 30 IU	100%
Vitamin K 25 µg	31%
Thiamin (Vitamin B1) 1.5 mg	100%
Riboflavin (Vitamin B2) 1.7 mg	100%
Niacin 20 mg	100%
Vitamin B6 2 mg	100%
Folic Acid 400 µg	100%
Vitamin B12 6 µg	100%
Biotin 30 µg	10%
Pantothenic Acid 10 mg	100%
Calcium 160 mg	16%
Iron 18 mg	100%
Phosphorus 110 mg	11%
Iodine 150 µg	100%
Magnesium 100 mg	25%
Zinc 15 mg	100%
Selenium 20 µg	29%
Copper 2 mg	100%
Manganese 2 mg	100%
Chromium 120 µg	100%
Molybdenum 75 µg	100%
Chloride 72 mg	2%
Potassium 80 mg	2%
Boron 150 µg	*
Nickel 5 µg	*
Silicon 2 mg	*
Tin 10 µg	*
Vanadium 10 µg	*
Lutein 250 µg	*

* Daily Value (DV) not established

Figure 12-23. A typical list of ingredients in a common multivitamin/mineral supplement.

I take supplements, but not in isolation. Just as a pharmaceutical product rarely cures a condition, an individual supplement won't either.

It's always interesting to hear thought leaders, usually sponsored by the pharmaceutical industry, warning of the waste and the potential 'danger' of supplements. It's sobering to consider that thousands of people die each year from taking prescription medications *as instructed* — to my knowledge, no one has died from a supplement. And yet we rarely hear from those thought leaders about the present and real dangers of prescription medication.

Taking supplements is often dismissed as causing 'expensive urine', to which I would add: I'm happy to have expensive blood, too. If the argument is that supplements' effects are often purely placebo, then it ignores the fact that placebo works equally and indiscriminately with both pharmaceutical products and vitamin supplements alike.

I'm always a little sceptical when so-called 'experts' dismiss alternative and complementary medicine, which focus on diet and exercise together with herbal and nutritional supplements, with the claim there's 'no evidence to support' a particular vitamin, herb, or nutritional approach. To me it indicates they have simply not kept up with the literature and clearly not read the studies, literally thousands of which have been published in peer-reviewed journals.[32] Sadly and disturbingly, nutritional and environmental medicine is barely covered during an undergraduate medicine degree, despite the fact that the WHO estimates at least 70 per cent of chronic degenerative diseases have a nutritional or environmental component. I believe that is a conservative estimate.

When you bother to read the medical literature beyond that sponsored by the food and pharmaceutical industries, there are so many evidence-based studies that show benefits of an integrative approach to medicine, incorporating nutritional advice, awareness of environmental toxins, and the importance of exercise, meditation, or mindfulness. Supplements are just part of that mix.

An integrative, holistic approach is not alternative medicine, it's just good medicine, and, with it, modern medicine and public health will change for the better.

Conclusion

The nutritional and environmental choices you make each day have the potential to nourish or harm your body and mind. Your choices affect your health, but also have the potential to change the world. In our democracies, we get to vote once every few years, but then have virtually no influence on public policy.

With every choice we make in how to nourish ourselves, we use what is arguably the most powerful vote in our modern world: how we spend our money. From what you eat and drink to your choice of personal-care products, homecare products, clothes, furnishing, or cosmetics, choose wisely, think ethically and sustainably, take control, and be the best you can be.

CHAPTER 13

Movement

The ability to move has been a significant factor in the evolution of our species — an understatement if ever there was one! As we stood on two feet, our perspective on the world changed. Even though our new posture presented us with significant structural challenges, such as balancing our head on a thin spine, our new view of the world literally and metaphorically extended our horizons and our opportunities.

Our mobility, sight, and dexterity, together with an expanded diet and unique ability to communicate, allowed us to redefine hunting and gathering in the animal kingdom. Even small movements, such as the ability to grasp things in our hands, allowed us to use weapons and tools with which to hunt, expanding our choices in foods. Where once humans made up a small fraction of all life on earth, we have moved from hunter-gatherer through the agricultural, scientific, and industrial revolutions into today's age of technology — and now we dominate almost all life on earth in one way or another, at least all life that we can see.

For almost the entire span of human history, movement as a matter of survival or necessity has been part of our daily ritual. During hunter-gatherer times, it allowed us to find food and shelter; in agricultural times, it enabled the physical burden of clearing, ploughing, and harvesting. During the industrial revolution, it meant we could work — all this was, of course, before the advent of the automobile, and our two legs were still our main means of transport. All that has changed, particularly over the last 40 years, with the technological revolution, which has meant that, more than any other time in human history, our lives revolve around inactivity.

Our transport is automated and our work leaves many people glued to desks and computers. In Australia, nearly 70 per cent of adults are either sedentary or have low levels of physical activity, and you can see the same pattern around the western world.[1] For leisure, a whole industry has been built around watching other people playing sport and exerting themselves, often to extremes. Sport, particularly team sport, has always been a means by which we channel our tribal instincts, but, nowadays, rather than taking part in it, we've adopted the global pastime of spending hours passively watching an endless stream of sport (amongst entertainment and news programs) on our screens at home, often while eating or drinking.

By building movement into your daily life, you have the simplest, cheapest, most accessible, and most effective way of improving your physical and mental health, not to mention also improving the outcomes of almost every treatment for any chronic degenerative diseases you may have developed on the way. In fact, there has never been a more important time to consciously and conscientiously move your body in your life long journey to be the best you can be.

Just as food and health have become commodities, so too it seems has the need to move. Each year in Australia, $8.5 billion is spent on gym memberships, sports equipment, and the latest fitness trends. Most people exercise to lose weight, but the real benefit to movement is that it improves every physical, mental, and emotional health measure. Almost every treatment for heart disease, cancer, high blood pressure, diabetes, and a myriad of other conditions including depression and anxiety, as well as your ability to get a consistently good night's sleep, are enhanced by exercise. The reality is that while our lives have become more sedentary, and because of the many stresses we face in the modern world, we need — now more than ever — to plan, and build, movement and exercise into our daily lives.

There are some basic aspects to any sustainable exercise plan:

- **Mobility and functional movement.** You should move, mobilise, and align joints and muscles in exercises that mimic and therefore strengthen the everyday functional movements of twisting, turning, bending, squatting, stretching, pulling, lunging, and pushing.
- **Core stability.** We still face challenges in our movement from balancing our 4.5-kilogram head on our spine and walking on two legs. The core muscles include everything except your arm and leg muscles, and are important for postural correction and joint stabilisation.
- **Endurance.** Throughout history, short bursts of extreme activity would not have been uncommon. Today, some high intensity, intermittent exercises combined with a steady, low-intensity activity such as walking mimics the hunt and gather. If walking or running are not appropriate or practical, try a lower impact activity such as cycling, swimming, or rowing — or better still, a combination of all three.
- **Maximal strength.** Safe load-bearing exercise is important for muscle development, neural development, bone density, and bone health.
- **Mindset.** Believe in your body and your program. Your body is capable of amazing things — you just need to trust yourself, whether starting out or elevating your already established routine.
- **Community and accountability.** Get a buddy, start a blog or social-media account, or document your progress in a diary or journal. Join a community that you connect with, and find peers or mentors who push you along, encourage you, and keep you accountable.

Furthermore, exercise shouldn't be seen as a bottled-up workout; rather, incorporate movement into your everyday activities. You can't sit down for eight hours, plonk yourself on a couch for three hours, exercise for 30 minutes, and think that is okay.

Here are three suggestions to incorporate more exercise or movement into your day:

- **Stay on feet as much as possible.** For every 30 minutes of sitting, walk around for five minutes. Even just go and fill up your stainless-steel water bottle.

- **Spend at least one hour a day standing at your desk.** A few books under your computer and keyboard can create a standing desk, and for that hour concentrate on having perfect posture and balanced breathing. As I write this book, I am alternating sitting and standing at my desk. It surprises me how much more energy I have and how much I move compared to when I just sit for hours. Remember the enzyme in the blood vessels of muscle that helps metabolises fat, the lipoprotein lipase I spoke about in Chapter 9: Postural Stress? It plays a critical role in metabolising fat, but a typical day of sitting will reduce its activity by 90–95 per cent.

- **Perform mobility work at your desk.** For instance: run a golf or tennis ball underneath your bare foot, massaging different muscles. This also helps with strength.

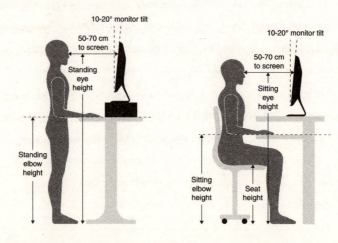

Figure 13-1. A balanced posture at the computer, when sitting and standing.

Why is exercise important?

Two essential and basic functions occur in the body on a microscopic level during movement. In the first, exercise increases the number of mitochondria, known as the powerhouses of our cells. Mitochondria are like microscopic 'batteries', and are found in cells throughout the body, including the brain. One of their many functions is to convert fat, carbohydrate, and protein into energy for the body. The greater the number of mitochondria in your cells, the better it is for your health. But as you age, they start dying off. Regular exercise increases mitochondrial number and activity. Without them, cells do not function optimally, and diseases follow.

In the second function, exercise stimulates the production of what's known as brain-derived neurotrophic factor (BDNF), a protein that supports the survival and growth of neurons or nerves. Exercise 'fertilises' your neurons, assists with memory and learning, and has been found to even help protect against dementia.[2] Regular exercise is key for memory, concentration, and mental sharpness.

Aerobic exercise means 'with oxygen'. This is where you increase your heart rate and breathing but not to the point that you can't do any more. Exercise such as long-distance running, hiking, or working out on many types of gym equipment (treadmill, stationary bike, rowing machine, step machine) is considered aerobic. It's worth mentioning that when you have reached a point of exhaustion, an aerobic exercise can also become anaerobic.

Anaerobic exercise means 'without oxygen'. This is where you quickly run out of breath, and includes exercise such as weight lifting to increase strength, sprinting, or climbing a long flight of stairs.

Aerobic	Anaerobic
Running, quick walking	Weight-lifting
Cycling	Sprinting
Swimming	Jumping
Flexibility	Other exercises that are short in duration and high in intensity

Figure 13-2. Aerobic and anaerobic exercises.

The health benefits of regular exercise and physical activity are hard to ignore, and these benefits are yours for the taking regardless of age, gender, or physical ability. Exercise combats disease, reduces inflammation, decreases unhealthy fats implicated in cardiovascular disease, bolsters your immune system, and reduces vulnerability to cancer. In fact, regular physical activity prevents and manages a wide range of health problems, including stroke, metabolic syndrome, type 2 diabetes, depression, arthritis, and so much more.

What are the other benefits of exercise?

- **Mood.** In the first instance, exercise stimulates brain chemicals (endorphins) that make you feel happier and more relaxed. Feeling better about your appearance also boosts your confidence and self-esteem. You don't just look healthier and feel healthier; you *are* healthier. Exercise and physical activity deliver oxygen and nutrients to your tissues, improving your metabolism and the efficiency of your cardiovascular system. When your heart and lungs, as well as the mitochondria in every cell, work more efficiently, you have more energy.
- **Sleep.** The better you sleep, the more physical, mental, and emotional energy and resilience you will have and the more likely you are to continue and enjoy your exercise. Regular physical activity helps you fall asleep faster and deepens your sleep. Just one note of caution: don't exercise too close to bedtime, because it elevates levels of the stress hormone cortisol, making you too energised to fall asleep. Be sure to cool down and calm down before bed.
- **Judgement.** Studies also show that you are less likely to give in to food cravings.[3] Exercise stimulates your physical and mental cognition, improving your ability to focus and be productive.[4]
- **Self-esteem.** Exercise gives you a greater sense of achievement.
- **Sex.** Regular physical activity enhances arousal for women and prevents erectile dysfunction in men because it improves the production of growth hormone, melatonin, and testosterone.

- **Weight loss.** Physical activity uses energy. The more intense the activity, the more mitochondria, the more energy you burn. If you don't have time for a full work-out, become more active during the day by taking the stairs instead of the lift, get off the bus one stop earlier, work in the garden or around the house, or walk the dog.
- **Function.** Exercise improves bone mineral content and density, joint stability, and flexibility and range of motion. These are keys to reducing injury and maximising general daily function — especially important as we age.

My exercise inspiration

Exercise needs to be interesting to keep you motivated. Over ten years ago, I found my own inspiration with one of Australia's leading personal trainers, Aaron McKenzie, who brings a holistic approach to fitness and nutrition based on functional movement, nutrient-dense food, and lifestyle.

Functional-movement exercise is about incorporating everyday movements into a work-out. It combines pushing and pulling, bending and stretching, twisting and turning. There's no jogging on a treadmill for hours wedged in between dozens of other runners or rows of fancy equipment. Instead, the focus is on stretching and flexibility, incorporating a wide variety of functional movements, and core-muscle strength.

'It's not just about working out in the gym,' explains McKenzie. A personal trainer since 1999, McKenzie has a holistic approach to health and believes many people push themselves too hard because they think exercise has to be difficult to get results. 'And often the fault is not with the exercise. It's with other areas of their life. They're not eating well, they're not sleeping and breathing well, and, as a consequence, they don't respond as well to exercise. People immediately think that *more* must be better, or I should push myself harder.'

McKenzie revolutionised my understanding of fitness. One of the most liberating concepts is that exercise performed in short 30–40 second bursts over 15–20 minutes three or four times a week — incorporating high-intensity intermittent training and some weight-bearing exercises — can boost your metabolism for 24 to 48 hours after the work-out.

The benefits are clearly long-lasting, even when compared to a ten-kilometre run, which I never enjoyed and which surprisingly only boosts the metabolism for up to six hours. For me, the focus on flexibility and stretching before the intense part of the work-out and on the core at the end of a session has been a revelation — and liberating, considering the postural stress of my working position.

Having said that, I understand why people take up long-distance running, cycling, or other endurance exercises. For many, it combines a physical challenge with a form of mindfulness. It's just that for the rest of us, *less* really is *more*.

Combining anaerobic and aerobic exercise

Your waistline is the most significant marker of risk for heart disease and diabetes. As we age, there is a loss of muscle mass, which is often replaced by fat, particularly around the internal organs, resulting in an increased waistline. While this is something that would seem fairly easy to recognise, it is not always as straightforward as that. There is a paradoxical condition, which I mentioned in Chapter 10: Sleep, called TOFI, meaning thin-outside-fat-inside, where a person appears not to be overweight, but their internal story is very different.

A study in 2015 from the Harvard School of Public Health showed that people who did 20 minutes of daily weight training had less of an increase in abdominal fat compared with individuals who spent the same amount of time just doing aerobic exercise.[5] This seems counter-intuitive, but, when you think about it, increasing muscle mass also increases mitochondrial number and activity. Remember, mitochondria are part of every cell and are essentially the power packs of cells. So, by doing weight-bearing exercise, you increase the amount of muscle and also the number and activity of the mitochondria — and more energy is burnt.

The Harvard study also showed that while aerobic exercise by itself was associated with less weight gain (because you lost both fat and muscle), anaerobic weight training reduced fat while at the same time building muscle mass. So, it's not simply about weight; it's also about the quality or type of weight you have or are losing. The beauty of incorporating both aerobic exercise and anaerobic weight training into your weekly routine is that you can combine reducing fat, building muscle, improving bone density, and building cardiovascular fitness.

When embarking on exercises that incorporate weights, dumbbells, or kettle bells, it is important to get proper instruction about correct technique. Engaging a qualified trainer or exercise physiologist who is focused on functional movements incorporated into weight-bearing and high-intensity intermittent exercise is a great investment. They can outline correct technique and tailor an exercise program personalised for you that is effective, safe, and sustainable.

Start with stretching

Flexibility and mobility are important components for our everyday lives but are also key in preparing the body before exercise: we need to stretch. Stretching reduces the incidence of injuries, which is important in making exercising more sustainable. The first part of a session should include a series of stretches moving through the whole body. This can also be a great opportunity to unwind and focus.

An excellent starting point for an effective stretching routine, and a great position to practise, is the 'resting squat', a posture that primates have used over millions of years. If you assume this position for just a few minutes each day, it benefits the spine, particularly the lumbar and sacral regions (at the base of the spine) and can help relieve back pain. If you have trouble doing it without support, you can grab onto a door frame and support the squat, slowly working up to doing it independently. The resting squat also helps the legs (particularly the thighs), strengthens the glutes (gluteus maximus) and hips, improves ankle mobility, and improves overall posture.

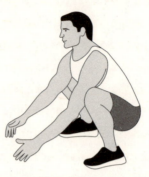

Figure 13-3. The resting squat. If you have problems with knees or ankles, holding onto something for support as you lower yourself to your own limit is helpful.

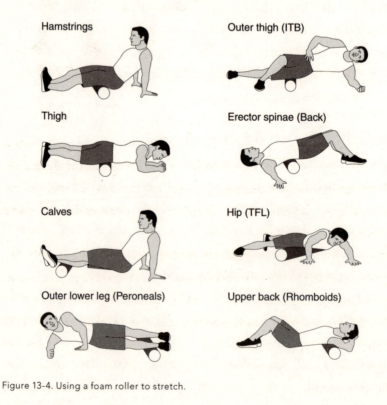

Figure 13-4. Using a foam roller to stretch.

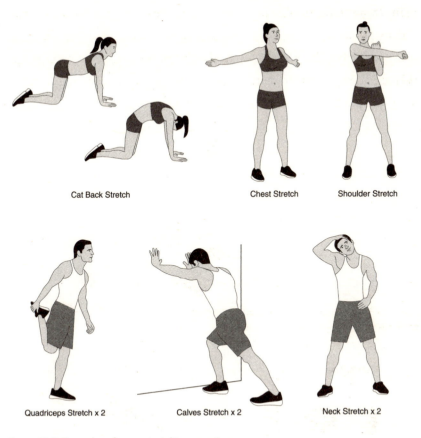

Cat Back Stretch Chest Stretch Shoulder Stretch

Quadriceps Stretch x 2 Calves Stretch x 2 Neck Stretch x 2

Figure 13-5. Examples of some stretching exercises.

In Chapter 9: Postural Stress, I outlined the benefits of going to the toilet in this squatting position, which has been assumed for thousands of years, facilitating our ancestors' bowel movements. It's nice to tie this excellent stretch in with the added benefits of an easier and more complete bowel movement.

The use of a foam roller is also an excellent way of stretching muscles and joints, moving backwards and forwards over the roller as you isolate a particular muscle group.

In addition, there are many other exercises that can be incorporated into your stretching routine.[6]

The work-out

High-intensity intermittent training might consist of three to four movements that use the whole body.[7] Getting your form right is important but does not need to be over-complicated. People need to work at their own level — some more intensely than others, with different emphases. The work-out itself can be as little as seven minutes or up to 20 minutes in duration. I found this particularly liberating and empowering. There are three to six sets of the movement with 30–40 seconds of activity, each followed by 20–30 seconds of rest.

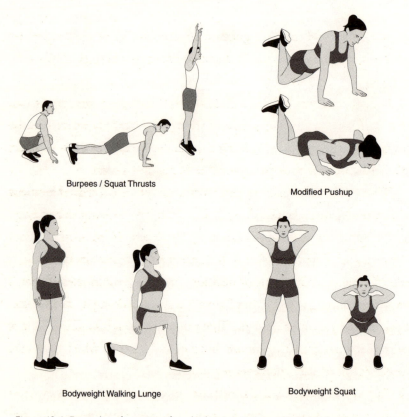

Burpees / Squat Thrusts

Modified Pushup

Bodyweight Walking Lunge

Bodyweight Squat

Figure 13-6. Examples of exercises for a high-intensity intermittent work-out.

When it comes to weight-bearing exercise, form is important. You can incorporate one or two of the movements to be weight bearing, also lasting for 30 to 40 seconds with a 20-to-30-second break.

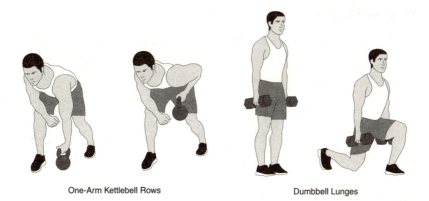

One-Arm Kettlebell Rows   Dumbbell Lunges

Figure 13-7. Examples of simple weight-bearing exercises.

After the work-out, it's good to incorporate some core corrective work to stimulate the smaller stabiliser muscles that keep the body well-aligned.

Lying on a foam roller is a great way to finish your exercise session. This is an opportunity to passively stretch and actively relax. Breathe slowly through your nose, holding the exhaled breath for a few seconds; this will switch on your parasympathetic nervous system.

When it comes to exercise and motivation, there is a critical moment when you decide to do it or leave it for another day. Going to bed early, around 9.30 p.m., and falling asleep by 10.00 p.m. helps in motivation. Being tired doesn't lend itself well to exercising. I have always found it helpful when that moment of decision arises to remind myself that 'I never regret doing exercise, but I always regret *not* doing it.' Don't over-think it. The answer is obvious. That's usually enough to get me out of bed rather than press the 'snooze' button, and it's true: when you make the effort to exercise, you never regret it!

You could even include exercise into everyday activities. You brush your teeth twice a day for two minutes each time — why not incorporate some slow squats into those four minutes, working on the large leg muscles while looking after the health of your mouth? I love multi-tasking!

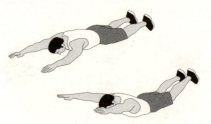

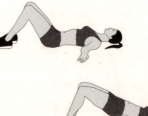

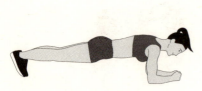

Plank

Superman / Extended Arms & Legs Lift

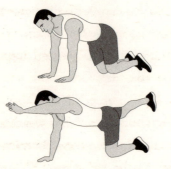

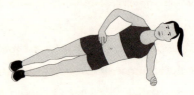

Swiss Ball Crunch

Hip Raise / Butt Lift / Bridge

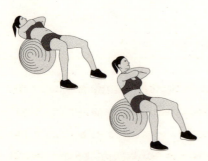

Bird Dogs / Alternating Reach & Kickback

Side Plank

Figure 13-8. Examples of exercises to strengthen the core muscles.

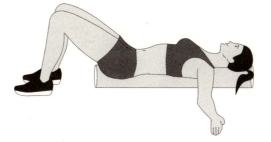

Figure 13-9. Using the foam roller to rest on after a work-out will stretch your back and shoulders.

Yoga and Pilates

Other options to increase your body's flexibility include yoga and Pilates. During my first ever yoga class, at university many years ago, the teacher advised me there was one key exercise sequence to build strength and flexibility that I should never forget, and I never have. It's called 'Salute to the Sun'. Apart from moving and stretching the whole body, it's also believed to be one of the most effective ways to balance hormones, and, if practised daily, can help balance your entire hormonal system. It's a combination of extension and flexion, lunges and weight-bearing, while coordinating the breath.

Each morning, one of the first things I do is ten rounds of 'Salute to the Sun', performed slowly and mindfully. I incorporate this stretching and strength exercise into the first three minutes of my 15-minute workout. Even if I wake feeling a bit stiff, by the end of my DIY yoga session I feel more flexible and energised — a great way to start a day.

If you want something more vigorous and aerobic, perform 'Salute to the Sun' more quickly; it can elevate your heart rate, giving you a more intense 'stretch', particularly on those days you don't do a full work-out. Yoga is a wonderful way to connect your mind and body, and to work on core strength, flexibility, and breathing.

It's worth getting proper instruction for proper technique, but, once you have it, it's yours for life. Here's a step-by-step instruction for a round of 'Salute to the Sun', coordinating movement and breath.

When your body arches open, or extends, inhale. When your body folds closed, or goes into flexion, exhale. Each round alternates the leg stretched in the lunge.

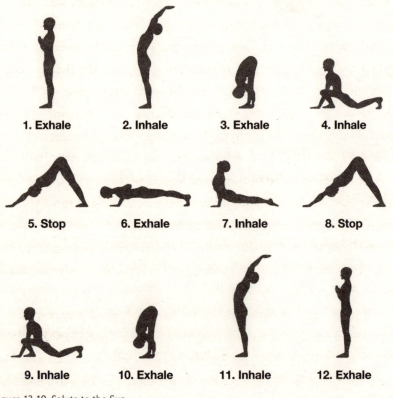

Figure 13-10. Salute to the Sun.

This is a great way to start each day, and incorporates so many positives that it's hard to ignore. Build it into your day.

The benefits of walking

Walking is an exercise that can be done over your entire life. In fact, it's a wonderfully accessible, social, health-giving, sustainable, weight-bearing, risk-free, and just-plain-free activity that has been the main form of exercise for all of human history.

As if that isn't reason enough to incorporate it into your own daily routine, research from the UK shows that walking speed is a better predictor of life expectancy over the next five years than blood pressure, cholesterol, or any other health indicator.[8] The research was based on participants aged 40–70 years answering a short questionnaire — 13 questions for men and 11 questions for women. The questionnaire is called the UK Longevity Explorer, and you can take the test online yourself (www.ubble.co.uk/risk-calculator/disclaimer.php).

One way to incorporate movement into your day and motivate yourself together with family and friends is with a pedometer to record the number of steps you and your 'friends' take each day. The results can be uploaded to a dashboard and shared with the group. This fusion of exercise, accountability, and community, facilitated through social media, is a great use of technology to educate and motivate yourself to get (and stay) active. The group checks each other's progress, with a healthy dose of competition thrown into the mix. The daily goal should be to walk 10,000 steps.

Where does '10,000 steps' come from? Originally attributed to a Japanese business slogan from the 1960s, the idea of 10,000 steps per day was investigated by researchers led by Dr Yoshiro Hatano. They looked at the typical steps per day of various lifestyles and established that 10,000 steps a day did in fact lead to better health.[9] Whatever the number's origin, it's a good place to start.

Conclusion

Build movement throughout each day. If you do want a workout, remember that less is more — a workout only needs to be ten minutes and you're done. You can walk your whole life, so keep practising. Our hunter-gather ancestors didn't work-out in a gym — they walked, ran in short bursts, and lifted things such as rocks, logs, and animals, and carried their young children. Simple stretches can be part of your day, too. Short bursts of intense activity are more effective and sustainable.

Incorporating and combining some weight-bearing exercise is a great way of stimulating muscle activity, improving bone density, burning energy, nurturing your mental and emotional wellbeing, controlling weight, and much more.

When deciding on the type of exercise that's right for you, ask these questions: Can you actually do it? Is it good for you? And most importantly, is the exercise sustainable? The key is to build movement, exercise, strength, and flexibility into your whole day and to become aware of the amount of time you are sedentary. The health benefits of moving are so well documented and above all are such an important part of being the best you can be.

CHAPTER 14

Thought

How you think is an important component of a fulfilled life. When you have a positive thought, it leads to positive feelings and a corresponding positive biochemistry throughout your body and mind. Even the act of smiling gives feedback to your brain to release neurotransmitters that affect the body's chemistry in a positive way. If you see someone you care deeply about, your body releases dopamine (the 'feel-good' hormone), oxytocin (the 'hugging' hormone), and growth hormone, all with the potential to help maintain good health or even to heal.

But negative thoughts brought on by a range of factors — including stress, poor diet, alcohol, caffeine, prescription and recreational drugs, medical conditions, or even just lack of sleep or exercise — create imbalances and deplete neurotransmitter levels as well. When you feel fearful or scared, the brain releases stress hormones such as cortisol and adrenaline, which are also inflammatory. A feeling of helplessness can also be bad for your health. The purpose of this book is to encourage and empower you to take control and be an active participant in your own health journey.

An essential part of this process is to build physical and mental resilience through an awareness of the various stresses that can compromise your body's balance or homeostasis, while incorporating the pillars of health into your daily life. This includes an awareness of how you think and how those thoughts may be affecting your wellbeing. How you think can be both a stress that compromises your health and a pillar that improves your health — it can even affect your genes.

Epigenetics

As discussed in Chapter 5: Emotional Stress, Bruce Lipton is a cellular biologist and the author of *The Biology of Belief*, a groundbreaking book on the new biology and science of epigenetics. Lipton is an all-time hero of mine, and his book changed the way I thought about thinking. Epigenetics challenges the widely held assumption that your genetic structure controls your health and, ultimately, your fate — a sort of genetic determinism.

There is no question that family genetics plays a role in health outcomes. I have certainly learned this lesson myself, in my own family. My uncle had prostate cancer at 60, as did my brother, as did I. If there is a history of cancer, heart disease, or Alzheimer's disease in your family, you need to take that seriously — there's a greater chance of you developing that disease, and the same is true of many other health conditions. But you need not feel that the locus of control is external and out of your reach; you need not become a victim to your family history. Lipton offers a very different understanding based on the emerging science of epigenetics.

The majority of genetic studies focus on the gene or DNA code, whereas epigenetics looks at the factors that control how and when each gene is expressed — a process that's still not entirely understood. Some genes are always expressed, but others are only expressed when triggered by a thought (a neurotransmitter), a toxin, or a nutrient. Epigenetics looks for the reason why particular genes are switched on and off. Mediating between our surroundings and our genes are the nervous and hormonal systems that adjust our biology in order to stay alive. Amazingly, how we interpret and react to our surroundings is a key determinant of how our inherited genetic code expresses itself.

Lipton explains it this way: 'I love eating hot Mexican food. I love the food to be so hot that perspiration pours out of me. But my friend gasps when eating the same food and asks: "How can you eat that stuff?" We're eating the same food, with the same spices, the same nervous system. But we have a very different interpretation. How you see the world and respond to the world is based on what you believe about the world. It's about your reaction to an event. If we believe we're victims of the world, we look at outside forces controlling us. But if you know that you're a master, you say, "This is what I will do," and set up a plan. You have to start behaving as if you're in that world. Your mind adjusts your biology and behaviour to conform to what you're saying and doing.'

I think this approach is both exciting and empowering. If you take control of your thinking, and for that matter, as I've already discussed, the nutrients and environmental toxins you are exposed to, you may be able to influence the way in which your own genes are expressed — and even passed on to future generations. Of course, many factors are beyond your control, such as a natural disaster or a random act of violence, but you can control your interpretation of these events, which influences your experience of it and gives you an internal locus of control. This has a dramatic impact on physical, mental, and emotional health.

We may not be able to change world events — or, perhaps more importantly, how they are reported — but we can certainly change the way we think about them, particularly when you realise how those thoughts have an impact on our health. Gaining a sense of personal control is a powerful tool in each and every one of our individual health journeys throughout life — it may be the most powerful tool of all.

Gratitude

The Roman philosopher Cicero said gratitude 'is not only the greatest but is also the parent of all the other virtues'. Psychologists are recognising that gratitude is more than feeling thankful for something; it is a deeper appreciation for someone (or something) that produces longer-lasting positivity and has a significant impact on our wellbeing, both individually and as a community.

Harvard Medical School defines gratitude as 'a thankful appreciation for what an individual receives, whether tangible or intangible. With gratitude, people acknowledge the goodness in their lives ... As a result, gratitude also helps people connect to something larger than themselves as individuals — whether to other people, nature, or a higher power.'[1]

Gratitude is a way to appreciate what you have rather than constantly searching for something new in the hopes it will make you happier, or thinking that you won't be happy or feel satisfied until every physical and material need is met. This 'search' is a powerful message in our society — we are encouraged to be good consumers rather than good citizens. As we are bombarded by images in the media of perceived 'beauty' and material 'pleasures', it's easy to lose sight of how much you really need and how much you actually have to be grateful for.

Psychologist Robert Emmons of the University of California, Davis, has done a great deal of research on gratitude. In one study, he investigated the role of a person's perception of their daily wellbeing and found that a conscious focus on gratitude had significant benefits for emotional wellbeing and interpersonal relationships.[2]

Participants in the study were divided into two groups, primed for 'gratitude' or 'hassle', and then asked to think of examples of these things in their recent lives. They were then asked to rate their own wellbeing. As the study progressed, people in the 'gratitude' group felt 25 per cent happier, were more optimistic about their lives and the future, and even did 1.5 hours more exercise a week. They also slept better. Given what I've already discussed about the benefits of a consistently good night's sleep, this reinforces the link between a good sleep routine and being positive.

Gratitude is important irrespective of age and a habit worth cultivating from childhood. Children who are encouraged to express gratitude have a more positive attitude to school and their families and friends.[3]

In a landmark study, researchers — including Professor Martin Seligman, who is considered the pioneer of positive psychology and the study of happiness — explored the effect of various positive-psychology interventions, and found the impact of a simple gratitude exercise had a greater impact than all the other interventions.[4] Participants were given a week to write and then deliver a letter of gratitude in person to someone who had been especially kind to them but had never been properly thanked. Interestingly, the benefits of this one-week exercise, which included feeling happier and less depressed, lasted for a month — a great 'return on investment'.

Clearly, studies such as these cannot prove cause and effect, but most of the studies published on this topic support an association between gratitude and an individual's wellbeing.

Robert Emmons proposes several theories about why expressing gratitude may be so important: it facilitates coping with stress, reduces toxic emotions resulting from self- or social comparisons, reduces materialistic craving, improves self-esteem, enhances accessibility to positive memories, enhances social relationships, motivates moral behaviour, and promotes physical health.[5]

Intuitively, we all know that genuinely expressing gratitude is an empowering experience for both the giver and receiver, so identify what you have to be grateful for and express that gratitude — regularly. Like any exercise, the benefits increase with time. It's often said that 'the best things in life are free', and practising gratitude on a daily basis is certainly one of the best.

The power of meditation

According to medical practitioner, psychotherapist, yoga teacher, and friend Swami Shankardev Saraswati, meditation can alter our perspective on life — giving us greater personal insight and control.[6] 'Meditation is a great experience when it is taught by an authentic and highly experienced teacher, and practised with sincerity. Although meditation does not necessarily remove the problems of life, it helps us to avoid creating more problems and complicating existing problems. It also supports a creative and intuitive approach to managing and sometimes solving existing problems. Over time, meditation brings deep personal insight. As we create an authentic connection with our inner world, our outer world also transforms; we find that we are naturally attracted to more positive habits, situations, activities, and relationships. Meditation also aids the healing process.'

Meditation practised regularly awakens our highest intelligence, unlocking and empowering the body's amazing ability to heal itself as well as restore and maintain health. It is our inner guide or 'guru', the wise part of us that knows what is best. When this wisdom is awakened, our body has a greater chance to harness the incredible power to heal itself.

Medical practitioner and senior lecturer at Monash University Craig Hassad lists the benefits of meditation and mindfulness:[7]

- improved mental health, including relief from depression, anxiety, panic disorder, stress, emotional dysregulation, and addictions
- improved sleep — 20 minutes of meditation is physiologically equivalent to two hours of sleep
- structural and functional changes in the brain, generation of new brain cells (neurogenesis) particularly for memory and higher brain functioning centres, prevention of dementia, and reduced activity in the amygdala (that part of our brain responsible for fear, particularly of things outside of our control).
- pain management, symptom control, improved physical and mental coping with major illnesses such as cancer, reduced wear-and-tear on the body, metabolic benefits, hormonal changes, possibly slower ageing, and improved genetic expression, function, and repair
- improved performance in sport, academic pursuits, and leadership
- deeper peace, insight, oneness, and, ultimately, transcendence.

As David Servan-Schreiber points out in his fabulous book *Anticancer: a new way of life*, meditation causes resonances that amplify our basic biological rhythms, which influence physiological functions including the regulation of blood-sugar levels, reduction of chronic inflammation, and better functioning of the immune system.[8] At birth, there is a perfect synchronisation of these rhythms, but, as we age, various stresses challenge this homeostasis. During meditation, there is re-synchronisation of different parts of the brain, similar to the synchronisation of those basic biological rhythms so vital for our health. The effects extend well beyond the time spent meditating. The regions of the brain that are associated with positive mood and optimism are considerably more active after practising mindfulness or meditation, even after only a few weeks' practice.

A PATIENT'S STORY — KATE

In her early 20s, while walking across a pedestrian crossing, a car hit Kate and she spent months lying on her back in a neck brace in hospital. For many years, her pain was 24/7, constant and unrelenting. Kate explained to me how bad things became:[9] 'My body was rejecting painkillers. I wasn't sleeping for more than three hours a night. Life was really challenging.'

'Challenging' indeed — Kate also had a very complicated medical history, including migraines, allergies, and glandular fever. When she was 18, she suffered toxic-shock syndrome, which resulted in both kidney and heart failure. Later, she contracted swine flu and pneumonia. She had already been through several near-death experiences through her various 'health challenges', and the car accident could have been the last straw.

After the road accident, she visited a range of medical practitioners, specialists, manual therapists, naturopaths, and nutritionists, and, over the years, she had been placed on a wide range of diets, including dairy- and gluten-free and Paleo. At the age of 27, she visited a physiotherapist who observed, 'You're not sleeping. Your body's not getting into parasympathetic mode. You're not absorbing nutrients. You're not going to heal.' The physiotherapist suggested she learn meditation to calm her nervous system. At the same time, in stark contrast, her neurosurgeon advised that the only way to resolve the chronic headaches and neck aches was a 'last resort' surgery, which Kate intuitively resisted.

After that discussion with her neurosurgeon, she decided to follow the advice of her physiotherapist and attended an introductory talk on meditation that explained its neuroscientific benefits. 'After my first meditation, I slept for 12 hours, and that was evidence straightaway that it made a big difference,' she said. Meditation unlocked the healing power of her body.

Today, Kate is sleeping well, absorbing her nutrients, and living relatively pain-free. She's on an empowering healing journey and finally enjoying good health. She moved from the corporate world and now teaches Vedic or transcendental-style meditation — which is simply sitting in a chair or on the floor with your eyes shut, focusing on your breath, and repeating a mantra.

Switching on your parasympathetic nervous system

The breath is central to the practice of yoga, meditation, and mindfulness. As I discussed at the end of Chapter 11: Breathing, the act of slowly inhaling air through the nose using the diaphragm, then exhaling and holding the exhaled breath momentarily for a few seconds, and repeating that for even only one to two minutes is a simple DIY way of switching on your parasympathetic nervous system. Even just doing this simple technique once can make a big difference. Try doing it a few times a day, and certainly before going to sleep.

What is the difference between mindfulness and meditation?

While meditation may be something you have promised yourself you would do and 'just haven't got around to', mindfulness is far more doable. It's gaining widespread acceptance and today is used in therapy, business, and education. Mindfulness is particularly useful after completing one activity and before beginning another. It's an 'exercise' you can incorporate into everyday life.

To some, shopping for food and then cooking may seem like menial tasks. But what if you focused on every aspect of them as an exercise in mindfulness? Good for the body, good for the mind, and, when you are really mindful, good for the environment. Even washing up could be seen as part of the same process.

If you feel you don't have enough time in your life, what about turning the activity of brushing and flossing your teeth, which should take two minutes twice a day, into an exercise in mindfulness and controlled breathing? Again, good for the body and mind.

Meditation and mindfulness can be practised for a few minutes or up to 30 minutes twice a day, depending on your own motivation and opportunity.

Meditation	Mindfulness
Connected with Buddhism, yoga, karma, gurus, spirituality, various religious orders, and more recently with New Age ideas. It comes from an ancient monastic tradition based on withdrawal from the world.	Related to psychology, education, scientific research, rational thought, and everyday language. Its values are not monastic, and integrate more easily into our modern world.
Requires the person meditating to sit or lie. But essentially just to be still.	Can happen in any daily activity by focusing on being present in the moment and aware of our surroundings.
Takes time (typically at least 20 minutes, but shorter periods are also practised).	Is an opportunity to stop and consciously quieten your mind for 15 seconds to two minutes throughout the day.
Focuses inwardly on the body.	Has a more expansive field of operation. It can be applied to any activity. It also relates to our actions, thoughts, emotions, and states of mind.

Figure 14-1. Differences between meditation and mindfulness.

There are many courses, teachers, online programs, and mobile apps to get you started.[10] As with other pillars of health, the key is commitment and 'giving it a go'. Create a benchmark. Inform and challenge yourself to experience how well you can feel. Set the bar high.

A new theory of wellbeing

When we think about what is important in life to us personally, or to our family and friends, happiness would have to come top of the list. But it is an elusive goal and it can be difficult to define what actually constitutes happiness.

Aristotle said happiness is a state of activity, which may be another way of saying, being engaged with life. While we are in the realm of the ancient Greeks, I'm also drawn towards another of their definitions of happiness: the joy that we might feel when striving for our potential. Reaffirming the message 'to be the best you can be'.

Researchers in the United States determined that in order to become happier, people need both a will and a way.[11] The fact that you are reading this book and have got to this chapter suggests you have the will to improve your health — and with this, hopefully, be happier.

My motivation for this book is to encourage you to be aware of the challenges we all face to our health and realise your potential to take control of it. The 'will' comes from motivation, our expectations, and how diligent we are, as well as an understanding that issues are rarely a simple yes or no, right or wrong — we need to have a tolerance of the ambiguity in life.

The 'way' is through the pillars, principles, and pointers I've provided you. Here's one last pointer to help you think.

Martin Seligman has made it his life's work to understand and promote optimism, happiness, positivity, and, most recently, wellbeing.[12] To that end, he has developed a model to identify the building blocks of wellbeing and satisfaction with life. He calls the model PERMAH:[13]

- **Positive emotion.** An essential part of wellbeing is experiencing happiness, joy, hope, love, and gratitude. When you are feeling positive, you can look back on the past with gladness, look into the future with hope, and enjoy and cherish the present — spending more time in appreciation for what you have rather than in expectation of what you might have had or are missing out on.

- **Engagement.** When you focus on doing the things you truly enjoy and care about, you can begin to engage completely with the present moment, using your strengths to meet challenges. Engagement is a sense of being blissfully absorbed in what you are doing, also called 'being in the flow'.

- **Relationship.** Everyone needs someone. We enhance our wellbeing and share it with others by building strong relationships with people around us — family, friends, co-workers, and neighbours. The longest and most comprehensive study of adult development ever performed, with over 75 years of data, found that close relationships were far more important than money or fame, and are better predictors of long and happy lives than social class, IQ, or genes.[14]

- **Meaning.** We are at our best when we dedicate time to something greater than ourselves. This might be religious faith, community work, family, politics, charity, or a professional or creative goal. Or even simple acts of kindness, which not only boost your own happiness but have a domino effect through anyone who sees the acts or receives the kindness. It can be as simple as holding open the door, smiling at someone, or giving a compliment.

- **Accomplishment/achievement.** Everyone needs to win sometimes. To achieve wellbeing and happiness, we must be able to look back on our life's accomplishments and say, 'I did it, and I did it as well as I could.' Accomplishing goals, achieving success, doing the best you can, and being the best you can be.

- **Health.** Everything is easier when all the pillars of health are present; incorporating health as a key component of wellbeing is a timely inclusion as we draw to the end of this book.

353

Conclusion

While it is often said, 'You are what you eat,' it is also becoming clear that 'how and what you think' has an equally dramatic impact on your health, your wellbeing, and, ultimately, your happiness.

Take control of your thoughts — harness the incredible healing powers of your own body and mind.

Conclusion

A Life Less Stressed: the five pillars of health and wellness is an exploration. I have uncovered and unravelled the stresses in life that can compromise health, and discovered the pillars of health and wellbeing that build resilience and help us to take control. While the chapters have separated out the various elements of stress and health, it's important to remember that each of these elements is actually inseparable: each interacts and then affects us to varying degrees as a whole person living on a whole planet.

The purpose of the book is to inform, inspire, and empower you. When incorporating changes into your life — starting today — there are some foundational concepts to remember to make the journey an easier one:

- **Internal locus of control.** You are the one who determines how you live your life, what you consume, the toxins you expose yourself to in your own home, the way you think and move — and this determines how your genes express themselves, which then shapes how healthy you can be. My goal is to empower you with knowledge and to give a framework or philosophy of health and its many challenges and opportunities so that the choices you make build resilience, health, and wellbeing.

- **Tolerance of ambiguity.** There is rarely one answer to a question. In the real world, there are always many contributing factors. We do not exist in isolation. We are all naturally drawn to certainty, as it makes the world so much easier to understand and believe in. But the reality is, we are surrounded by ambiguity, alternative viewpoints, and different approaches to almost every question. Above all, there is still a great deal we do not yet know. A tolerance of ambiguity is an important trait in a world constantly changing with conflicting priorities as you strive to take and maintain control of your health.

- **Benchmark yourself.** Listen to your body and mind. Commit to changes for a period of time that at least gives you a chance to experience just how different you can actually feel. Then when you start to make compromises, you will have something useful and meaningful to compare your health and wellbeing with.

The five pillars build the physical, mental, and emotional resilience needed to simply be well. Start here:

- **Sleep.** Make it a priority. From your health's perspective, it is the most important part of the day. If you haven't been sleeping well, you have some catching up to do. Commit to a consistently good night's sleep and be patient. Sleep is the springboard to every health journey.

- **Breathing.** Don't forget there is a difference between just breathing and breathing well, particularly when you sleep. Using your nose and engaging the diaphragm are key components of breathing well. Remember, holding the exhaled breath for a few seconds over one to two minutes is a simple yet effective way of switching on the 'rest and digest' part of your nervous system. It is a mindful practice that is easy to do several times a day.

- **Nutrition.** Experiment for a few months and at least give yourself something to gauge how well you can feel. Avoid processed food, sugar, and seed oils; measure quantities to familiarise yourself with how much you eat; get to know what 'low-carbohydrate' means; try to restrict or avoid all gluten and dairy for at least a few weeks or months; go alcohol-free for a period of weeks or months. Keep in mind that it is the first week of avoidance that is the most difficult. Then focus on lots of vegetables in a wide variety of colours; be sure to include healthy fats because your body needs them, they are a great source of energy, and they will ensure you won't get hungry; eat quality, ethically grown protein and get to know what moderate protein intake means; drink clean, filtered water in reusable containers; use quality salt that contains 50–60 trace elements; respect your gut biome and feed your friends, not your foes.

- **Movement.** It's surprising how little you need to do to make a difference, and you'll sleep better, too. Don't sit for hours at your desk or in front of the TV. Get up and move throughout the day. Exercise improves every measure of physical, mental, and emotional health, and also improves almost every treatment for chronic degenerative diseases.

- **Thought.** Be grateful for what you have and the people that surround you; nurture the relationships you are a part of. Practise gratitude and be positive. Engage in and find meaning in your work and life. Practise mindfulness, even for just a few minutes throughout the day. Give meditation a go; the potential benefits to overcome chronic disease and build your health and wellbeing can be profound. Practise random acts of kindness and empathy.

So much of our relationship with our environment is adversarial, from the exploitation of earth's resources, animals, and vegetation, to the assault on the microbes in our bodies and in our soils. Something has to change. We share our bodies with trillions of microbes, many of which have not even been identified, and the way we engage with them in a symbiotic relationship is critically important to our health and wellbeing, and will undoubtedly be the next frontier in medical research and healthcare. The same is true of how we nurture and replenish our soils and how we grow our food.

The importance of this symbiotic relationship with microbes is a metaphor for a wider sustainable, peaceful, and healthier future. We also share our planet with billions of people, the vast majority of whom we also don't know — and yet the manner in which we engage with each other and our planet, hopefully also in a 'symbiotic' way, is just as important to our planet's long-term health and wellbeing.

We should always aim to leave the world in a better condition than we found it — for our future generations.

Above all, there are so many lessons to be learned from the past: How did we evolve as an individual living within a tribe or community? What did we eat for hundreds of thousands of years that allowed us to get to this point in our evolution? What is our relationship with the rest of the world, large and small, seen and unseen?

The many stresses we surround ourselves with are also having an impact on our health and that of our only planet: industrial agriculture, processed foods, chemical soup, and electromagnetic fields to name but a few.

We have a right not to be poisoned, and we should demand that right. We live in a world that has been dominated by a free-market economy where money talks and profit is king. The time of 'economic rationalism' must surely give way to a period of 'planning rationalism', where human and planetary health and sustainability are the driving force, and profit really is the *bottom* line.

It is up to us as individuals and communities to ensure we steer the future in the right direction. We are all, every living organism and every atom, connected — so we are all affected by choices we make and the decisions we take. If we are waiting for the change to come from governments and regulatory bodies, we may be waiting a long time.

Human ingenuity and our technological society will undoubtedly move forward and develop in new and exciting ways. But renewable, clean, cheap energy; zero waste; and how we as individuals and as a society choose to spend our money will drive that change. In those choices, we need to reward sustainable, environmentally conscious industries in the everyday choices we make.

I'm an optimist. We live in an exciting time, with access to, and the democratisation of, information and knowledge like never before. In addition, our unique ability to communicate and share information has always distinguished our journey through human history. Our ability to communicate today with one another is unprecedented. It is said 'with knowledge comes power'. Our ability to communicate that knowledge will help us all make choices that will shape our collective future.

If you have one goal in life, it should be to fulfil your potential — as a person, in relationships, through the work you do, and as part of a community, locally and globally. In order to fulfil your potential, take control of your health, build resilience in your life and that of our planet — and let's all be the best we can be.

Be well.

ACKNOWLEDGEMENT

Expressing Gratitude

I'd like to thank my patients for putting their trust in me. As any health practitioner knows, we take on a big responsibility — our patients' health — and we can learn so much from our patients' individual stories. I know I have. Yet there's so much that I never get a chance to say to my patients in their visits to my dental practice. It's not just about knowing where to start but deciding where to finish, and, in that way, writing this book has some similarities.

So, in a sense, this book is for my patients, as well as all people who feel they are affected by stress.

I have worked in partnership in the same dental practice as my brother, Dr Joshua Ehrlich, for almost 40 years. I have always thought that if I could convince my brother to incorporate a new direction into our practice, then it was a good idea. I want to thank him for his love and support. After 40 years of working together, not to mention having shared our lives, we are closer than ever. Over 20 years ago, we were fortunate to be joined by another dentist and partner, Dr Craig Wilson, who has similarly been supportive and encouraging and brought a new perspective to our professional-health journey; while not related, I often describe him as a 'brother from another mother', and he has always provided a great balance to our collective dynamic. Over ten years ago, Dr Yin Yin Teoh, whom I consider a 'sister from another mister', joined us as well, and I would like to thank my whole professional family for their support and encouragement.

In recent years, my nephew Dr Lewis Ehrlich (Josh's son) has become part of that family. Having literally been exposed to much of what I discuss in the book throughout his life, his own interest in health — not only as a dentist, but also as a qualified holistic health coach and personal trainer — has brought a whole new energy and enthusiasm for health, which has affected us all. It's exciting for us all to be working together with still so much to learn. I have often said that the more I learn, the more I realise I don't know, and working as a team enriches the journey.

I would also like to thank Dr Michelle Woolhouse, my co-host for three years in our podcast *The Good Doctors*. Together, we explored many of the issues discussed in this book. Our time of working together was also a rewarding and stimulating period of my life. I learned a great deal and thank her for sharing her knowledge so generously with me.

The writing of the book, my first, has been a stimulating and rewarding experience. Jennifer Fleming — author, broadcaster, producer, and one of my wonderful patients — guided me through the early stages, while introducing me to the discipline of trying to contain my desire to say too much, all at once. I would also like to thank Karen Pittar and Rhonda Mackay for their editorial assistance in the earlier drafts.

My dear friends Eric Moses, David Saul, Mark Ninio, and Gary Zamel have all been great sounding boards for me over many years and offered great feedback, encouragement, grounding, and some wonderful insights.

I have also greatly enjoyed working with my editor David Golding. I would like to thank him, Stephanie Siriwardene, Allison Colpoys, Marika Webb-Pullman, Cora Roberts, Sarah Braybrooke, Mick Pilkington, and everyone else at Scribe Publications for helping me bring my ideas to print. I have learned a great deal from the experience.

I would also like to thank Trina Johnson and Amanda Hosey from Fruitful Creative for their work on the images. Also, Alison Caddick for providing the index.

The Australian Dental Association offers its members a fabulous library facility and, through that, access to every scientific journal in any field from any year. It is a fantastic service, and I would sincerely like to thank the ADA in general, but, specifically, Penny Comans, the Library Manager, for her wonderful assistance and support over the entire time of writing, and, of course, for helping hunt down the almost 300 references you find in this book.

My own family have been a great source of inspiration and encouragement. I would like to thank my wife, my best friend, my dance and life partner, Annie Wilson, whose enthusiasm for life and people is inspirational and infectious. As well as that, her expertise in higher education, specifically in learning and teaching, together with her support and encouragement, both personal and professional, has always been a great source of strength for me. My life has been so enriched by you, Annie.

Speaking of enriching my life, I would also like to thank my two daughters, Lydia and Sofie. Both have been supportive and inspirational. They encouraged me to start my own podcast five years ago and then went on to produce and promote it. I would literally not have done it without them and have learned so much and got to interview some amazing and inspirational people.

They have also embraced the messages espoused in this book and are a daily reminder to me of how to find a good balance in health, and of how to incorporate environmentally responsible and ethical decisions, which have just become part of their everyday life. Lydia assisted me in research for this book and continues to produce and promote our new podcast series, *Unstress*. Sofie, while studying for a Bachelor of Health Sciences (Nutrition), has also coordinated the practice's health messaging on social media, and I look forward to working with her in our practice soon. Both are holistic health coaches, and I am their best and biggest client so far.

Finally, I'd like to thank you for reading this book.

Notes

Introduction

1   World Health Organisation (WHO), 'The Top 10 Causes of Death', www.who.int/
    mediacentre/factsheets/fs310/en/index2.html

Chapter 1: An Integrative, Holistic Approach to Health

1   WHO, 'Pharmaceutical Industry', www.who.int/trade/glossary/story073/en/

2   PwC, 'From Vision to Decision: Pharma 2020', www.pwc.com/gx/en/pharma-life-
    sciences/pharma2020/assets/pwc-pharma-success-strategies.pdf

3   WHO & Health Action International, *Understanding and Responding to
    Pharmaceutical Promotion: a practical guide*, www1.paho.org/hq/dmdocuments/2011/
    drug-promotion-manual-CAP-3-090610.pdf

4   Health Action International, 'The Promotion of Medicines and Patient Health', www.
    politicsofmedicines.org/articles/promotion-of-medicines-and-patient-health?print=1

5   WHO, *Global Health and Ageing*, October 2011, www.who.int/ageing/publications/
    global_health.pdf

6   WHO, 'Health through Safe Drinking Water and Basic Sanitation', www.who.int/
    water_sanitation_health/mdg1/en/; UN Water, 'Facts and Figures', www.unwater.org/
    water-cooperation-2013/water-cooperation/facts-and-figures-/en/

Chapter 2: A Personal Journey

1   Harvard Medical School, 'Past Deans of the Faculty of Medicine', hms.harvard.edu/
    about-hms/facts-figures/past-deans-faculty-medicine

2   Australasian Society of Oral Medicine and Toxicology, 'Response to the "Dental
    Amalgam and Mercury in Dentistry" Report of an NHMRC Working Party', May
    1999, asomat.com/downloads/ASOMAT-response-to-NHMRC-review.pdf

3   National Health and Medical Research Council (NHMRC), 'Dental Amalgam and
    Mercury in Dentistry', February 1999, asomat.com/downloads/NHMRC-Amalgam-
    Review.pdf

4   NHMRC, 'Dental Amalgam: filling you in', www.nhmrc.gov.au/_files_nhmrc/
     publications/attachments/d18_dental_amalgam_filling_you_in_131223.pdf

5   UN Environmental Program, Minamata Convention on Mercury, www.
     mercuryconvention.org

6   Allan Savory, 'Episode 22: Holistic Health', *The Good Doctors*, thegooddoctors.com.
     au/health-podcast/holistic-health-allan-savory/

Chapter 3: Big Pharma, Big Profits

1   Kelly Brownell & Kenneth Warner, 'The Perils of Ignoring History: Big Tobacco
     played dirty and millions died. How similar is Big Food?', *The Milbank Quarterly*,
     March 2009, 87(1), pp. 259–94; Rohit Malik, 'Catch Me If You Can: Big Food using
     Big Tobacco's playbook? Applying the lessons learned from Big Tobacco to attack
     the obesity epidemic', Food and Drug Law Seminar Paper, 6 December 2010, nrs.
     harvard.edu/urn-3:HUL.InstRepos:8965631

2   Naomi Oreskes & Erik Conway, *Merchants of Doubt: how a handful of scientists
     obscured the truth on issues from tobacco smoke to global warming*, Bloomsbury, 2011

3   Vincent Parry, 'The Art of Branding a Condition', *Medical Marketing and Media*,
     May 2003, 38(5), pp. 42–5, www.darkpharma.nl/uploads/7/3/2/8/7328594/
     theartofbrandingacondition.pdf

4   WHO, 'Spending on Health: a global overview', www.who.int/mediacentre/
     factsheets/fs319/en/

5   Bloomberg, 'The World's Healthiest Countries', 2012, urpsmla.org/IMG/pdf_
     WORLDS_HEALTHIEST_COUNTRIES_V2.pdf

6   Australian Institute of Health and Welfare, 'Health Expenditure Australia 2013–14',
     www.aihw.gov.au/publication-detail/?id=60129552713

7   John Abramson, *Overdosed America: the broken promise of American medicine*,
     HarperCollins, 2004

8   Kathleen Strong et al., 'Preventing Chronic Diseases: how many lives can we save?',
     The Lancet, 29 October 2005, 366(9496), pp. 1578–82

9   Samuel Epstein, *National Cancer Institute and American Cancer Society: criminal
     indifference to cancer prevention and conflicts of interest*, 2011

10   Glinda Cooper, Berrit C. Stroehla, 'The Epidemiology of Autoimmune Diseases',
     Autoimmunity Reviews, May 2003, 2(3), pp. 119–25

11   WHO, 'The Global Burden of Disease', 2004, www.who.int/healthinfo/global_
     burden_disease/GBD_report_2004update_full.pdf

12   B. Hill, 'Allergies', Australian Society of Clinical Immunology and Allergy Annual
     Conference, November 2003

13   Baade et al. 'Trends in Incidence of Childhood Cancer in Australia, 1983–2006',
     British Journal of Cancer, 2010 2 February 2010, 102(3), pp. 620–6; Surveillance,

Epidemiology, and End Results Program, 'SEER Cancer Statistics Review 1975–2012, SEER 9 Areas, Ages 0–19', seer.cancer.gov/archive/csr/1975_2012/browse_csr.php?sectionSEL=29&pageSEL=sect_29_table.02.html

14 M.G. Sawyer et al., 'The Mental Health of Young People in Australia: key findings from the child and adolescent component of the national survey of mental health and well-being', *Australian and New Zealand Journal of Psychiatry*, December 2001, 35(6), pp. 806–14

15 Elizabeth Mumpfer, 'Can Awareness of Medical Pathophysiology in Autism Lead to Primary Care Autism Prevention Strategies?', *North American Journal of Medicine and Science*, July 2013, 6(3), pp. 134–144

16 National Commission of Audit, 'Mental Health', 2014, www.ncoa.gov.au/report/appendix-vol-2/10-8-mental-health.html

17 Australian Bureau of Statistics, 'National Survey of Mental Health and Wellbeing: summary of results, 2007', www.abs.gov.au/AUSSTATS/abs@.nsf/Lookup/4326.0Main+Features12007

18 Australian Bureau of Statistics, 'Australian Social Trends, March 2009', www.abs.gov.au/AUSSTATS/abs@.nsf/allprimarymainfeatures/9045D0375B862263CA2575E40018B10C?opendocument

19 Fairfax Media & Lateral Economics, *The Herald/Age–Lateral Economics Index of Australia's Wellbeing*, December 2011, lateraleconomics.com.au/wp-content/uploads/2014/02/Fairfax-Lateral-Economics-Index-of-Australias-Wellbeing-Final-Report.pdf

20 American Psychiatric Association, *Diagnostic and Statistical Manual of Mental Disorders, Fifth Edition*, 2013, dsm.psychiatryonline.org/doi/book/10.1176/appi.books.9780890425596

21 Allen Frances, 'Opening Pandora's Box: the 19 worst suggestions for *DSM-5*', *Psychiatric Times*, 11 February 2010, 27(9)

22 Arline Kaplan, 'DSM-V Controversies', *Psychiatric Times*, 1 January 2009, www.psychiatrictimes.com/articles/dsm-v-controversies

23 Peter Gotzsche, *Deadly Medicines and Organised Crime: how Big Pharma has corrupted healthcare*, Radcliffe Publishing, 2013

24 Martin Keller et al., 'Efficacy of Paroxetine in the Treatment of Adolescent Depression: a randomised, controlled trial', *Journal of the American Academy of Child and Adolescent Psychiatry*, July 2001, 40(7), pp. 762–72

25 Access to Medicine Foundation, 'The Access to Medicine Index 2014', p. 58 and p. 61, accesstomedicinefoundation.org/media/atmf/2014-Access-to-Medicine-Index.pdf

26 Sammy Almashat et al., 'Rapidly Increasing Criminal and Civil Monetary Penalties Against the Pharmaceutical Industry: 1991 to 2010', 16 December 2010, www.citizen.org/our-work/health-and-safety/rapidly-increasing-criminal-and-civil-monetary-penalties-against

27   Ross Walker, 'Episode 4: Cholesterol: Your Heart, Your Health', *The Good Doctors*, thegooddoctors.com.au/health-podcast/cholesterol-heart-health-with-dr-ross-walker/

28   Ray Moynihan & Alan Cassels, *Selling Sickness: how the world's biggest pharmaceutical companies are turning us all into patients*, Nation Books, 2006

29   Max Nisen, 'The 10 Best Selling Prescription Drugs in the United States', *Business Insider*, 29 June 2012, www.businessinsider.com.au/10-best-selling-blockbuster-drugs-2012-6

30   Michael Eades, 'Absolute Risk versus Relative Risk: why you need to know the difference', www.proteinpower.com/drmike/statins/absolute-risk-versus-relative-risk-need-know-difference/; P.S. Sever et al., 'Prevention of Coronary and Stroke Events with Atorvastatin in Hypertensive Patients Who Have Average or Lower-than-average Cholesterol Concentrations, in the Anglo-Scandinavian Cardiac Outcomes Trial–Lipid Lowering Arm (ASCOT-LLA): a multicentre randomised controlled trial', *The Lancet*, 5 April 2003, 361(9364), pp. 1149–58

31   Thomas Bodenheimer, 'Uneasy Alliance: clinical investigators and the pharmaceutical industry', *The New England Journal of Medicine*, 2000, 342(20), pp. 1539–44

32   Uffe Ravnskov, *Ignore the Awkward!: how the cholesterol myths are kept alive*, 2010; Jonny Bowden & Stephen Sinatra, *The Great Cholesterol Myth: why lowering your cholesterol won't prevent heart disease — and the statin-free plan that will*, Far Winds Press, 2012

33   AllTrials, Petition, www.alltrials.net/petition/

34   Ben Goldacre, *Bad Pharma: how drug companies mislead doctors and harm patients*, Faber and Faber, 2012

35   Lisa Bero et al., 'Factors Associated with Findings of Published Trials of Drug–Drug Comparisons: why some statins appear more efficacious than others', *PLoS Medicine*, 5 June 2007, 4(6), p. e184.

36   R.E. Kelly Jr et al., 'Relationship between Drug Company Funding and Outcomes of Clinical Psychiatric Research', *Psychological Medicine*, November 2006, 36(11), pp. 1647–56

37   Marcia Angell, *The Truth about the Drug Companies: how they deceive us and what to do about it*, Random House, 2005

38   Howard Markel, 'Patents, Profits, and the American People: the Bayh–Dole Act of 1980', *The New England Journal of Medicine*, 29 August 2013, 369(9), pp. 794–6

39   Max Nisen, 'The 10 Best Selling Prescription Drugs in the United States', op. cit.

40   Huseyin Naci et al., 'Industry Sponsorship Bias in Research Findings: a network meta-analysis of LDL cholesterol reduction in randomised trials of statins', *The British Medical Journal*, 3 October 2014, (349), g5741

41   C. Glenn Begley & John Ioannidis, 'Reproducibility in Science: improving the standard for basic and preclinical research', *Circulation Research*, 2 January 2015, 116(1), pp. 116–26

4. The Food Pyramid and Other Myths

1   Kurt Lande & Warren Sperry, 'Human Atherosclerosis in Relation to the Cholesterol Content of the Blood Serum', *Archives of Pathology and Laboratory Medicine*, 1936, 22, pp. 301–12

2   John Yudkin, 'Diet and Coronary Thrombosis', *The Lancet*, 27 July 1957, 270(6987), pp. 155–62

3   John Yudkin, 'The Causes and Cure of Obesity', *The Lancet*, 19 December 1959, 274(7112), pp. 1135–8

4   John Yudkin, *Pure, White, and Deadly: the problem of sugar*, Davis-Poynter, 1972

5   Cristin Kearns et al., 'Sugar Industry and Coronary Heart Disease Research: a historical analysis of internal industry documents', *JAMA Internal Medicine*, 1 November 2016, 176(11), pp. 1680–5

6   Ancel Keys, 'Atherosclerosis: a problem in newer public health', *Journal of the Mt Sinai Hospital, New York*, July–August 1953, 20(2), pp. 118–39

7   Jacob Yerushalmy & Herman Hilleboe, 'Fat in the Diet and Mortality from Heart Disease: a methodologic note', *New York State Journal of Medicine*, 15 July 1957, 57(14), pp. 2343–54

8   Denise Minger, *Death by Food Pyramid: how shoddy science, sketchy politics, and shady special interests have ruined our health*, Primal Blueprint Publishing, 2013; Denise Minger, 'The Truth about Ancel Keys: we've all got it wrong', 22 December 2011, deniseminger.com/2011/12/22/the-truth-about-ancel-keys-weve-all-got-it-wrong/

9   Sandra Jones, 'Fast Food Loses Tick but Can the Heart Foundation Regain Its Credibility?', theconversation.com/fast-food-loses-tick-but-can-the-heart-foundation-regain-its-credibility-3475

10   Richard de Shazo et al., 'The Autopsy of Chicken Nuggets Reads "Chicken Little"', *The American Journal of Medicine*, November 2013, 126(11), pp. 1018–19

11   Jane Cowan, 'McDonalds Gets Tick of Approval', www.abc.net.au/worldtoday/content/2007/s1841333.htm

12   Sandra Jones, 'Fast Food Loses Tick but Can the Heart Foundation Regain Its Credibility?', op. cit.

13   Health Star Rating System, 'About Health Star Ratings', 23 December 2016, healthstarrating.gov.au/internet/healthstarrating/publishing.nsf/Content/About-health-stars

14   Health Star Rating System, 'Acknowledgements', 6 December 2014, healthstarrating. gov.au/internet/healthstarrating/publishing.nsf/Content/Acknowledgements

15   Katinka Day, 'Dishonest Health Star Ratings on Milo and Kellogg's Cereals', *Choice*, 15 February 2016, www.choice.com.au/food-and-drink/nutrition/food-labelling/articles/nestle-milo-kelloggs-cereals-misuse-health-star-ratings

16   Elizabeth Pulgaron & Alan Delamater, 'Obesity and Type 2 Diabetes in Children:

epidemiology and treatment', *Current Diabetes Reports*, August 2014, 14(8), p. 508

17   David Maahs et al., 'The Epidemiology of Type 1 Diabetes', *Endocrinology and Metabolism Clinics of North America*, September 2010, 39(3), pp. 481–497

18   Goodarz Danaei et al., 'National, Regional, and Global Trends in Fasting Plasma Glucose and Diabetes Prevalence since 1980: systematic analysis of health examination surveys and epidemiological studies with 370 country-years and 2.7 million participants', *The Lancet*, June 2011, 378(9785), pp. 31–40

19   James DiNicolantonio et al., 'Added Fructose: a principal driver of type 2 diabetes mellitus and its consequences', *Mayo Clinic Proceedings*, March 2015, 90(3), pp. 372–81

20   S.M. de la Monte & J.R. Wands, 'Alzheimer's Disease Is Type 3 Diabetes: evidence reviewed', *Journal of Diabetes Science and Technology*, November 2008, 2(6), pp. 1101–13

21   Alzheimer's Disease International, *The Global Impact of Dementia: an analysis of prevalence, incidence, cost, and trends*, World Alzheimer Report 2015, London 2015

22   Centres for Disease Control and Prevention, *2014 National Diabetes Statistics Report*, www.cdc.gov/diabetes/data/statistics/2014statisticsreport.html

23   Nidhi Bansal, 'Prediabetes Diagnosis and Treatment: a review', *World Journal of Diabetes*, 15 March 2015, 6(2), pp. 296–303

24   Lydia Bazzano et al., 'Effects of Low-Carbohydrate and Low-Fat Diets: a randomised trial', *Annals of Internal Medicine*, September 2014, 161(5), pp. 309–18; Hu et al., 'Effects of Low-Carbohydrate Diets versus Low-Fat Diets on Metabolic Risk Factors: a meta-analysis of randomised controlled clinical trials', *American Journal of Epidemiology*, 1 October 2012, 176 (Supplement 7), pp. S44–S54

25   American Diabetes Association, 'The Cost of Diabetes', www.diabetes.org/advocacy/news-events/cost-of-diabetes.html

26   Juhee Kim et al., 'Trends in Overweight from 1980 through 2001 among Preschool-aged Children Enrolled in a Health Maintenance Organisation', *Obesity*, July 2006, 14(7), pp. 1107–12

27   Harvard School of Public Health, 'Healthy Eating Plate and Healthy Eating Pyramid', www.hsph.harvard.edu/nutritionsource/pyramid-full-story/

28   USDA, Interactive DRI Calculator for Healthcare Professionals, www.nal.usda.gov/fnic/interactiveDRI/

5. Emotional Stress

1   Lynne Casey & Rachel Pui-Tak Liang, *Stress and Wellbeing in Australia Survey 2014*, Australian Psychological Society, www.psychology.org.au/Assets/Files/2014-APS-NPW-Survey-WEB-reduced.pdf

2   Hans Selye, *The Stress of Life*, McGraw-Hill, 1956

3 Yuval Noah Harari, *Sapiens: a brief history of humankind*, Vintage, 2014

4 Alain de Botton, *The News: a user's manual*, Pantheon, 2014

5 Elissa Epel et al., 'Accelerated Telomere Shortening in Response to Life Stress', *Proceedings of the National Academy of Sciences of the United States of America*, 7 December 2004, 101(49), pp. 17312–15

6 Claudia Dreifus, 'Finding Clues to Ageing in the Fraying Tips of Chromosomes', *The New York Times*, 3 July 2007, www.nytimes.com/2007/07/03/science/03conv.html

7 Dean Ornish et al., 'Effect of Comprehensive Lifestyle Changes on Telomerase Activity and Telomere Length in Men with Biopsy-proven Low-risk Prostate Cancer: five-year follow-up of a descriptive pilot study', *Lancet Oncology*, October 2013, 14(11), pp. 1112–20; Elizabeth Fernandez, 'Lifestyle Changes May Lengthen Telomeres, A Measure of Cell Ageing', 16 September 2013, www.ucsf.edu/news/2013/09/108886/lifestyle-changes-may-lengthen-telomeres-measure-cell-aging

8 Nessa Carey, *The Epigenetics Revolution: how modern biology is rewriting our understanding of genetics, disease, and inheritance*, Columbia University Press, 2013

9 Bruce Lipton, *The Biology of Belief: unleashing the power of consciousness, matter, and miracles*, Hay House, 2008

10 Kelly McGonigal, 'How to Make Stress Your Friend', www.ted.com/talks/kelly_mcgonigal_how_to_make_stress_your_friend

11 Abiola Keller et al., 'Does the Perception that Stress Affects Health Matter?: the association with health and mortality', *Health Psychology*, September 2012, 31(5), pp. 677–84

12 Hermann Nabi et al., 'Increased Risk of Coronary Heart Disease among Individuals Reporting Adverse Impact of Stress on Their Health: the Whitehall II prospective cohort study', *European Heart Journal*, September 2013, 34(34), pp. 2697–705; Safiya Richardson et al., 'Meta-analysis of Perceived Stress and Its Association with Incident Coronary Heart Disease', *The American Journal of Cardiology*, 15 December 2012, 110(12), pp. 1711–16

13 Kelly Turner, *Radical Remission: surviving cancer against all odds*, HarperCollins, 2014

6. Nutritional Stress

1 Kathleen Strong et al., 'Preventing Chronic Diseases: how many lives can we save?', op. cit.

2 WHO, 'Preventing Chronic Diseases: a vital investment', 2005, www.who.int/chp/chronic_disease_report/full_report.pdf

3 William Doe, 'The Intestinal Immune System', *Gut*, December 1989, 30(12), pp. 1679–85

4 David Perlmutter & Kristin Loberg, *Grain Brain: the surprising truth about wheat, carbs, and sugar — your brain's silent killers*, Little, Brown & Company, 2013

5   Simone Peters et al., 'Randomised Clinical Trial: gluten may cause depression in subjects with non-coeliac gluten sensitivity — an exploratory clinical study', *Alimentary Pharmacology and Therapeutics*, May 2014, 39(10), pp. 1104–12; Stephen Genuis & Rebecca Lobo, 'Gluten Sensitivity Presenting as a Neuropsychiatric Disorder', *Gastroenterology Research and Practice*, 2014, (5); Marios Hadjivassiliou et al., 'Gluten Sensitivity: from gut to brain', *Lancet Neurology*, March 2010, 9(3), pp. 318–30

6   Continence Foundation of Australia, 'Bristol Stool Chart', www.continence.org.au/pages/bristol-stool-chart.html

7   Michael Holick & T.C. Chen, 'Vitamin D Deficiency: a worldwide problem with health consequences', *The American Journal of Clinical Nutrition*, April 2008, 87(4), pp. 1080S–6S

8   John Ioannidis, 'More than a Billion People Taking Statins?: potential implications of the new cardiovascular guidelines', *Journal of the American Medical Association*, February 2014, 311(5), pp. 463–4

9   Samuel Epstein, *National Cancer Institute and American Cancer Society*, op. cit.; Surveillance, Epidemiology, and End Results Program, 'SEER Cancer Statistics Review 1975–2012, SEER 9 Areas, Ages 0–19', op. cit.

10 Sanne Peters et al., 'Incorporating Added Sugar Improves the Performance of the Health Star Rating Front-of-pack Labelling System in Australia', *Nutrients,* 5 July 2017, 9(7)

11 NHMRC, 'Eat for Health: Australian dietary guidelines', 2013, p. 104

12 Janet James et al., 'Preventing Childhood Obesity by Reducing Consumption of Carbonated Drinks: cluster randomised controlled trial', *The British Medical Journal*, 2004, (328), pp. 1237

13 Cynthia Kenyon, 'The First Long-lived Mutants: discovery of the insulin/IGF-1 pathway for ageing', *Philosophical Transactions of the Royal Society of London, Series B, Biological Sciences*, 12 January 2011, 366(1561), pp. 9–16

14 A.R. Gaby, 'Adverse Effects of Dietary Fructose', *Alternative Medicine Review*, December 2005, 10(4), pp. 294–306

15 George Bray et al., 'Consumption of High-fructose Corn Syrup in Beverages May Play a Role in the Epidemic of Obesity', *The American Journal of Clinical Nutrition*, April 2004, 79(4), pp. 537–43

16 WHO, 'WHO Calls on Countries to Reduce Sugars Intake among Adults and Children', 4 March 2015, www.who.int/mediacentre/news/releases/2015/sugar-guideline/en/

17 Lydia Bazzano et al., 'Effects of Low-Carbohydrate and Low-Fat Diets: a randomised trial', op. cit.

18 William Davis, *Wheat Belly: lose the wheat, lose the weight, and find your path back to health*, Rodale, 2014

19 Lisa Kucek et al., 'A Grounded Guide to Gluten: how modern genotypes and processing impact wheat sensitivity', *Comprehensive Reviews in Food Science and Food Safety*, May 2015, 14(3), pp. 285–302

20 Alessio Fasano et al., 'Zonulin, a Newly Discovered Modulator of Intestinal Permeability, and its Expression in Coeliac Disease', *The Lancet*, 2000, 355(9214), pp. 1518–19

21 Alessio Fasano, 'Zonulin and Its Regulation of Intestinal Barrier Function: the biological door to inflammation, autoimmunity, and cancer', *Physiological Reviews*, 2011, 91(1), pp. 151–76; Alessio Fasano, 'Zonulin, Regulation of Tight Junctions, and Autoimmune Diseases', *Annals of the New York Academy of Sciences*, July 2012, 1258(1), pp. 25–33

22 Vikas Kumar et al., 'Dietary Roles of Non-starch Polysaccharides in Human Nutrition: a review', *Critical Reviews in Food Science and Nutrition*, October 2012, 52(10), pp. 899–935

23 Rod Taylor et al., 'Reduced Dietary Salt for the Prevention of Cardiovascular Disease: a meta-analysis of randomised controlled trials', *American Journal of Hypertension*, August 2011, 24(8), pp. 843–53; Katarzyna Stolarz-Skrzypek et al., 'Fatal and Nonfatal Outcomes, Incidence of Hypertension, and Blood Pressure Changes in Relation to Urinary Sodium Excretion', *Journal of the American Medical Association*, 4 May 2011, 305(17), pp. 1777–85

24 H. Joe Wang et al., 'Alcohol, Inflammation, and Gut–Liver–Brain Interactions in Tissue Damage and Disease Development', *World Journal of Gastroenterology*, 21 March 2010, 16(11), pp. 1304–13

7. Environmental Stress

1 Duncan Cameron et al., 'A Sustainable Model for Intensive Agriculture', Grantham Centre for Sustainable Futures, University of Sheffield, December 2015, grantham. sheffield.ac.uk/engagement/policy/a-sustainable-model-for-intensive-agriculture/

2 Global Change Courses, 'Land Degradation', University of Michigan, www. globalchange.umich.edu/globalchange2/current/lectures/land_deg/land_deg.html

3 Nikos Alexandratos & Jelle Bruinsma, *World Agriculture Towards 2030/2050: the 2012 revision*, Food and Agriculture Organisation of the UN, 2012, www.fao.org/docrep/016/ap106e/ap106e.pdf

4 Allan Savory, *Holistic Management: a new framework for decision making*, Island Press, 1999

5 Allan Savory, 'How to Fight Desertification and Reverse Climate Change', www.ted. com/talks/allan_savory_how_to_green_the_world_s_deserts_and_reverse_climate_change

6 Food and Agriculture Organisation of the UN, *Global Food Losses and Food Waste: extent, causes, and prevention*, 2011, www.fao.org/docrep/014/mb060e/mb060e.pdf

7   Jonathan Foley, 'It's Time to Rethink America's Corn System', *Scientific American*, 5 March 2013, www.scientificamerican.com/article/time-to-rethink-corn/

8   'US Could Feed 800 Million People with Grain that Livestock Eat', *Cornell Chronicle*, 7 August 1997, www.news.cornell.edu/stories/1997/08/us-could-feed-800-million-people-grain-livestock-eat

9   Emily Cassidy et al., 'Redefining Agricultural Yields: from tonnes to people nourished per hectare', *Environmental Research Letters*, September 2013, 8(3)

10 Australian Academy of Science, *The Science of Climate Change: questions and answers*, 2015, www.science.org.au/learning/general-audience/science-booklets-0/science-climate-change

11 Yuval Noah Harari, *Sapiens*, op. cit.

12 David Coady et al., 'How Large Are Global Energy Subsidies?', International Monetary Fund, 2015, www.imf.org/external/pubs/ft/wp/2015/wp15105.pdf

13 Wi-fi in Schools Australia, 'Governments and Authorities Around the World', www.wifi-in-schools-australia.org/p/worldwide.html

14 Charalabos Papageorgiou et al., 'Effects of Wi-fi Signals on the p300 Component of Event-related Potentials during an Auditory Hayling Task', *Journal of Integrative Neuroscience*, June 2011, 10(2), pp. 189–202; Argiro Maganioti et al., 'Wi-fi Electromagnetic Fields Exert Gender-related Alterations on EEG', 6th International Workshop on Biological Effects of Electromagnetic Fields, 2010

15 Julian Cribb, *The Poisoned Planet: how constant exposure to man-made chemicals is putting your life at risk*, Allen and Unwin, 2014

16 Physicians for Social Responsibility, 'The Need for Chemical Reform in the United States', www.psr.org/resources/the-need-for-chemical-reform-in-the-us.pdf

17 Marc Cohen, '10 Toxic Truths', Global Spa and Wellness Summit, New Delhi, 2013, mams.rmit.edu.au/3s4wbamg1ekt.pdf

18 Theo Colborn et al., *Our Stolen Future: are we threatening our fertility, intelligence, and survival? — a scientific detective story*, Plume, 1997

19 UN Environmental Program and the WHO, '*State of the Science of Endocrine-disrupting Chemicals — 2012*, 2013, www.who.int/ceh/publications/endocrine/en/

20 Stephen Trumble et al., 'Blue Whale Earplug Reveals Lifetime Contaminant Exposure and Hormone Profiles', *Proceedings of the National Academy of Sciences*, 15 October 2013, 110(42), pp. 16922–26

21 Halima Kazem, 'US Residents Monitor Fukushima Radiation', *Al Jazeera*, 19 January 2014, www.aljazeera.com/humanrights/2014/01/us-residents-monitor-fukushima-radiation-201411911450378232.html

22 International Program on the State of the Ocean, 'Latest Review of Science Reveals Ocean in Critical State from Cumulative Impacts', 2013, www.stateoftheocean.org/research.cfm

23 Food and Agriculture Organisation of the UN, *World Review of Fisheries and Aquaculture Report 2012*, www.fao.org/docrep/016/i2727e/i2727e.pdf

24 Jenna Jambeck et al., 'Plastic Waste Inputs from Land into the Ocean', *Science*, 13 Feb 2015, 347(6223), pp. 768–71

25 Matthew Evans, *The Real Food Companion*, Murdoch, 2010

26 Matthew Evans, *What's the Catch*, SBS TV, 2014, www.sbs.com.au/programs/whats-the-catch

27 Julian Cribb, *The Poisoned Planet*, op. cit.

8. Dental Stress

1 Susanna Paju et al., '*Porphyromonas gingivalis* May Interfere with Conception in Women', *Journal of Oral Microbiology*, June 2017, 9(1)

2 Satheesh Mannem & Vijay Chava, 'The Relationship between Maternal Periodontitis and Preterm Low Birth Weight: a case-control study', *Contemporary Clinical Dentistry*, April–June 2011, 2(2), pp. 88–93

3 Rosario Guiglia et al., 'Osteoporosis, Jawbones, and Periodontal Disease', *Medicinia Oral Patologia Oral y Cirugia Bucal*, January 2013, 18(1), pp. e93–e99

4 Michael Karin, 'Innate Immunity Gone Awry: linking microbial infections to chronic inflammation and cancer', *Cell*, 2006, 124(4), pp. 823–35

5 Scott Peterson et al., 'The Dental Plaque Microbiome in Health and Disease', *PLOS One*, March 2013, 8(3), www.ncbi.nlm.nih.gov/pmc/articles/PMC3592792/

6 Koichiro Matsuo & Jeffrey Palmer, 'Anatomy and Physiology of Feeding and Swallowing — Normal and Abnormal', *Physical Medicine and Rehabilitation Clinics of North America*, November 2008, 19(4), pp. 691–707

7 Weston A. Price, *Nutrition and Physical Degeneration: a comparison of primitive and modern diets and their effects*, Price-Pottenger Nutrition Foundation, 2009

8 Daniel Garliner, *Myofunctional Therapy*, Saunders, 1981

9 Robert Little, 'Stability and Relapse of Mandibular Anterior Alignment: University of Washington studies', *Seminars in Orthodontics*, September 1999, 5(3), pp. 191–204

10 Rafael Roda et al., 'Review of Temporomandibular Joint Pathology, Part I: classification, epidemiology, and risk factors', *Medicina Oral, Patologia Oral, y Cirugia Bucal*, 2007, (12), pp. E292–8, scielo.isciii.es/pdf/medicorpa/v12n4/06.pdf

11 Mats Hanson, 'Amalgam: hazards in your teeth', *Journal of Orthomolecular Psychiatry*, September 1983, 12(3), pp. 194–201; B. Nilsson & B. Nilsson, 'Mercury in Dental Practice, I: the working environment of dental personnel and their exposure to mercury vapour', *Swedish Dental Journal*, 1986, 10(1–2), pp. 1–14

12 J.F. Fisher, 'Elemental Mercury and Inorganic Mercury Compounds: human health aspects', WHO, 2003, apps.who.int/iris/handle/10665/42607

13   Peter Goering et al., 'Toxicity Assessment of Mercury Vapour from Dental
      Amalgams', *Fundamental and Applied Toxicology*, 1992, 19(3), pp. 319–29; National
      Research Council Committee on the Toxicological Effects of Methylmercury,
      'Chemistry, Exposure, Toxicokinetics, and Toxicodynamics' in *Toxicological Effects
      of Methylmercury*, National Academic Press, 2000, www.ncbi.nlm.nih.gov/books/
      NBK225779/

14   Leszek Hahn et al., 'Whole Body Imaging of the Distribution of Mercury Released
      from Dental Fillings into Monkey Tissues', *The FASEB Journal*, November 1990,
      4(14), pp. 3256–60

15   L. Friberg, 'Environmental Health Criteria 118: inorganic mercury', WHO, 1991

16   Patrick Stortebecker, 'Mercury Poisoning from Dental Amalgam through a Direct
      Nose–Brain Transport', *The Lancet*, 27 May 1989, 333(8648), p. 1207

17   N.D. Boyd, 'Mercury from Dental "Silver" Tooth Fillings Impairs Sheep Kidney
      Function', *The American Journal of Physiology*, October 1991, 261(4), pp. R1010–R1014

18   Boyd Haley, 'The Relationship of the Toxic Effects of Mercury to Exacerbation of the
      Medical Condition Classified as Alzheimer's Disease', *Medical Veritas*, 2007, (4), pp.
      1510–24

19   Dental Amalgam Mercury Solutions, 'Alzheimer's Disease and Other Autoimmune
      Degenerative Conditions: the mercury connection', amalgam.org/education/scientific-
      evidenceresearch/alzheimers-disease-autoimmune-degenerative-conditions-mercury-
      connection/

20   Per Hultman et al., 'Adverse Immunological Effects and Autoimmunity Induced by
      Dental Amalgam and Alloy in Mice', *The FASEB Journal*, December 1994, 8(14), pp.
      1183–90

21   Anne Summers et al., 'Mercury Released from Dental "Silver" Fillings Provokes an
      Increase in Mercury- and Antibiotic-Resistant Bacteria in Oral and Intestinal Flora of
      Primates', *Antimicrobial Agents and Chemotherapy*, April 1993, 37(4), pp. 825–34

22   Magnus Nylander et al., 4th International Symposium on Epidemiology in
      Occupational Health, Como, Italy, September 1985; Diana Echeverria et al.,
      'Behavioural Effects of Low-level Exposure to Hg⁰ among Dentists', *Neurotoxicology
      and Teratology*, 1995, 17(2), pp. 161–8

23   G. Drasch et al., 'Mercury Burden of Human Foetal and Infant Tissues', *European
      Journal of Paediatrics*, August 1994, 153(8), pp. 607–10

24   Australasian Integrative Medicine Association, 'Position Paper on Mercury Amalgam',
      2011, www.mercuryfreedentistry.com.au/images/letters/AIMA%20POSITION%20
      PAPER%20ON%20DENTAL%20AMALGAM.pdf

25   International Academy of Oral Medicine and Toxicology, 'The Scientific Case Against
      Amalgam', iaomt.org/wp-content/uploads/The-Case-Against-Amalgam.pdf

26   Yurdanur Ucar & William Brantley, 'Biocompatibility of Dental Amalgams',
      International Journal of Dentistry, 2011

27   NHMRC, 'Dental Amalgam: filling you in', op. cit.

28   Vera Stejskal, 'Metals as a Common Trigger of Inflammation Resulting in Non-specific Symptoms: diagnosis and treatment', *Israel Medical Association Journal*, 2014, 16(2), pp. 753–8; Vera Stejskal et al., 'Metal-induced Inflammation Triggers Fibromyalgia in Metal-allergic Patients', *Neuroendocrinology Letters*, 2013, 34(6), pp. 559–65

29   Masayuki Inoue, 'The Status Quo of Metal Allergy and Measures against It in Dentistry', *Journal of Japan Prosthodont Society*, 1993, 37(6), pp. 1127–38

30   Maki Hosoki & Keisuke Nishigawa, 'Dental Metal Allergy' in Young Suck Ro (ed.), *Contact Dermatitis*, InTech, 2011; Matt Kaplan, 'Infections May Trigger Metal Allergies', *Nature*, 2 May 2007, www.nature.com/news/2007/070430/full/news070430-6.html; Anthony Goon & C.L. Goh, 'Metal Allergy in Singapore', *Contact Dermatitis*, March 2005, 52(3), pp. 130–2

31   Robert Rietschel et al., 'Detection of Nickel Sensitivity Has Increased in North American Patch-test Patients', *Dermatitis*, 2008, 19(1), pp. 16–19

32   Jacob Thyssen & Torkil Menne, 'Metal Allergy: a review on exposures, penetration, genetics, prevalence, and clinical implications', *Chemical Research in Toxicology*, 15 February 2010, 23(2), pp. 309–18

33   Elizabeth Valentine-Thon et al., 'LTT-MELISA Is Clinically Relevant for Detecting and Monitoring Metal Sensitivity', *Neuroendocrinology Letters*, 2006, 27(Suppl. 1), pp. 17–24

34   Elizabeth Valentine-Thon & Hans-Walter Schiwara, 'Validity of MELISA for Metal-sensitivity Testing', *Neuroendocrinology Letters* 2003, 24(1–2), pp. 57–64

35   MELISA Foundation, www.melisa.org

36   Stefano Eramo et al., 'Oestrogenicity of Bisphenol A Released from Sealants and Composites: a review of the literature', *Annali di Stomatologia*, 2010, 1(3–4), pp. 14–21

37   Stepan Podzimek et al., 'Immune Markers in Oral Discomfort Patients before and after Elimination of Oral Galvanism', *Neuroendocrinology Letters*, 2013, 34(8), pp. 802–8

38   Paul Connett et al., *The Case Against Fluoride: how hazardous waste ended up in our drinking water and the bad science and powerful politics that keep it there*, Chelsea Green, 2010

39   Anna Choi et al., 'Developmental Fluoride Neurotoxicity: a systematic review and meta-analysis', *Environmental Health Perspectives*, October 2012, 120(10), pp. 1362–8

40   Marianne Empson et al., 'Prevalence of Thyroid Disease in an Older Australian Population', *International Medical Journal*, July 2007, 37(7), pp. 448–55

41   Cancer Australia, 'Thyroid Cancer Statistics', 2013, thyroid-cancer.canceraustralia.gov.au/statistics

42   Samuel Epstein, *National Cancer Institute and American Cancer Society*, op. cit.

43   Childsmile Program, www.child-smile.org.uk

9. Postural Stress

1   Shwetha Nair et al., 'Do Slumped and Upright Postures Affect Stress Responses?: a randomised trial', *Health Psychology*, June 2015, 34(6), pp. 632–41

2   James Levine, 'Sick of Sitting', *Diabetologia*, August 2015, 58(8), pp. 1751–8

3   Lionel Bey & Marc Hamilton, 'Suppression of Skeletal Muscle Lipoprotein Lipase Activity during Physical Inactivity: a molecular reason to maintain daily low-intensity activity', *Journal of Physiology*, 1 September 2003, 551(Pt 2), pp. 673–682

4   David Dunstan, 'Sitting is Deadly', *Catalyst*, ABC TV, 2012, www.abc.net.au/catalyst/stories/3568627.htm

5   Ryan Falck et al., 'What Is the Association between Sedentary Behaviour and Cognitive Function?: a systematic review', *British Journal of Sports Medicine*, 1 May 2017, (51), pp. 800–11

6   Happy Body at Work, www.happybodyatwork.com.au

7   Bernard Duvivier et al., 'Breaking Sitting with Light Activities vs Structured Exercise: a randomised crossover study demonstrating benefits for glycaemic control and insulin sensitivity in type 2 diabetes', *Diabetologia*, March 2017, 60(3), pp. 490–8

8   Kenneth Hansraj, 'Assessment of Stresses in the Cervical Spine Caused by Posture and Position of the Head', *Surgical Technology International*, 2014, (25), pp. 277–9

9   David Simons et al., *Myofascial Pain and Dysfunction: The Trigger Point Manual, vol. 1: upper half of body*, Lippincott, Williams & Wilkins, 1999

10   Access Economics, 'The High Price of Pain: the economic impact of persistent pain in Australia', November 2007, www.painaustralia.org.au/images/pain_australia/MBF%20Economic%20Impact.pdf

11   Ron Ehrlich et al., 'The Effect of Jaw Clenching on the Electromyographic Activities of Two Neck and Two Trunk Muscles', *Journal of Orofacial Pain*, 1999, 13(2), pp. 115–20

12   T. Miyahara et al. 'Modulations of Human Soleus H reflex in Association with Volumetric Clenching of Teeth', *Journal of Neurophysiology*, September 1996, 76(3), pp. 2,033–41

13   Ron Ehrlich et al., 'Electromyographic Activity in Walking Subjects with and without Prosthetic Devices' in Fay Horak & Marjorie Woollacott (eds), *Posture and Gait: control mechanisms*, University of Oregon Books, 1992

14   Dov Sikirov, 'Comparison of Straining during Defecation in Three Positions: results and implications for human health', *Digestive Diseases and Sciences*, July 2003, 48(7), pp. 1201–5

15   Ryuji Sakakibara et al., 'Influence of Body Position on Defecation in Humans', *Lower Urinary Tract Symptoms*, 2010, 2(1), pp. 16–21

10. Sleep

1   Carol Worthman, 'Developmental Cultural Ecology of Sleep' in Mona El-Sheikh (ed.), *Sleep and Development: familial and socio-cultural considerations*, Oxford Press, 2011

2   Lasse Dissing-Olesen et al., 'New Brain Lymphatic Vessels Drain Old Concepts', *EBioMedicine*, August 2015, 2(8), pp. 776–7; Nadia Jessen et al., 'The Glymphatic System: a beginner's guide', *Neurochemical Research*, December 2015, 40(12), pp. 2,583–99

3   Lulu Xie et al., 'Sleep Drives Metabolite Clearance from the Adult Brain', *Science*, 18 October 2013, 342(6158), pp. 373–7; Hedok Lee et al., 'The Effect of Body Posture on Brain Glymphatic Transport', *The Journal of Neuroscience*, 5 August 2015, 35(31), pp. 11,034–44

4   Vinod Kumar, 'Melatonin: a master hormone and a candidate for universal panacea', *Indian Journal of Experimental Biology*, May 1996, 34(5), pp. 391–402

5   Walter Pierpaoli et al., *The Melatonin Miracle: nature's age-reversing, disease-fighting, sex-enhancing hormone*, Pocket Books, 1996

6   Freda DeKeyser Ganz, 'Sleep and Immune Function', *Critical Care Nurse*, April 2012, 32(2), pp. e19–e25

7   Nikolaus Netzer et al., 'Women with Sleep Apnoea Have Lower Levels of Sex Hormones', *Sleep and Breathing*, January 2003, 7(1), pp. 25–9

8   Monica Anseren & Sergio Tufik, 'The Effects of Testosterone on Sleep and Sleep-disordered Breathing in Men: its bidirectional interaction with erectile function', *Sleep Medicine Reviews*, October 2008, 12(5), pp. 365–79

9   Hans Van Dongen et al., 'The Cumulative Cost of Additional Wakefulness: dose-response effects on neurobehavioral functions and sleep physiology from chronic sleep restriction and total sleep deprivation', *Sleep*, 15 March 2003, 26(2), pp. 117–26

10   National Sleep Foundation, '2005 Sleep in America Poll', sleepfoundation.org/sites/default/files/2005_summary_of_findings.pdf

11   Gary Wittert, 'The Relationship between Sleep Disorders and Testosterone in Men', *Asian Journal of Andrology*, 2014, 16(2), pp. 262–5

12   Roseanne Armitage, 'The Effects of Antidepressants on Sleep in Patients with Depression', *The Canadian Journal of Psychiatry*, November 2000, 45(9), pp. 803–9

13   American Academy of Sleep Medicine, *International Classification of Sleep Disorders, Second Edition*, 2005.

14   M.G. Sawyer et al., 'The Mental Health of Young People in Australia', op. cit.

15   David Lawrence et al., 'The Mental Health of Children and Adolescents: report on

the second Australian child and adolescent survey of mental health and wellbeing', August 2015, www.health.gov.au/internet/main/publishing.nsf/content/mental-pubs-m-child2

16 Sarah Holden et al. 'The Prevalence and Incidence, Resource Use and Financial Costs of Treating People with Attention Deficit/Hyperactivity Disorder (ADHD) in the United Kingdom (1998 to 2010)', *Child and Adolescent Psychiatry and Mental Health*, 11 October 2013, 7(1), p. 34

17 Centres for Disease Control and Prevention, 'ADHD Data and Statistics', 18 July 2017, www.cdc.gov/ncbddd/adhd/data.html

18 Jim Papadopolous, 'Episode 68: Sleeping Disorders in Children', *The Good Doctors*, thegooddoctors.com.au/health-podcast/sleep-disorders-dr-jim-papadopolous/

19 Sanjeev Mehta et al., 'Non-invasive Means of Measuring Hepatic Fat Content', *World Journal of Gastroenterology*, 14 June 2008, 14(22), pp. 3476–83

20 Max Hirshkowitz et al., 'National Sleep Foundation's Sleep Time Duration Recommendations: methodology and results summary', *Sleep Health*, March 2015, 1(1), 40–3

21 Nicole Bijlsma, *Healthy Home, Healthy Family: is where you live affecting your health?*, Joshua Books, 2010

22 Ketema Paul et al., 'Influence of Sex on Sleep Regulatory Mechanisms', *Journal of Women's Health*, September 2008, 17(7), pp. 1201–8

23 Kelly Baron et al., 'Exercise to Improve Sleep in Insomnia: exploration of the bidirectional effects', *Journal of Clinical Sleep Medicine*, 15 August 2013, 9(8), pp. 819–24

24 Terri Weaver & Ronald Grunstein, 'Adherence to Continuous Positive Airway Pressure Therapy: the challenge to effective treatment', *Proceedings of the American Thoracic Society*, 15 February 2008, 5(2), pp. 173–8

25 C.L. Phillips et al., 'Health Outcomes of Continuous Positive Airway Pressure versus Oral Appliance Treatment for Obstructive Sleep Apnoea: a randomised controlled trial', *American Journal of Respiratory and Critical Care Medicine*, 15 April 2013, 187(8), pp. 879–87

26 Kate Sutherland & Peter Cistulli, 'Mandibular Advancement Splints for the Treatment of Sleep Apnoea Syndrome', *Swiss Medical Weekly*, September 2011, (141), p. w13276

27 Thomas Roth et al., 'Insomnia: pathophysiology and implications for treatment,' *Sleep Medicine Reviews*, February 2007, 11(1), pp. 71–9

28 Jodie Harris et al., 'A Randomised Controlled Trial of Intensive Sleep Retraining (ISR): a brief conditioning treatment for chronic insomnia', *Sleep*, 1 January 2012, 35(1), pp. 49–60; Arthur Spielman & Paul Glovinsky, 'What a Difference a Day Makes', *Sleep*, January 2012, 35(1), pp. 11–12

11. Breathing

1   Tania Clifton-Smith & Janet Rowley, 'Breathing Pattern Disorders and Physiotherapy: inspiration for our profession', *Physical Therapy Reviews*, 2011, 16(1), pp. 75–86

2   Buteyko Institute of Breathing and Health, www.buteyko.info

3   Christina Zelano et al., 'Nasal Respiration Entrains Human Limbic Oscillations and Modulates Cognitive Function', *The Journal of Neuroscience*, 7 December 2016, 36(49), pp. 12,448–67, www.jneurosci.org/content/36/49/12448

4   Tania Clifton-Smith & Janet Rowley, 'Breathing Pattern Disorders and Physiotherapy', op. cit.

5   National Kidney Foundation, 'Medications to Treat Bed-wetting', www.kidney.org/patients/bw/BWmeds

6   Tsung-Wei Huang & Tai-Horng Young, 'Novel Porous Oral Patches for Patients with Mild Obstructive Sleep Apnoea and Mouth Breathing: a pilot study', *Journal of Otolarnygology — Head and Neck Surgery*, February 2015, 152(2), pp. 369–73

12. Nutrition

1   Weston A. Price, *Nutrition and Physical Degeneration*, op. cit.

2   Sally Fallon & Mary Enig, *Nourishing Traditions: the cookbook that challenges politically correct nutrition and the diet dictocrats*, NewTrends, 2001

3   Weston A. Price Foundation, www.westonaprice.org

4   Price-Pottenger Nutrition Foundation, price-pottenger.org

5   Nutrition Coalition, 'Saturated Fats: do they cause heart disease?', www.nutrition-coalition.org/saturated-fats-do-they-cause-heart-disease/

6   Irena Macri, 'Making Sense of Healthy Cooking Oils and Fats', *Eat Drink Paleo*, 6 January 2014, eatdrinkpaleo.com.au/making-sense-of-healthy-cooking-oils-fats/

7   NHMRC, 'Protein', *Nutrient Reference Values for Australia and New Zealand*, 9 April 2014, www.nrv.gov.au/nutrients/protein

8   Chris Kresser, 'Liver: nature's most potent superfood,' 11 April 2008, chriskresser.com/natures-most-potent-superfood/

9   Mayo Clinic, 'Pregnancy Nutrition: foods to avoid during pregnancy', www.mayoclinic.org/healthy-lifestyle/pregnancy-week-by-week/in-depth/pregnancy-nutrition/art-20043844

10   Ransom Myers & Boris Worm, 'Extinction, Survival, or Recovery of Large Predatory Fishes', *Philosophical Transactions B*, 29 January 2005, 360(1453), pp. 13–20

11   Matthew Evans, *What's the Catch*, op. cit.

12   Berkley Wellness, 'Sardines: a good source of Omega-3s', 6 May 2013, www.berkeleywellness.com/healthy-eating/food/article/sardines-good-source-omega-3s

13 Diane Feskanich et al., 'Milk, Dietary Calcium, and Bone Fractures in Women: a 12-year prospective study', *American Journal of Public Health*, June 1997, 87(6), pp. 992–7

14 Physicians Committee for Responsible Medicine, 'Milk Consumption and Prostate Cancer', www.pcrm.org/health/health-topics/milk-consumption-and-prostate-cancer

15 'Putting the Polish on those Humble Beans', www.westonaprice.org/health-topics/ food-features/putting-the-polish-on-those-humble-beans/

16 Sarah Britton, 'The Life-changing Loaf of Bread', *My New Roots*, 12 February 2013, www.mynewroots.org/site/2013/02/the-life-changing-loaf-of-bread/

17 Nora Gedgaudas, *Primal Body, Primal Mind: beyond the Paleo diet for total health and a longer life*, Healing Arts, 2010

18 Christian Allan & Wolfgang Lutz, *Life Without Bread: how a low-carbohydrate diet can save your life*, Keats, 2000

19 Michael Gershon, *The Second Brain: the scientific basis of gut instinct and a groundbreaking new understanding of nervous disorders of the stomach and intestines*, HarperCollins, 1998

20 Sandor Katz, *The Art of Fermentation: an in-depth exploration of essential concepts and processes from around the world*, Chelsea Green, 2012

21 Sunitha George et al., 'A Perception on Health Benefits of Coffee', *Critical Reviews in Food Science and Nutrition*, May 2008, 48(5), pp. 464–86

22 Masood Butt & Muhammad Sultan, 'Coffee and Its Consumption: benefits and risks', *Clinical Reviews in Food Science and Nutrition*, April 2011, 51(4), pp. 363–73

23 Michael Holick & T.C. Chen, 'Vitamin D Deficiency: a worldwide problem with health consequences', op. cit.

24 Jean-Claude Souberbielle et al., 'Vitamin D and Musculoskeletal Health, Cardiovascular Disease, Autoimmunity, and Cancer: recommendations for clinical practice', *Autoimmune Reviews*, September 2010, 9(11), pp. 709–15

25 The Chemical Maze, chemicalmaze.com

26 Nicole Bijlsma, www.buildingbiology.com.au; Nicole Bijlsma, *Healthy Home, Healthy Family*, op. cit.

27 Michael Mosley & Mimi Spencer, *The FastDiet: lose weight, stay healthy, and live longer with the simple secret of intermittent fasting*, Atria, 2015

28 National Health Service, 'Vitamins and Minerals', www.nhs.uk/Conditions/vitamins-minerals/Pages/vitamins-minerals.aspx

29 Environmental Working Group, 'The Dirty Dozen', www.ewg.org/foodnews/dirty_dozen_list.php

30 Environmental Working Group, 'The Clean Fifteen', www.ewg.org/foodnews/clean_fifteen_list.php

31 Markets and Markets, 'Wellness Supplements Market Worth 249.4 Billion USD by 2020', www.marketsandmarkets.com/PressReleases/wellness-supplements.asp

32 Lesley Braun & Marc Cohen, *Herbs and Natural Supplements: an evidence-based guide, volume 2*, Elvsevier, 2014; Joseph Pizzorno & Michael Murray, *Textbook of Natural Medicine*, Elvsevier, 2012

13. Movement

1 Australian Bureau of Statistics, 'Australian Health Survey: Physical Activity, 2011–2012', www.abs.gov.au/ausstats/abs@.nsf/Lookup/4364.0.55.004main+features12011-12

2 Linda Teri et al., 'Exercise Interventions for Dementia and Cognitive Impairment: the Seattle protocols', *The Journal of Nutrition Health and Ageing*, July 2008, 12(6), pp. 391–4

3 Bliss Hanlon et al., 'Neural Response to Pictures of Food after Exercise in Normal-weight and Obese Women', *Medicine and Science in Sports and Exercise*, October 2012, 44(10), pp. 1864–70

4 Sarah Mullane et al., 'Acute Effects on Cognitive Performance Following Bouts of Standing and Light-intensity Physical Activity in a Simulated Workplace Environment', *Journal of Science and Medicine in Sport*, May 2017, 20(5), pp. 489–93

5 Rania Mekery et al., 'Weight Training, Aerobic Physical Activities, and Long-term Waist Circumference Change in Men', *Obesity*, February 2015, 23(2), pp. 461–7

6 WorkoutLabs, workoutlabs.com

7 ibid.

8 Andrea Ganna & Erik Ingelsson, 'Five-year Mortality Predictors in 498,103 UK Biobank Participants: a prospective population-based study', *The Lancet*, 8 August 2015, 386(9993), pp. 533–40

9 Catrine Tudor-Locke et al., 'Revisiting "How Many Steps Are Enough?"', *Medicine and Science in Sports and Exercise*, July 2008, 40(7 Suppl.), pp. S537–43

14. Thought

1 Harvard Medical School, 'In Praise of Gratitude', *Harvard Mental Health Letter*, November 2011, www.health.harvard.edu/newsletter_article/in-praise-of-gratitude

2 Robert Emmons & Michael Mccullough, 'Counting Blessings versus Burdens: an experimental investigation of gratitude and subjective well-being in daily life,' *Journal of Personality and Social Psychology*, February 2003, 84(2), pp. 377–89

3 Jeffrey Froh et al., 'Being Grateful Is Beyond Good Manners: gratitude and motivation to contribute to society among early adolescents', *Motivation and Emotion*, June 2010, 34(2), pp. 144–57

4 Martin Seligman et al., 'Positive Psychology Progress: empirical validation of interventions', *American Psychologist*, July–August 2005, 60(5), pp. 410–21

5 Robert Emmons & Anjali Mishra, 'Why Gratitude Enhances Wellbeing: what we know, what we need to know' in Kennon Sheldon et al. (eds), *Designing Positive Psychology: taking stock and moving forward*, New York University Press, 2011

6 Big Shakti, www.bigshakti.com

7 Craig Hassad, 'The Health Benefits of Meditation and Being Mindful', www.monash.edu/health-wellbeing

8 David Servan-Schreiber, *Anticancer: a new way of life*, Scribe, 2010

9 Kate Cliff, 'Episode 47: Meditation: Patient Story and Mind–Body Medicine', *The Good Doctors*, thegooddoctors.com.au/health-podcast/kate-cliff-meditation/

10 Big Shakti, op. cit.; Address Stress, www.addressstress.com; Headspace, www.headspace.com

11 Sonja Lyubomirsky et al., 'Becoming Happier Takes Both a Will and a Proper Way: an experimental longitudinal intervention to boost wellbeing', *Emotion*, April 2011, 11(2), pp. 391–402

12 Martin Seligman, *Learned Optimism: how to change your mind and your life*, Knopf, 1990; *Authentic Happiness: using the new positive psychology to realise your potential for lasting fulfilment*, Free Press, 2002; *Flourish: a visionary new understanding of happiness and wellbeing*, Free Press, 2011

13 Hagai Avisar, 'The Perma Model', Positive Psychology Melbourne, 18 June 2015, positivepsychologymelbourne.com.au/the-perma-model/

14 Harvard Study of Adult Development, www.adultdevelopmentstudy.org

Index

Academy of Nutrition and Dietetics 74

Access to Medicine Foundation 46

addictions 348

additives 39, 106, 130–2, 167; *see also* preservatives

ADHD 42, 44, 46, 105, 232, 239–40

adrenal glands 87, 88, 110

adrenaline 83, 87, 89, 100, 170, 188, 343; and caffeine 307, 316

ageing, cellular 98; and exercise 204; and fructose 117; and meditation 348; and sleep 229; and zinc 294

agriculture, animal 141–3, 283; and greenhouse gases 145–6; industrialised 121, 126–7, 131, 138, 139–41, 283, 358; and legumes 294; sustainable model of 140–1

agricultural revolution 1, 92–3, 109, 277, 325; *see also* grain

alcohol, and breathing disorders 267; and detoxing 316; and general health 298, 308–9, 316, 357; and negative thoughts 343; and oral cancer 197; overconsumption of 133–4; and sleep 242, 247, 251; in western diet 106

allergies 42; and bedding 249; and breathing 263, 267–8; defined 187–8; and dairy 289;

and dental stress 171; environmental toxins 213, 235, 262–3, 313; and food 122, 125, 251, 263, 270; and metal 189–91; and sleep 249; and sunscreen 311; and home care 313; types of 188–9; *see also* grains

AllTrials campaign 52, 53

Alzheimer's disease 46, 185, 229, 307, 344

ambiguity, and serotonin 100; psychological tolerance of 352, 355–6

American Diabetics Association 69, 70; International Diabetes Federation 72–3

American Heart Foundation 69, 70

American Society of Nutrition 74

amino acids 281–2, 304

amygdala 263, 348

anaemia 107

anaphylactic reaction 188

animal ethics 128, 283, 284, 287–8

antibiotics, in farming practices 128, 139, 142, 285; in fish farming 158, 287, 288; in humans 11, 139, 282, 285, 319; resistance to 4–5, 139, 185, 319

anti-anxietics 45

antidepressants, and Big Pharma 44–5, 46, 53, 54; and side effects 24, 108, 232; and western medicine 11